ROGER A. BRUMBACK, M.D.
DEPARTMENT OF PATHOLOGY
940 STANTON L. YOUNG BLVD.
OUHSC---P.O. BOX 26901
OKLAHOMA CITY, OK 73190

The Renal Biopsy

OTHER MONOGRAPHS IN THE SERIES MAJOR PROBLEMS IN PATHOLOGY

Published

Whitehead: *Mucosal Biopsy of the Gastrointestinal Tract, 3rd ed.*
Azzopardi: *Problems in Breast Pathology*
Katzenstein & Askin: *Surgical Pathology of Non-neoplastic Lung Disease, 2nd ed.*
Frable: *Thin-Needle Aspiration Biopsy*
Wigglesworth: *Perinatal Pathology*
Jaffe: *Surgical Pathology of Lymph Nodes and Related Organs*
Wittels: *Surgical Pathology of Bone M. rrow*
Finegold: *Pathology of Neoplasia in Children and Adolescents*
Taylor: *Immunomicroscopy*
Wolf & Neiman: *Disorders of the Spleen*
Fu & Reagan: *Pathology of the Uterine Cervix, Vagina and Vulva*
LiVolsi: *Surgical Pathology of the Thyroid*

Forthcoming

Virmani, Atkinson & Fenoglio: *Pathology of the Heart*
Whitehead: *Mucosal Biopsy of the Gastrointestinal Tract, 4th ed.*
Mackay, Lukeman & Ordonez: *Tumors of the Lung*
Hendrickson & Kempson: *Surgical Pathology of the Uterine Corpus, 2nd ed.*
Nash & Said: *Pathology of Acquired Immune Deficiency*
Frable: *Fine Needle Aspiration Biopsy, 2nd ed.*
Mackay & Ordonez: *Soft Tissue Tumors*
Crissman & Zarbo: *Surgical Pathology of the Upper Aerodigestive Tract Mucosa*
Vardiman & Variokojis: *Pathology of Myeloproliferative Disorders*
Henson & Albores-Saavedra: *Pathology of Incipient Neoplasia, 2nd ed.*
Azzopardi: *Pathology of the Breast, 2nd ed.*
Fox, Young & Buckley: *Pathology of the Ovary and Fallopian Tube*
Ellis, Auclair & Gnepp: *Pathology of the Salivary Glands*
Fox: *Pathology of the Placenta, 2nd ed.*
Jaffe: *Surgical Pathology of the Lymph Nodes, 2nd ed.*
Lack: *Surgical Pathology of the Adrenal Glands*
Lloyd: *Surgical Pathology of the Pituitary Gland*
Kornstein: *Pathology of the Anterior Mediastinum*

Liliane J. Striker, M.D.
National Institutes of Health
Bethesda, Maryland

Jean L. Olson, M.D.
Associate Professor, Department of Pathology
Johns Hopkins School of Medicine
Baltimore, Maryland

Gary E. Striker, M.D.
Director, Kidney, Urologic and Hematology Division
National Institutes of Health
Bethesda, Maryland

The Renal Biopsy

Volume 8 in the Series
MAJOR PROBLEMS IN PATHOLOGY

Second Edition

JAMES L. BENNINGTON, M.D.,
Consulting Editor
Chairman, Department of Pathology
Children's Hospital of San Francisco
San Francisco, California

1990
W.B. SAUNDERS COMPANY
Harcourt Brace Jovanovich, Inc.
Philadelphia London Toronto Montreal Sydney Tokyo

W. B. SAUNDERS COMPANY
Harcourt Brace Jovanovich, Inc.

The Curtis Center
Independence Square West
Philadelphia, PA 19106

Library of Congress Cataloging in Publication Data

Striker, Liliane J.

The renal biopsy/Liliane J. Striker and Jean L. Olson and Gary E. Striker.—2nd ed.

p. cm.—(Major problems in pathology; v. 8)

Rev. ed. of: Use and interpretation of renal biopsy/Gary E. Striker, Leonard J. Quadracci, Ralph E. Cutler. 1978.

ISBN 0–7216–3040–5

1. Kidneys—Diseases—Diagnosis. 2. Kidneys—Biopsy. I. Olson, Jean L. II. Striker, Gary E., 1934– III. Striker, Gary E., 1934– Use and interpretation of renal biopsy. IV. Title. V. Series.
[DNLM: 1. Biopsy, Needle. 2. Kidney—pathology. 3. Kidney Diseases—diagnosis. W1 MA492X v. 8/WJ 302 S917u]

RC904.S75 1990

616.6′10758—dc20

DNLM/DLC

for Library of Congress 89–70252
CIP

Editor: Richard Zorab
Designer: Maureen Sweeney
Production Manager: Linda R. Turner
Manuscript Editor: Wendy Andresen
Illustration Coordinator: Brett MacNaughton
Indexer: Linda Van Pelt

The Renal Biopsy, Second Edition ISBN 0–7216–3040–5

Copyright © 1990, 1978 by W. B. Saunders Company.
All rights reserved. No part of this publication may be reproduced or transmitted in any form or by any means, electronic or mechanical, including photocopy, recording, or any information storage and retrieval system, without permission in writing from the publisher.

Printed in the United States of America.

Last digit is the print number: 9 8 7 6 5 4 3 2 1

Preface

The approach used in this text is intended to be very practical, that is, to provide a guide to the interpretation of renal biopsies. The assumption is made that the reader is primarily interested in this text to aid in the interpretation of renal biopsies, rather than seeking a reference text on renal diseases. There are a number of splendid clinical and pathologic anatomy texts to meet the latter needs, and only those aspects of renal disease that are pertinent to renal biopsy interpretation are included herein. Similarly, the references that are listed at the end of each section are representative rather than inclusive. We have deliberately chosen to restrict the number of references and instead have provided a list of more comprehensive reference texts of renal diseases on page iv.

The first edition of *The Renal Biopsy* had a similar title and appeared under the authorship of one of the current contributors (G.E.S.), but the present edition bears little other similarity. Thus, while we have elected to use the diagrams and a few illustrations from the first edition of this book, the focus, format, and text have been completely redirected.

The patient population from which the authors draw their experience reflects that of Western Europe (Hôpital Tenon, Dr. Liliane Morel-Maroger Striker), the Atlantic Seaboard (Johns Hopkins University, Dr. Jean Olson), and the Pacific Northwest (University of Washington, Dr. Gary Striker). The age range is similarly broad, encompassing infancy to advanced age. Finally, the breadth of experience encompasses nearly 15,000 renal biopsies over a period of almost 25 years. There is no particular geographic focus, but few tropical diseases are covered in this text.

The wise consultation and advice of many clinicians and pathologists in guiding and shaping our approaches to renal biopsy interpretation are gratefully acknowledged. It is possible to mention but a few, such as Drs. G. Richet and J.P. Mery (Paris), R.H. Heptinstall (Maryland), and B.H. Scribner and E.P. Benditt (Washington).

LILIANE J. STRIKER, M.D.
JEAN L. OLSON, M.D.
GARY E. STRIKER, M.D.

REFERENCE TEXTS

1. The Nephrotic Syndrome. JS Cameron and RJ Glassock (eds). Marcel Dekker, New York, 1988.
2. Pathology of Glomerular Disease. S Rosen (ed). Churchill Livingstone, New York, 1983.
3. Pathology of the Kidney, 3rd ed. RH Heptinstall (ed). Little, Brown, & Company, Boston, 1983.
4. Pediatric Nephrology. P Royer, R Habib, H Mathieu, and M Broyer (eds). WB Saunders Company, Philadelphia, 1974.
5. Renal Biopsy Pathology with Diagnostic and Therapeutic Implications. BH Spargo, AE Seymour, and NG Ordonez (eds). John Wiley & Sons, New York, 1980.
6. Renal Disease: Classification and Atlas of Glomerular Diseases. J Churg, LH Sobin, et al (eds). Igaku-Shoin, Tokyo, 1980.
7. Renal Pathology with Clinical and Functional Correlations. CC Tisher and BM Brenner (eds). JB Lippincott, Philadelphia, 1989.

Contents

Chapter

1

ROLE OF THE RENAL BIOPSY IN THE EVALUATION OF RENAL DISEASE

Renal biopsy provides one of the few objective measurements of the type, nature, site, extent, and state of evolution of renal diseases. There are surely many imperfections in our current ability to interpret and understand the changes revealed at biopsy. However, many techniques that have previously been restricted to the research laboratory await application by the inventive, insightful pathologist. The purpose of this chapter is to provide an approach to renal biopsy using currently available methods and to explore the questions that can now be addressed by means of renal biopsy.

The single purpose of the diagnosis must be kept in mind—that is, to provide sufficient accurate information on which to base an approach to both a treatment plan and prognosis. Thus it is no longer justified to examine a renal biopsy specimen by other than the most modern and sophisticated methods available to modern pathologists. These include, at the very minimum, detailed light and immunofluorescence microscopic studies using various stains or probes for immune reactants and other foreign proteins indicated by the particular clinical and laboratory picture. Electron microscopic evaluation of a sufficient sample of the various compartments is required in certain categories of disease and provides information of interest in most renal biopsies. It is only after this type of study that one can render an opinion that does justice to the patient, to the clinician, and to the tissue obtained at considerable expense and a certain amount of risk.

Accurate interpretation requires detailed knowledge of the structure and function of a normal kidney, from infancy to adulthood. In addition, it is necessary to have an appreciation of the general responses of tissues to injury and those that are particular to the kidney. Finally, each compartment must be assessed separately and in the most quantitative manner available for the observations at hand.

The basic features that can be assessed are as follows:

LIGHT MICROSCOPY
- Glomeruli
  - Normal (Figs. 1–1 and 1–2)
  - Cellular change
    - Epithelial (spreading) (Figs. 1–3, 1–4, and 1–5)
    - Endothelial (swelling) (Figs. 1–6, 1–7, and 1–8)
  - Increased cellularity (proliferation)
    - Intraglomerular
      - Mesangial/endothelial (Figs. 1–9 and 1–10)
      - Inflammatory cell infiltrate (Figs. 1–11 and 1–12)
    - Extraglomerular
      - Epithelial
        - Synechia (cellular, Figs. 1–13, 1–14, and 1–15)
        - Crescent (Figs. 1–16 and 1–17)

- Extracellular matrix (sclerosis)
  - Obsolescence (Figs. 1–18 and 1–19)
  - Peripheral basement membrane (vascular loop)
    - Thickening (Figs. 1–20 and 1–21)
    - Wrinkling and thickening (Figs. 1–22 and 1–23)
    - Splitting (Figs. 1–24 and 1–25)
  - Mesangial spaces (Figs. 1–26 and 1–27)
  - Bowman's space/capsule
- Other
  - Necrosis
  - Deposits (see immunofluorescence, below)

Tubules
- Normal (Figs. 1–28 and 1–29)
- Cellular changes
  - Necrosis/regeneration/hyaline droplets and so on (Fig. 1–30)
- Basement membrane changes
  - Thickening/duplication/deposits (Fig. 1–31)
- Other
  - Atrophy/dilation/casts

Interstitium
- Normal (see Fig. 1–28)
- Edema (Fig. 1–32)
- Infiltrate (Fig. 1–33)
- Fibrosis (Fig. 1–34)

Blood Vessels
- Normal (Figs. 1–35 and 1–36)
- Cellular changes
  - Intima
    - Proliferation (Figs. 1–37 and 1–38)
    - Inflammatory cell infiltrate (Figs. 1–39 and 1–40)
    - Deposits
      - Fibrin (Figs. 1–41 and 1–42)
      - Hyalin/amyloid/and so on (Figs. 1–43 and 1–44)
  - Media
    - Cellular changes
      - Hyperplasia/hypertrophy/infiltrates (Figs. 1–45 and 1–46)
    - Extracellular matrix changes
      - Basement membrane
      - Elastin
      - Interstitial collagen (Figs. 1–47 and 1–48)
  - Adventitia
    - Cellular changes
      - Hyperplasia/infiltrates
    - Extracellular matrix changes
      - Hyperplasia/infiltrates
      - Fibrosis
    - Total vascular wall
      - Inflammation, necrosis (Figs. 1–39 and 1–40)

IMMUNOFLUORESCENCE MICROSCOPY

Deposits
- Glomeruli
  - Basement membrane
    - Linear (Figs. 1–49 and 1–50)
    - Granular (subepithelial, post-streptococcal) (Figs. 1–51 and 1–52)
    - Granular (subepithelial, membranous glomerulonephritis) (Figs. 1–53 and 1–54)
    - Subendothelial (membranoproliferative glomerulonephritis type I) (Figs. 1–55 and 1–56)
    - Intramembranous (membranoproliferative glomerulonephritis type II) (Figs. 1–57 and 1–58)
    - Subendothelial (systemic lupus erythematosus) (Figs. 1–59 and 1–60)
  - Mesangium (Fig. 1–61)
- Tubular Basement Membranes
  - Linear (Fig. 1–62)
  - Granular (Fig. 1–63)
- Interstitium
- Blood Vessels (Fig. 1–64)

ELECTRON MICROSCOPY

Glomerular
- Cellular changes
  - Epithelial/endothelial/mesangial (see Figs. 1–5 and 1–8)
- Extracellular matrix changes
  - Increase/duplication/thinning/interruption
- Deposits
  - Location: mesangial, subepithelial, subendothelial, intramembranous, Bowman's space/capsule

The changes need to be integrated within the framework of the overall laboratory and clinical work-up. The diagnosis is the sum of all of these data.

GLOSSARY OF DESCRIPTIVE TERMS

Terms Relating to Distribution/Structure

Diffuse. Involving all or almost all glomeruli.

Focal. Involving less than 50% of glomeruli.

Segmental. Involving portions of individual glomeruli.

Sclerosis. Increase in extracellular matrix. The sclerotic areas stain positively with periodic acid-Schiff (PAS), Masson's trichrome, and periodic acid-silver methenamine (PASM).

Text continued on page 34

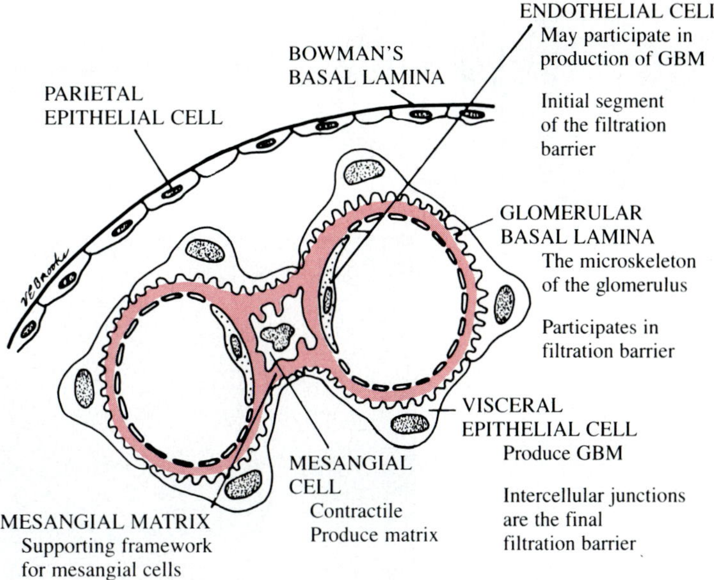

Figure 1–1. Normal. Diagram of a normal glomerulus.

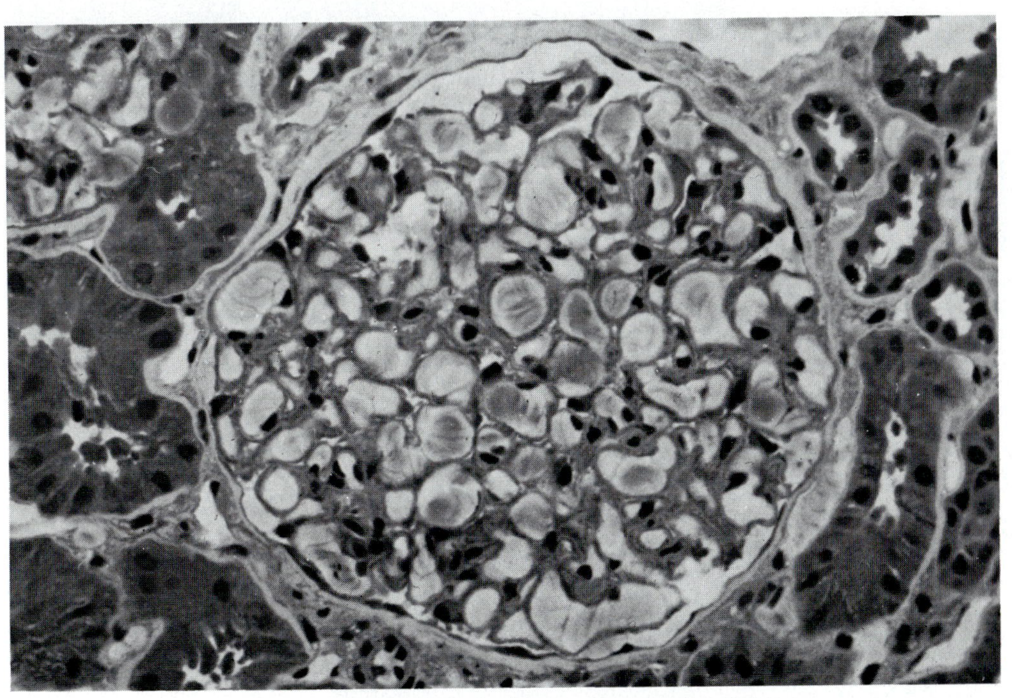

Figure 1–2. Normal. Normal glomerulus. (H&E, ×300.)

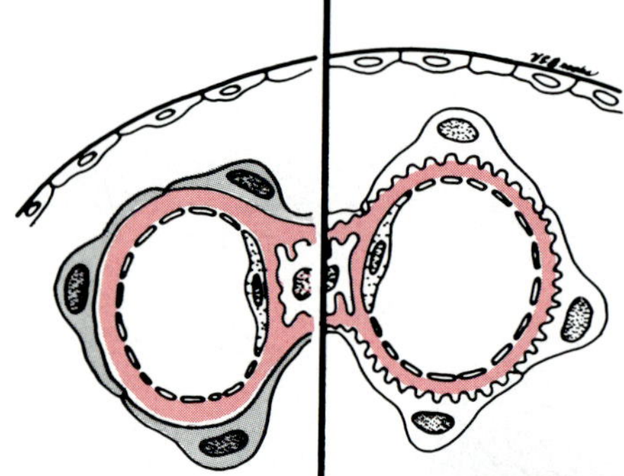

Figure 1–3. Cellular change, podocyte spreading. Diagram of glomerular visceral epithelial cell cytoplasmic spreading.

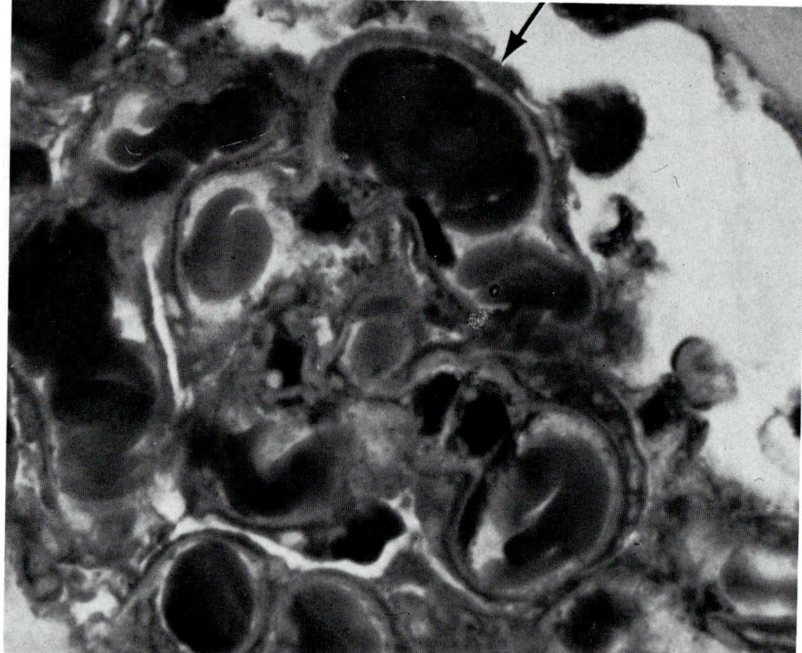

Figure 1–4. Epithelial cell change, podocyte spreading. There is a thickened, continuous layer of epithelial cell cytoplasm covering the urinary side of the glomerular basement membrane. (H&E, ×1200.)

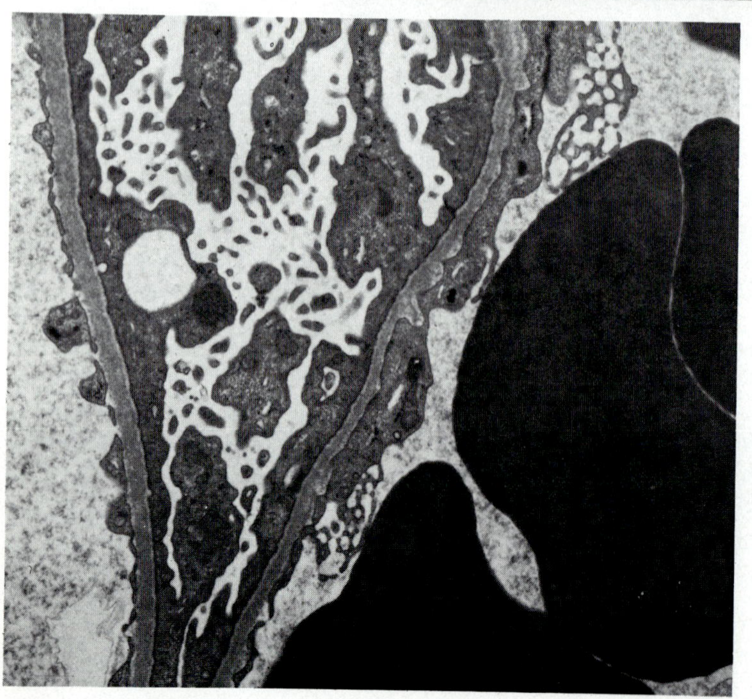

Figure 1–5. Epithelial cell change, podocyte spreading. The epithelial cell cytoplasm has lost its complex interdigitations.

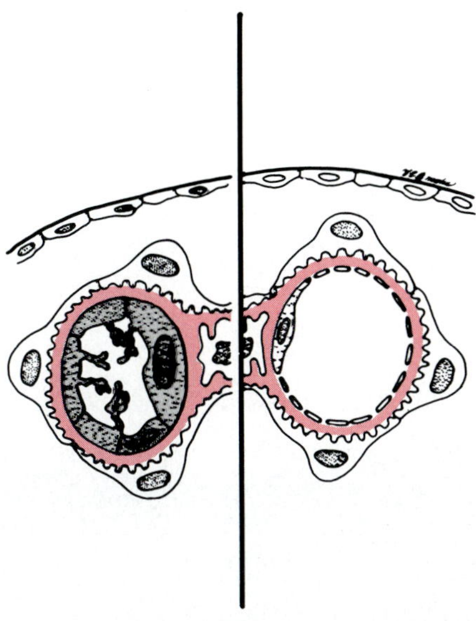

Figure 1–6. Endothelial cell change, swelling. Diagram of endothelial cell injury, manifested by swelling, surface irregularities, and hypercellularity.

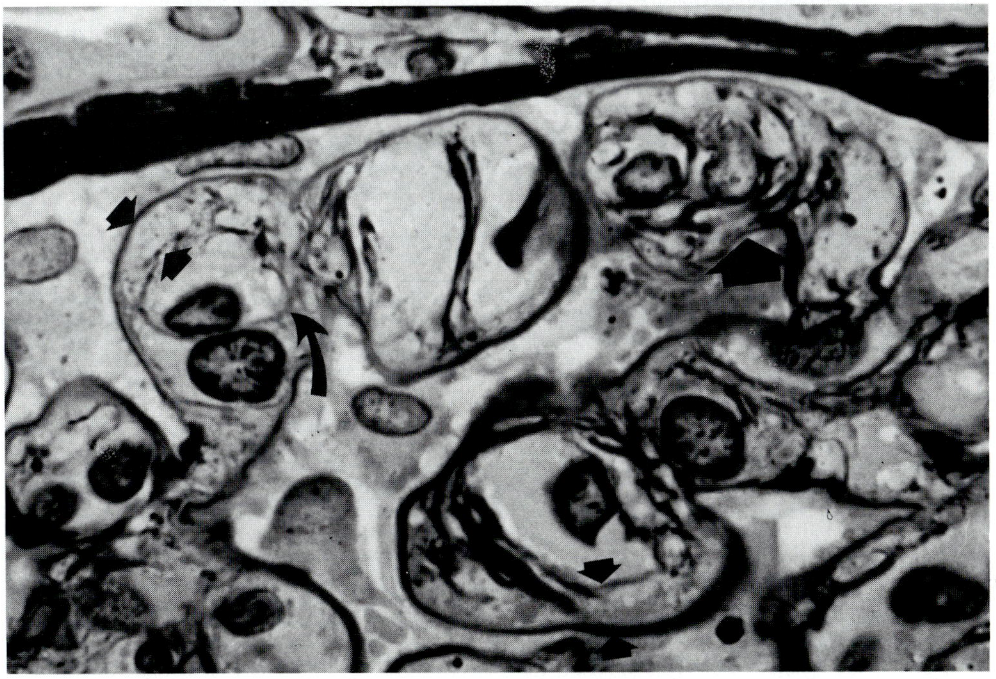

Figure 1–7. Endothelial cell change, swelling. The endothelial cell cytoplasm is prominent (curved arrow), and the subendothelial spaces are markedly thickened (arrows). (PASM, ×1200.)

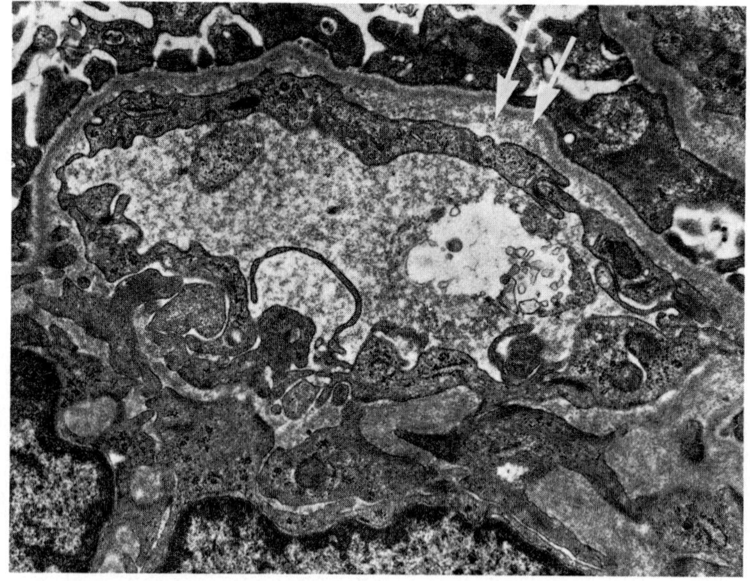

Figure 1–8. Endothelial cell change, swelling. At higher magnification, the endothelial cell cytoplasm is markedly thickened and no longer is highly fenestrated. (×2000.)

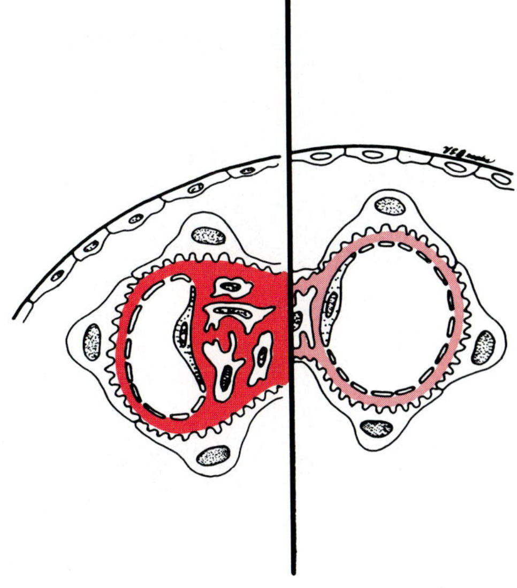

Figure 1–9. Hypercellularity, mesangial. Diagram of mesangial cell hypercellularity. Note that although this diagram depicts hypercellularity limited to the mesangium, it is often impossible to differentiate mesangial cells from endothelial cells.

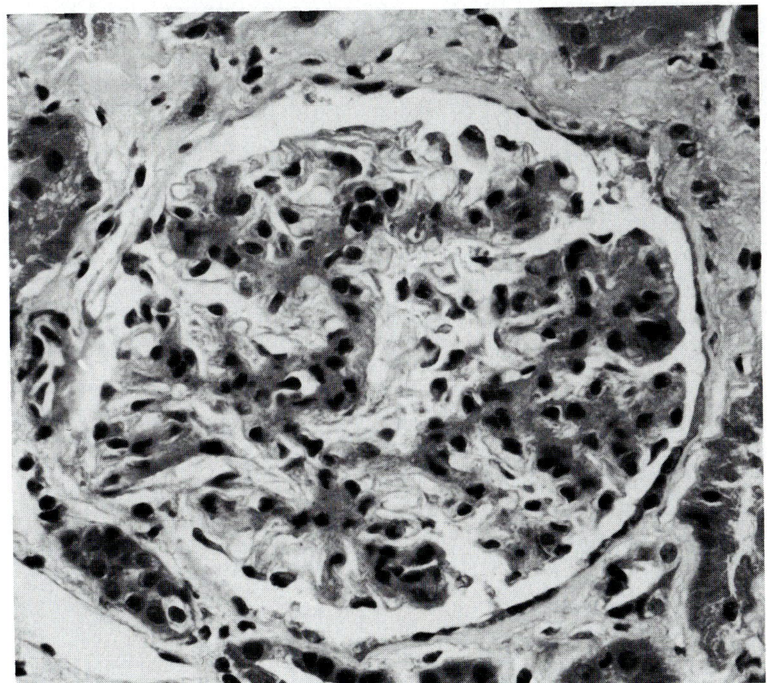

Figure 1–10. Hypercellularity, mesangial. The centrolobular (mesangial) regions contain an increased number of nuclei. (H&E, ×300.)

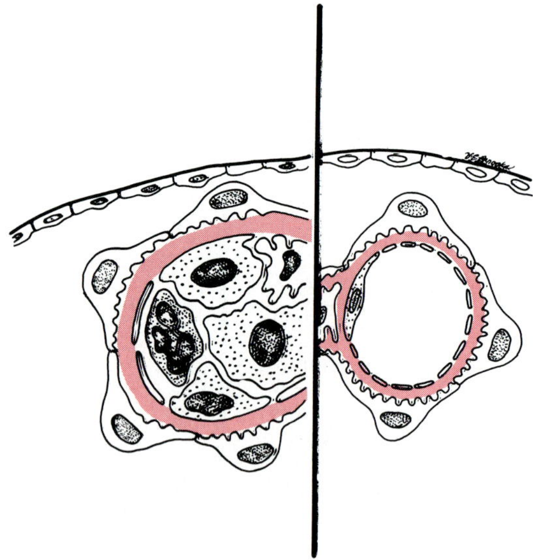

Figure 1–11. Hypercellularity, inflammation. Diagram of inflammatory cell infiltration by neutrophils and macrophages, accompanied by proliferation of resident glomerular cells.

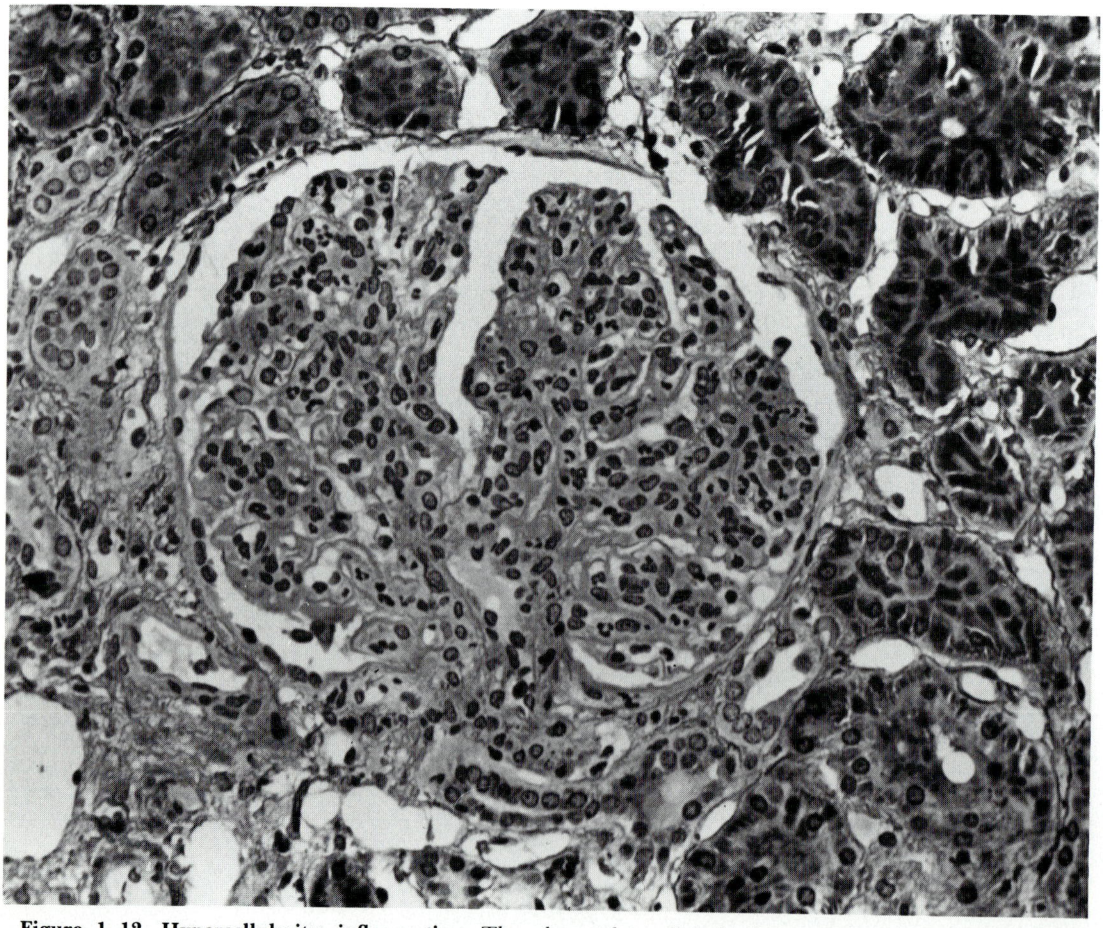

Figure 1–12. Hypercellularity, inflammation. The glomerular cellularity is greatly increased. Many of the intraglomerular cells are neutrophils. (PASM, ×300.)

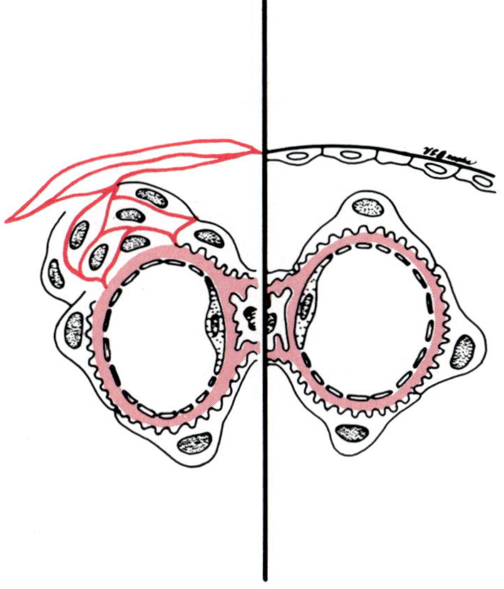

Figure 1–13. Hypercellularity, epithelial, synechia. Diagram of segmental epithelial cell proliferation, resulting in the formation of a synechia.

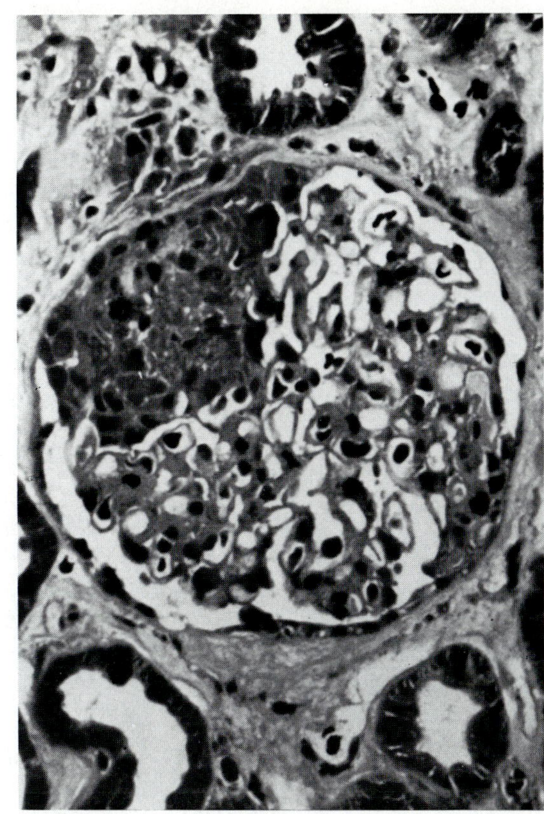

Figure 1–14. Hypercellularity, epithelial, synechia. There is a localized area of epithelial cell proliferation between 1 and 3 o'clock. Note the cellular response in the interstitium adjacent to the synechia. (Masson's trichrome, ×300.)

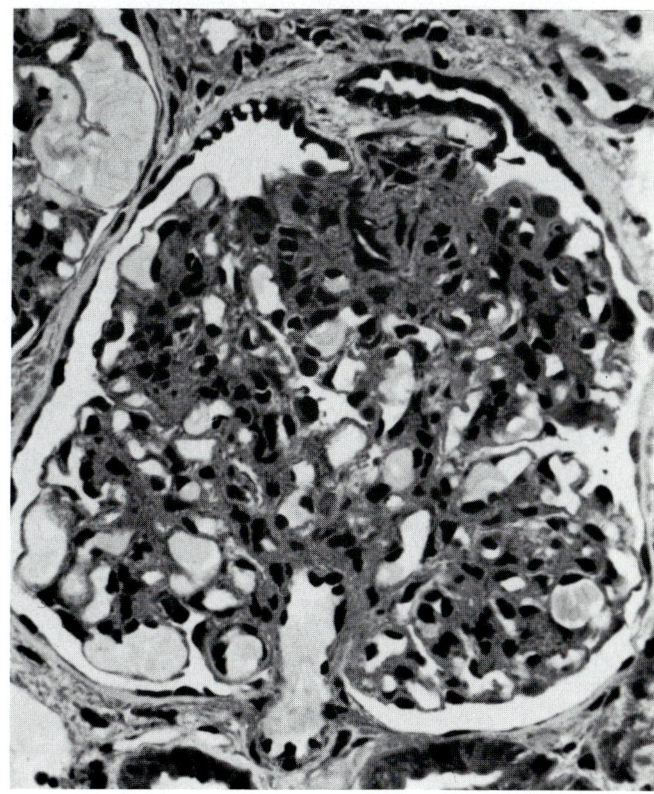

Figure 1–15. Hypercellularity, epithelial, synechia (organized). The synechia is composed of connective tissue, which forms a bridge between the basement membrane of the glomerulus and that of Bowman's capsule. (Masson's trichrome, ×300.)

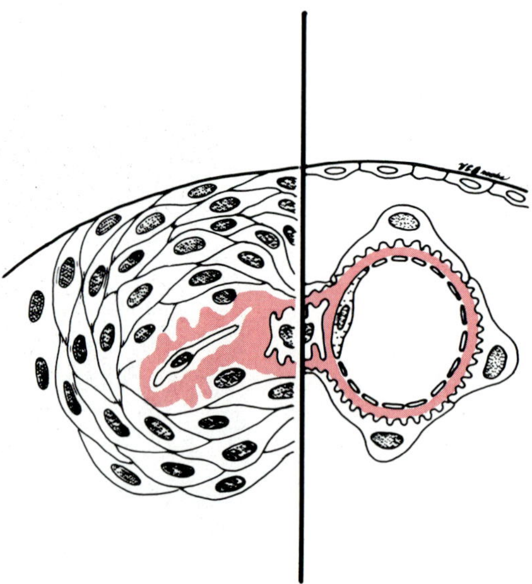

Figure 1–16. Hypercellularity, epithelial, diffuse (crescent). Diagram of diffuse epithelial cell proliferation.

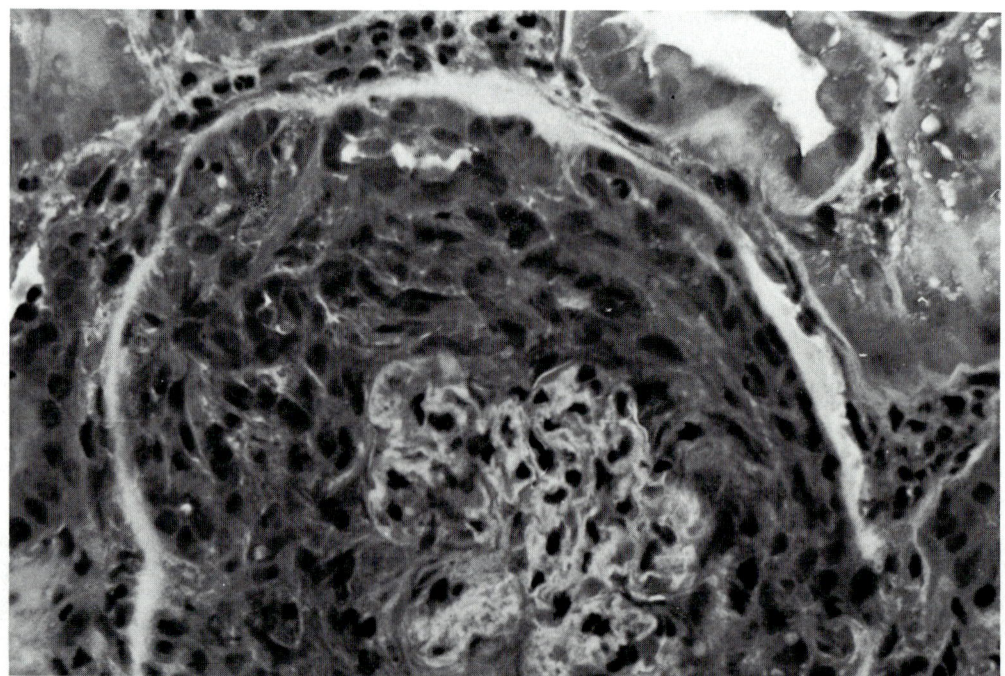

Figure 1–17. Hypercellularity, epithelial, diffuse (crescent). Bowman's space is completely filled with cells. There is an admixture of glomerular epithelial cells and inflammatory cells. (H&E, ×300.)

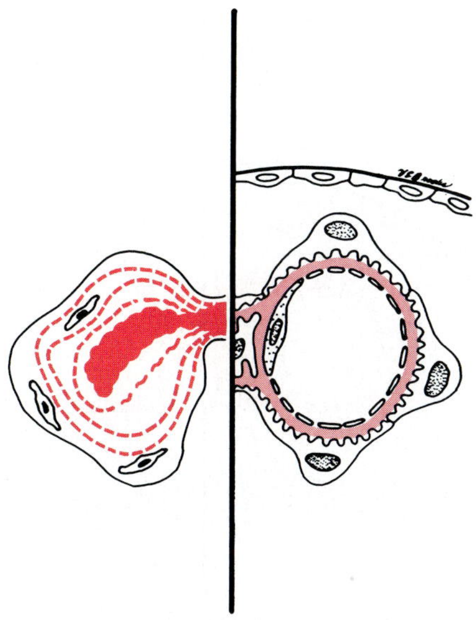

Figure 1–18. Sclerosis, obsolescence. Diagram of a fibrotic, shrunken (i.e., obsolescent) glomerulus.

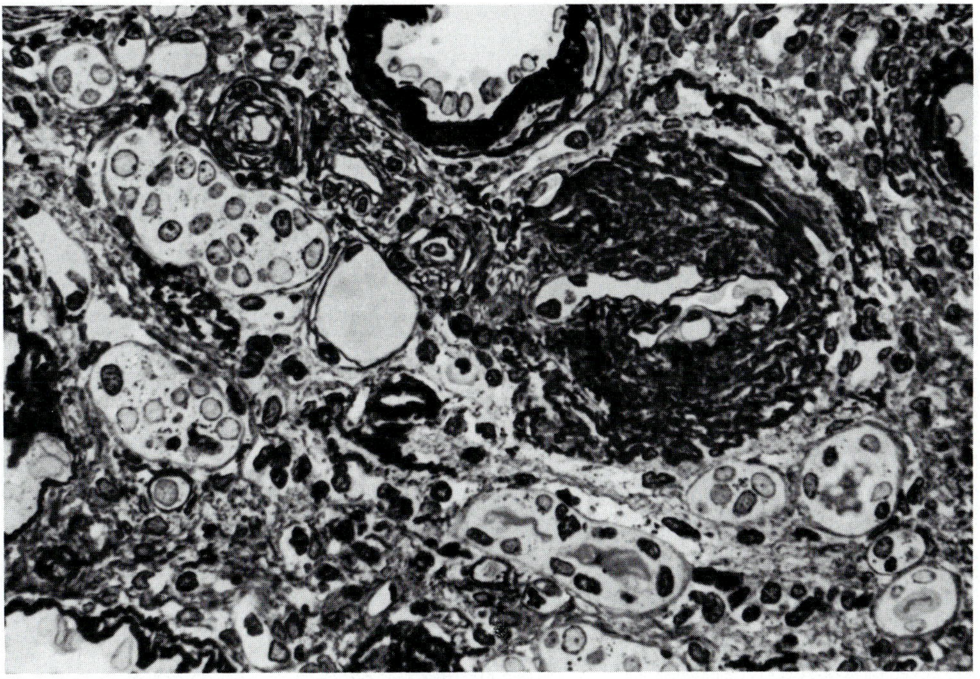

Figure 1–19. Sclerosis, obsolescent glomerulus. Organization of the crescent results in complete fibrosis (i.e., obsolescent glomerulus). Fragments of Bowman's capsule can still be recognized (top), but the capsule has been interrupted over most of its perimeter. (PASM, ×150.)

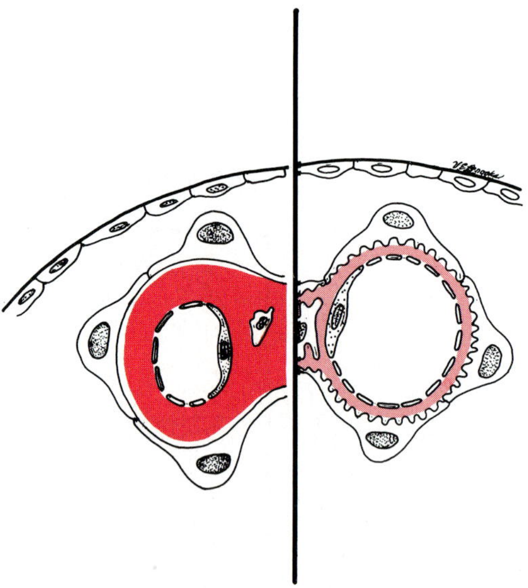

Figure 1–20. Glomerular basement membrane, thickening. Diagram of diffuse thickening of the glomerular basement membrane and an increase in the amount of the mesangial matrix.

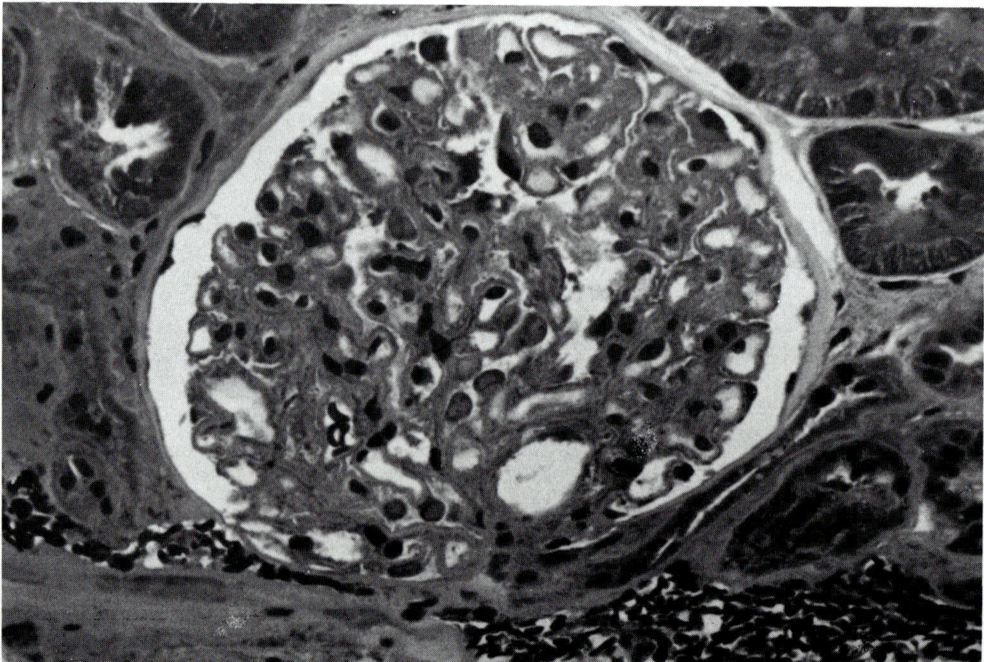

Figure 1–21. Glomerular basement membrane, thickening. The glomerular basement membranes are uniformly and diffusely thickened. They have a stiff appearance, and the number of patent vascular loops is diminished. (H&E, ×300.)

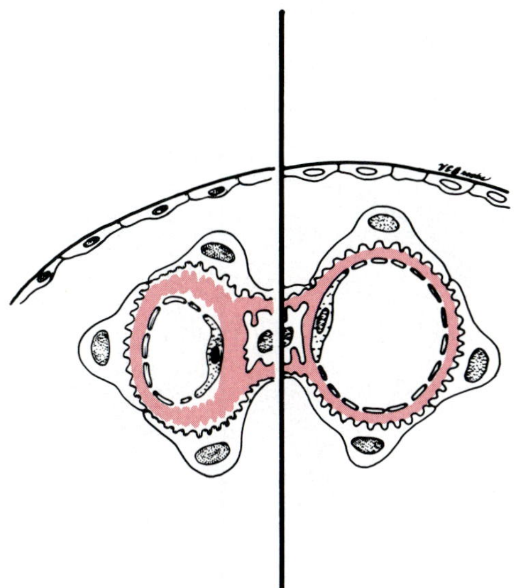

Figure 1–22. Glomerular basement membrane, collapse. Diagram of wrinkling of the glomerular basement membrane. This change is most marked near the mesangial region and results in narrowing of the lumen.

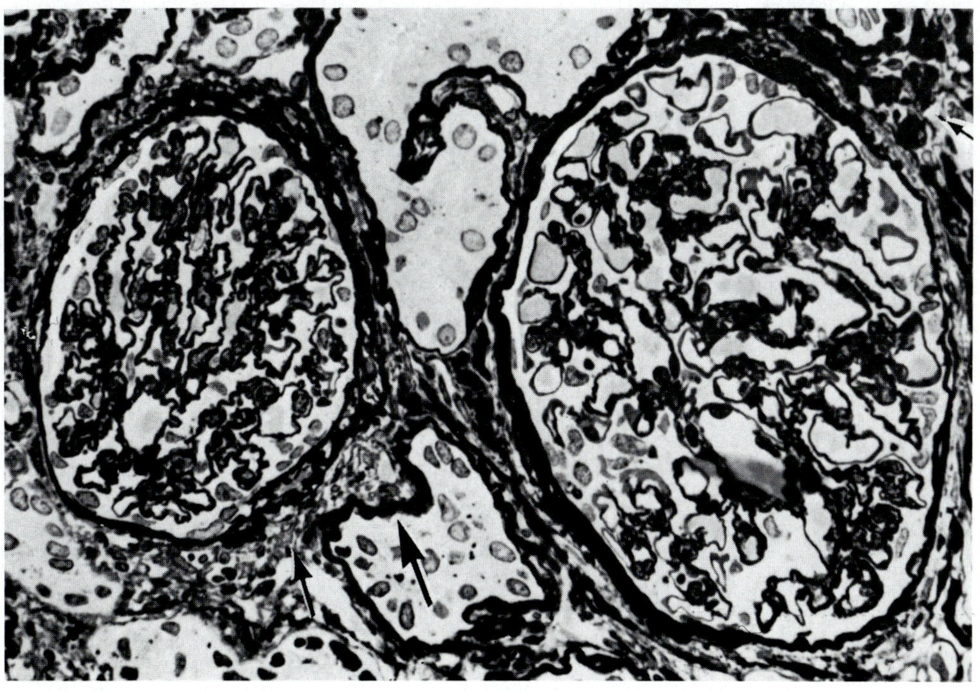

Figure 1–23. Glomerular basement membrane, collapse. The glomerulus on the right is less affected. That on the left reveals diffuse wrinkling and collapse of the tufts. (PASM, ×250.)

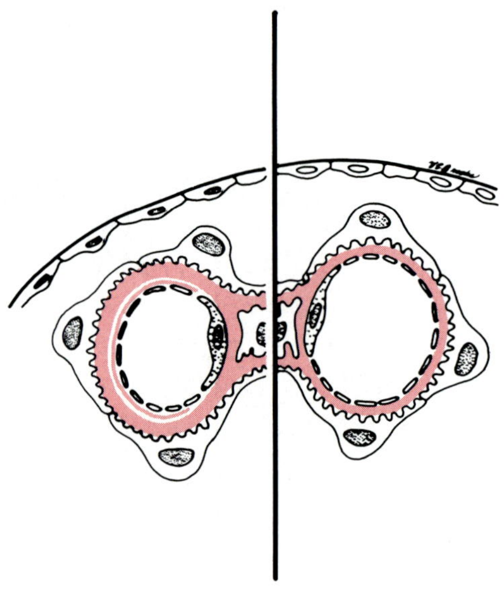

Figure 1–24. Glomerular basement membrane, duplication. Diagram of the formation of a second layer of basement membrane in the subendothelial space.

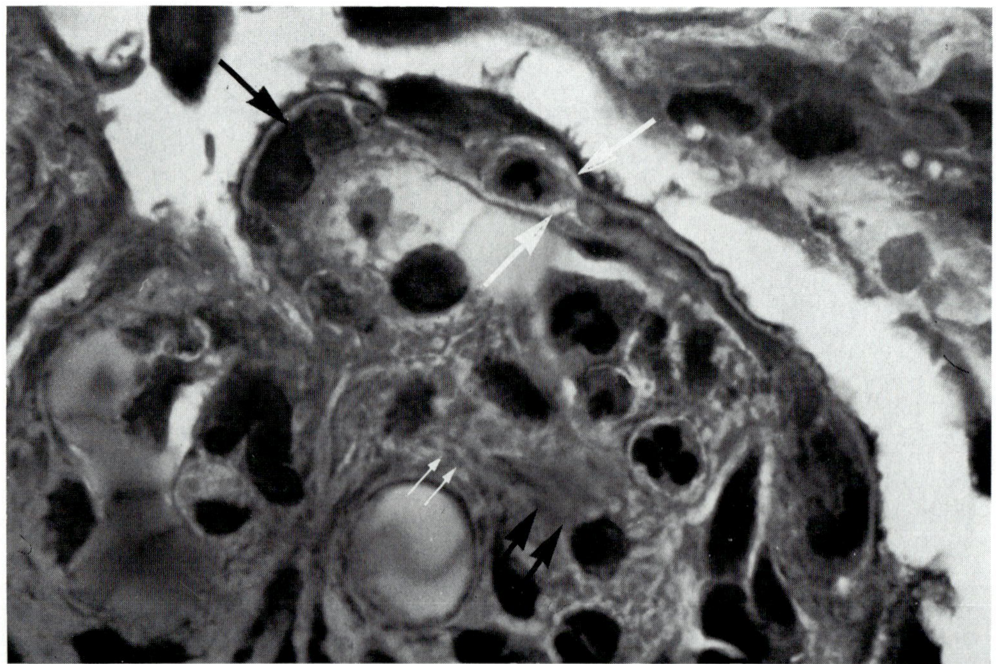

Figure 1–25. Glomerular basement membrane, duplication. There is marked widening of the peripheral glomerular wall, resulting from the formation of two layers of basement membrane (large, light arrows) and the interposition of cell cytoplasm between these two laminae. The amount of matrix within the mesangium is also increased (double arrows, light and dark), and deposits are found in the subendothelial regions (dark arrow). (H&E, ×1200.)

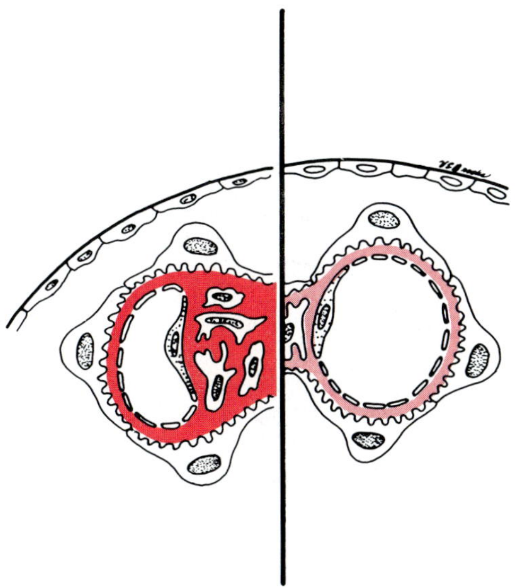

Figure 1–26. Mesangial matrix, sclerosis. Diagram of mesangial sclerosis. Note that the sclerosis is frequently preceded by mesangial proliferation.

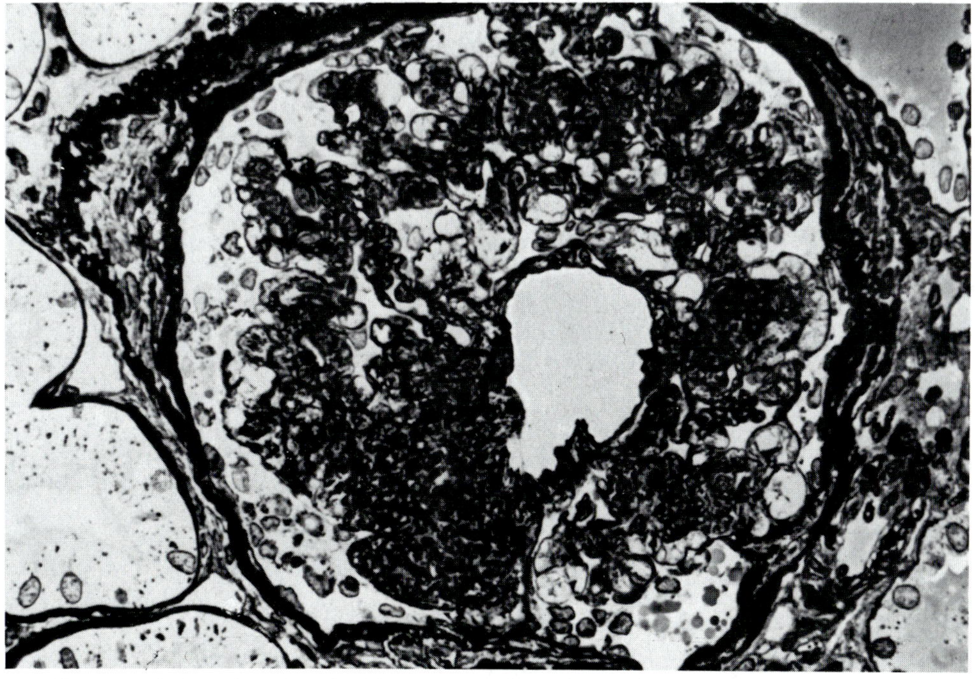

Figure 1–27. Mesangial matrix, sclerosis. The most prominent feature is an increase in the amount of mesangial matrix. The vascular spaces are severely compromised. Although all mesangial regions are involved, those near the vascular pole (bottom) are most sclerotic. (PASM, ×300.)

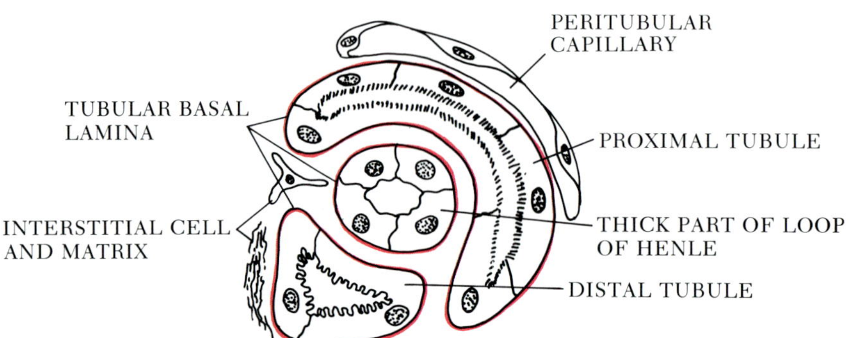

Figure 1–28. Normal, tubules and interstitium. Diagram of the tubulo-interstitial compartment.

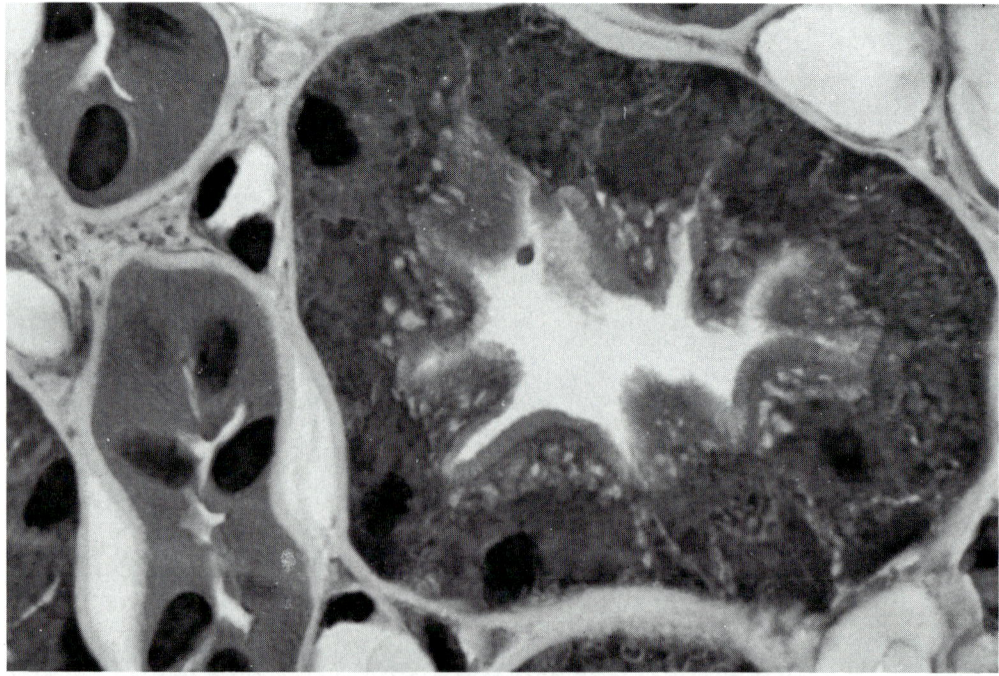

Figure 1–29. Normal, tubules and interstitium. The morphology of the tubules and interstitium is well preserved in this methacrylate-embedded specimen. (H&E, ×1200.)

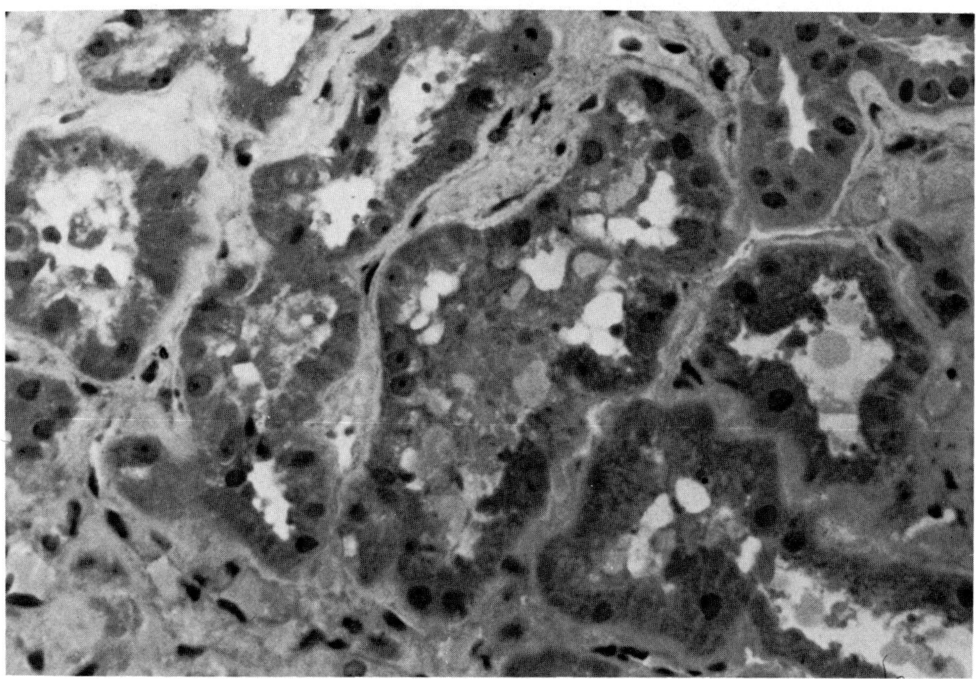

Figure 1–30. Tubules, cell injury. The proximal tubular epithelium shows changes varying from vacuolation to frank necrosis. (H&E, ×300.)

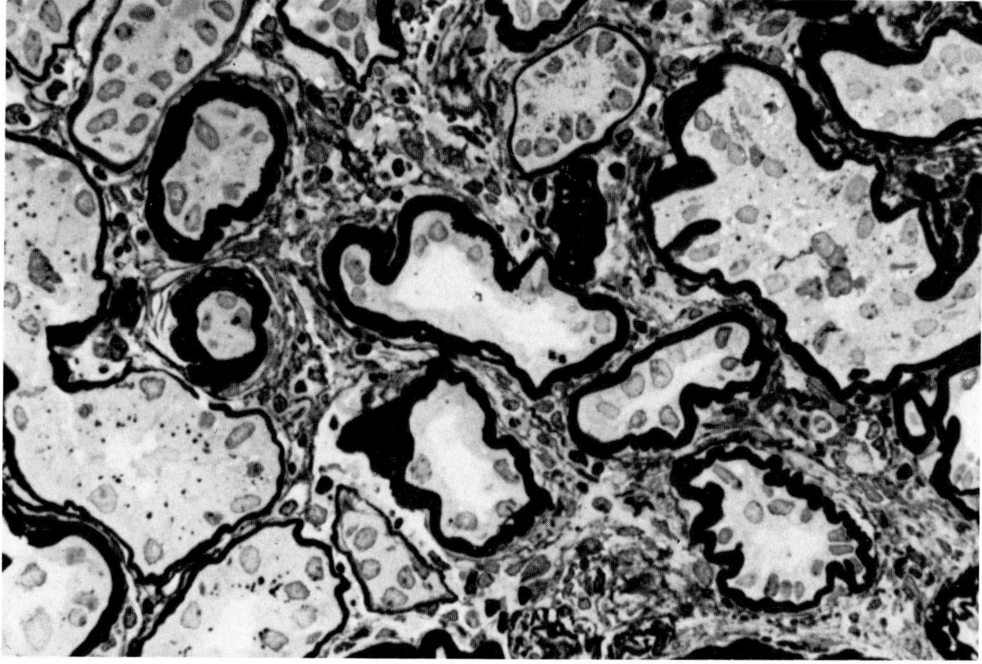

Figure 1–31. Tubules, basement membrane thickening. The tubular basement membranes are diffusely thickened. In the area of interstitial fibrosis, the tubular epithelium is atrophied and the basement membrane thickening is accentuated. (PASM, ×300.)

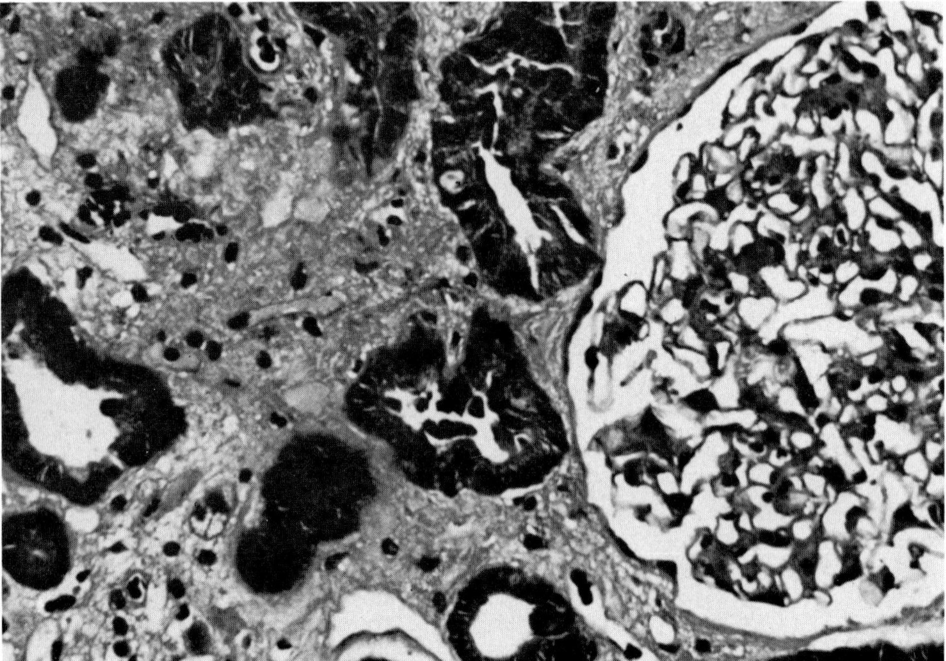

Figure 1–32. Interstitium, edema. The interstitial spaces are filled with fluid, separating capillaries from the tubules. (Masson's trichrome, ×300.)

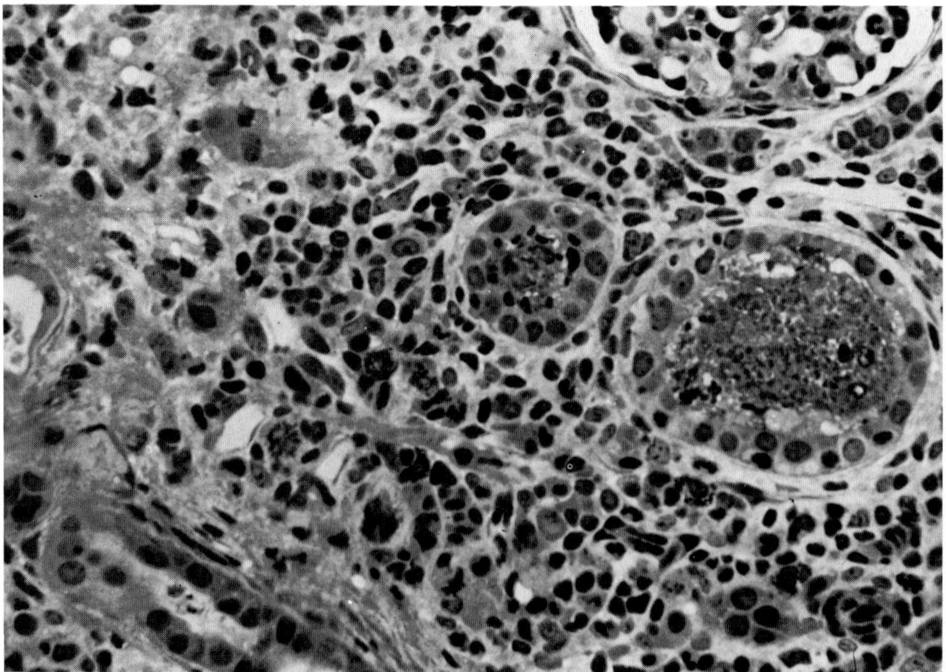

Figure 1–33. Interstitium, inflammation. The interstitium is widened and distorted by a dense infiltrate of mononuclear inflammatory cells. (H&E, ×250.)

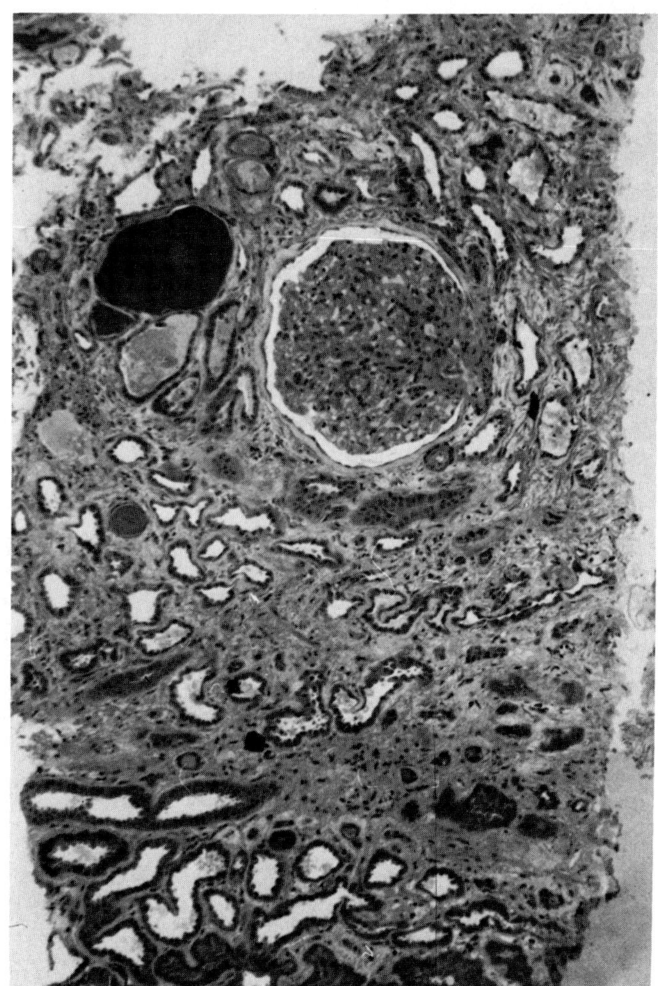

Figure 1–34. Interstitium, fibrosis. The fibrosis is diffuse and the encased tubules are atrophic. The fibrotic zones are irregularly distributed. (H&E, ×100.)

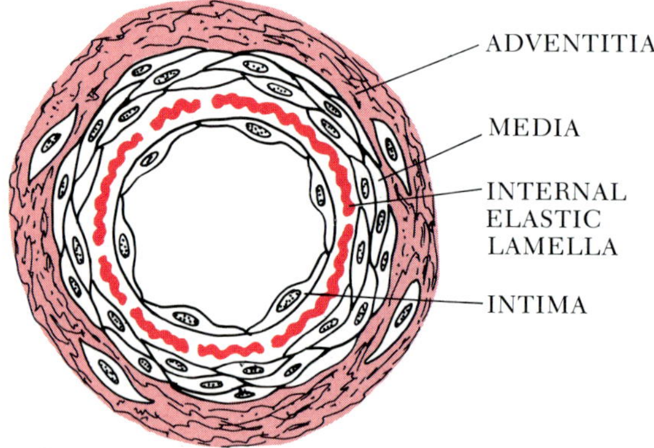

Figure 1–35. Artery, normal. Diagram of a normal artery.

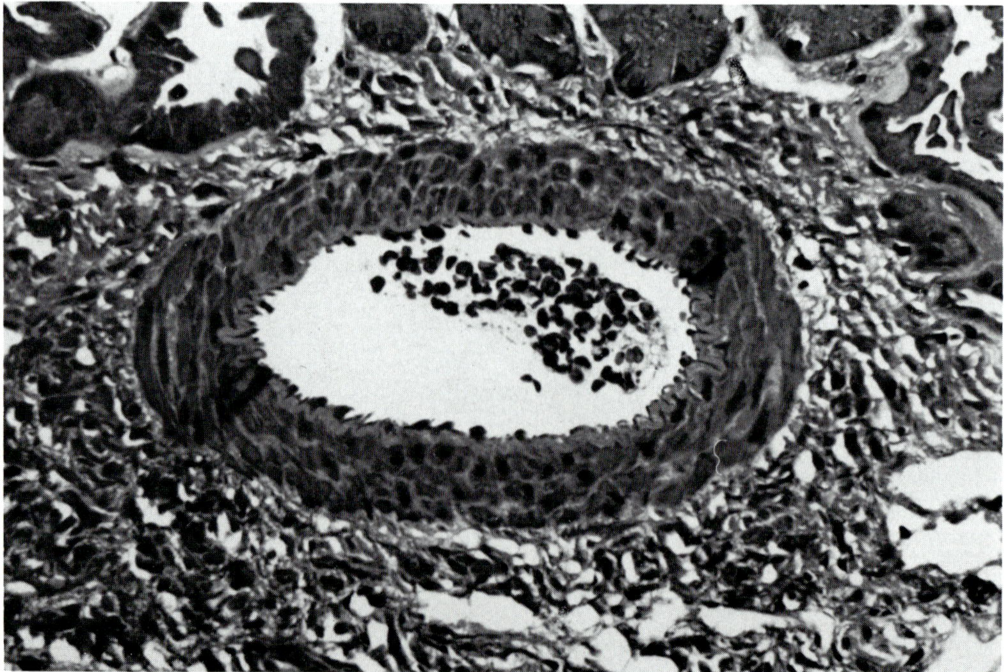

Figure 1–36. Artery, normal. Normal artery. (H&E, ×300.)

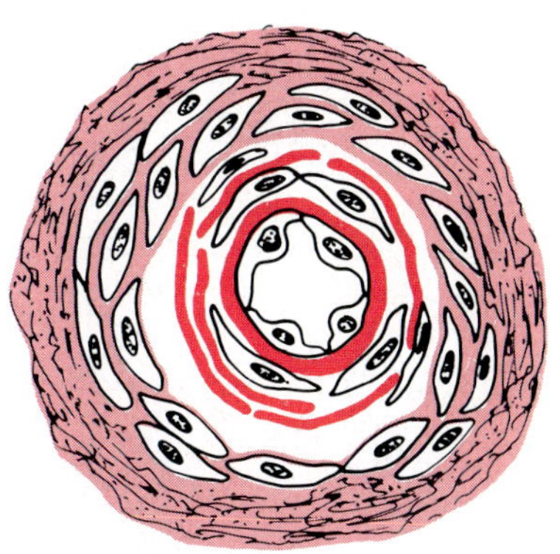

Figure 1–37. Intima, proliferation. Diagram of intimal proliferation. Also present is an increase in the amount of extracellular matrix.

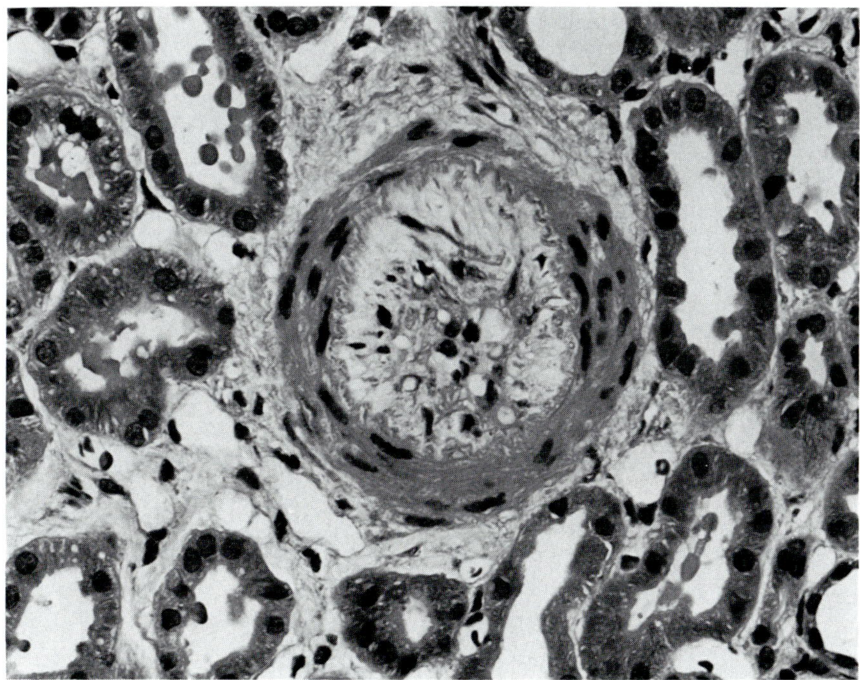

Figure 1–38. Intima, proliferation. The intimal region is markedly widened and contains an increased number of cells. (H&E, ×200.)

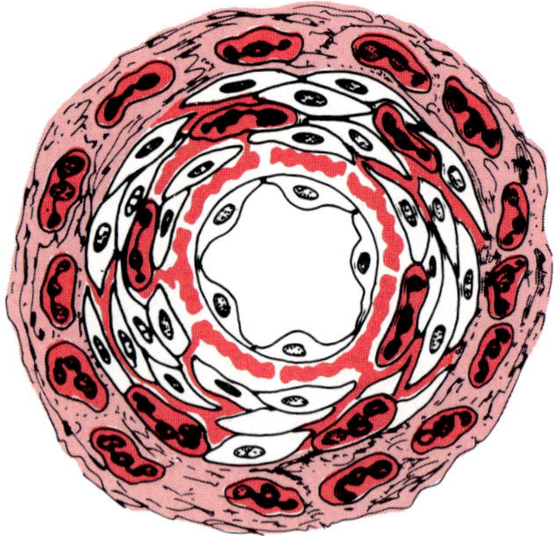

Figure 1–39. Intima, inflammatory cell infiltrate. Diagram of infiltration of the vascular wall with inflammatory cells.

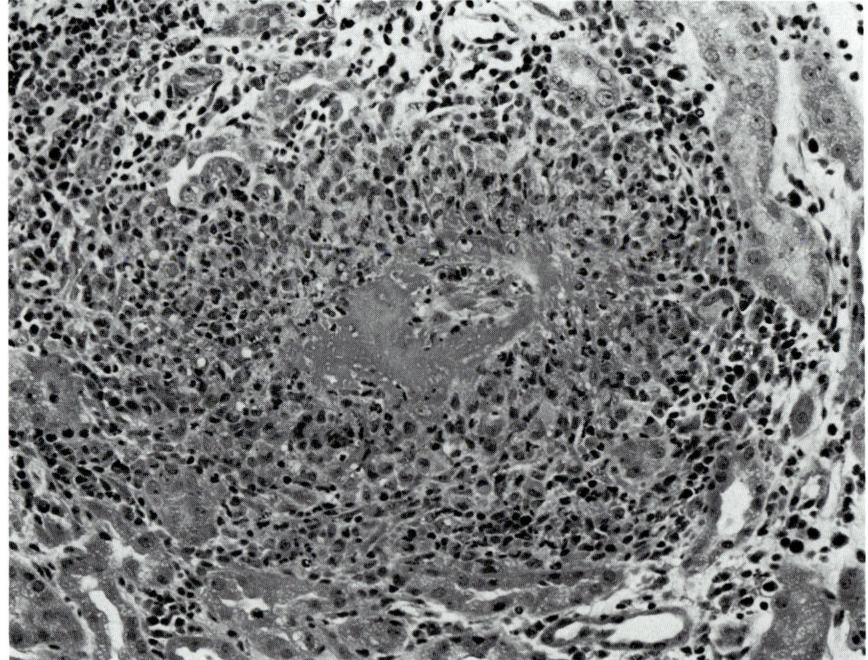

Figure 1–40. Intima, inflammatory cell infiltrate. The entire thickness of the vessel wall is infiltrated with a dense mass of inflammatory cells. The lumen is nearly obliterated, and the architecture of the blood vessel is difficult to appreciate. (H&E, ×100.)

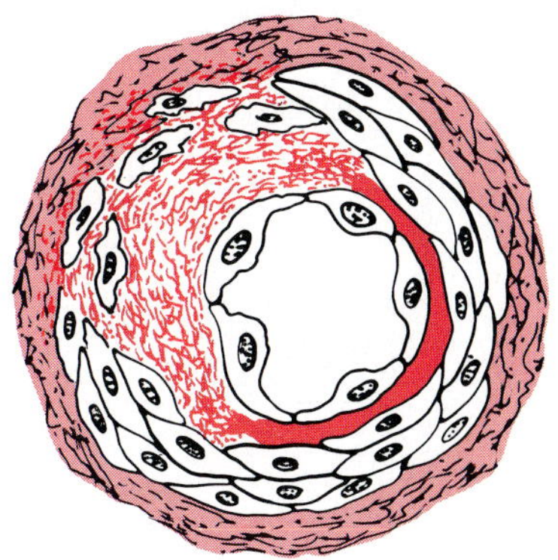

Figure 1–41. Intima, fibrin deposits. Diagram of disruption of the vascular wall and deposition of fibrin in the damaged area.

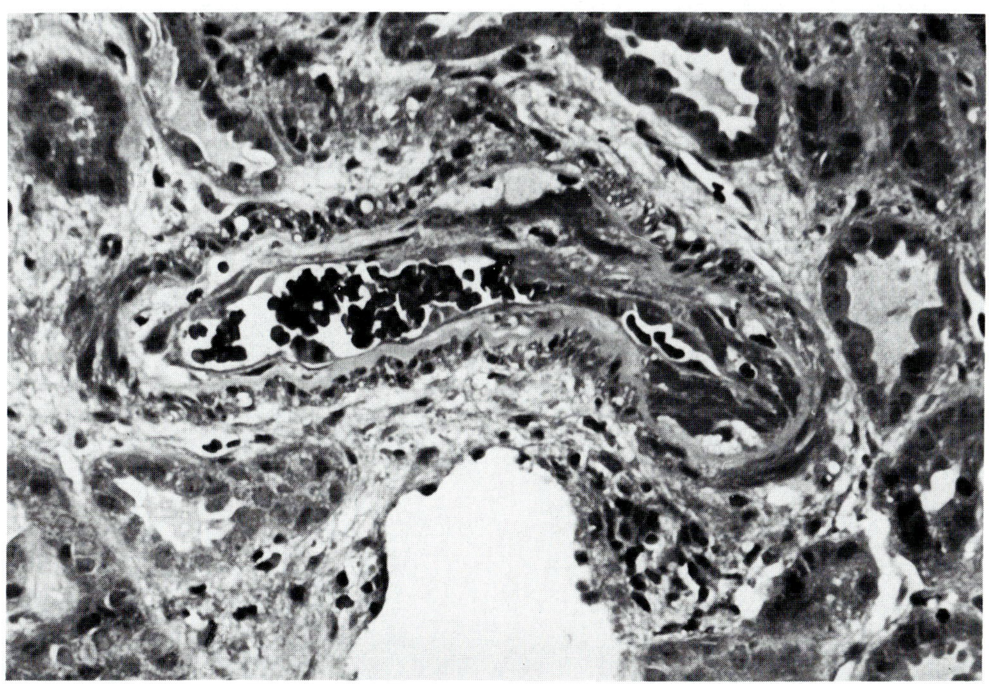

Figure 1–42. Intima (and media), fibrin deposits. The intima and media are disrupted (right center), and there is a mass of bright deposit consisting of fibrin. (Masson's trichrome, ×200.)

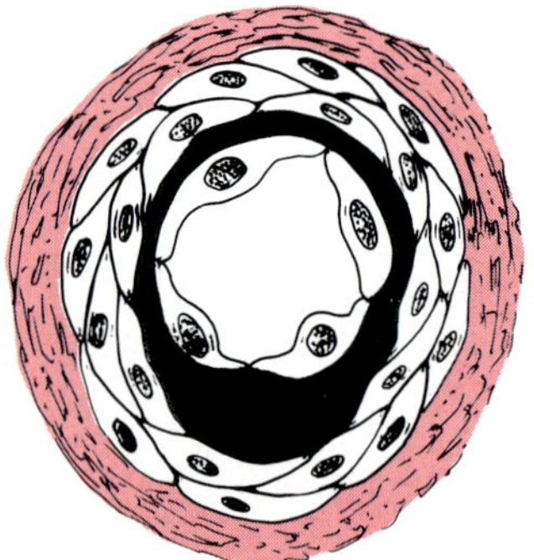

Figure 1–43. Intima, hyalin deposits. Diagram of a large hyalin deposit in the subintima.

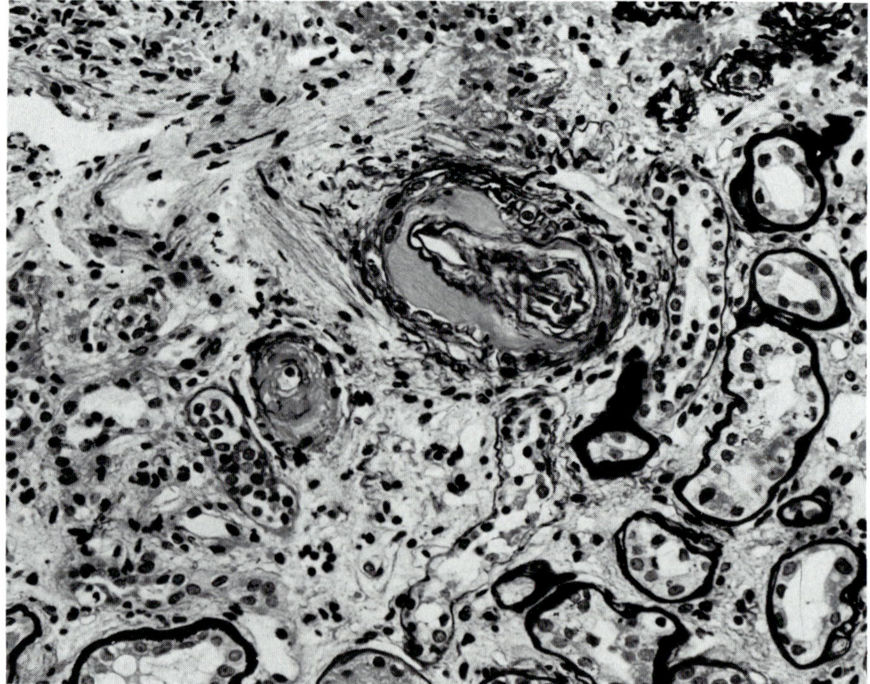

Figure 1–44. Intima (and media), hyalin deposits. There are hyalin deposits in both the arteriole (left center) and the small artery. (PASM, ×100.)

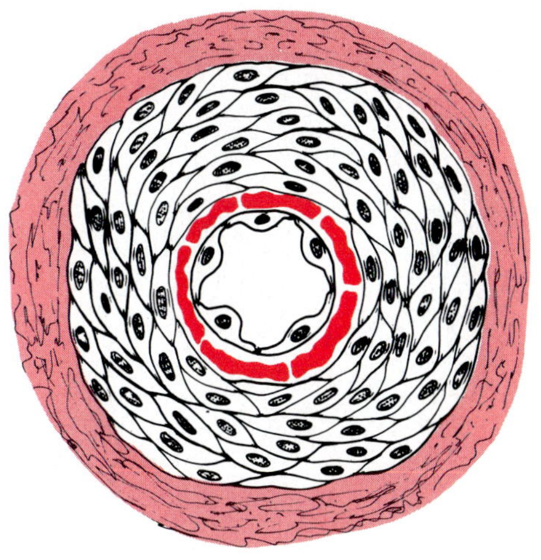

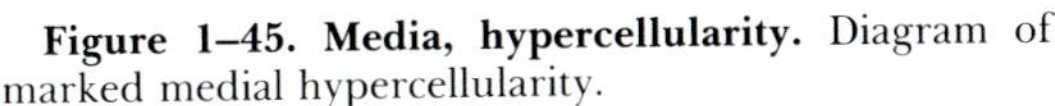

Figure 1–45. Media, hypercellularity. Diagram of marked medial hypercellularity.

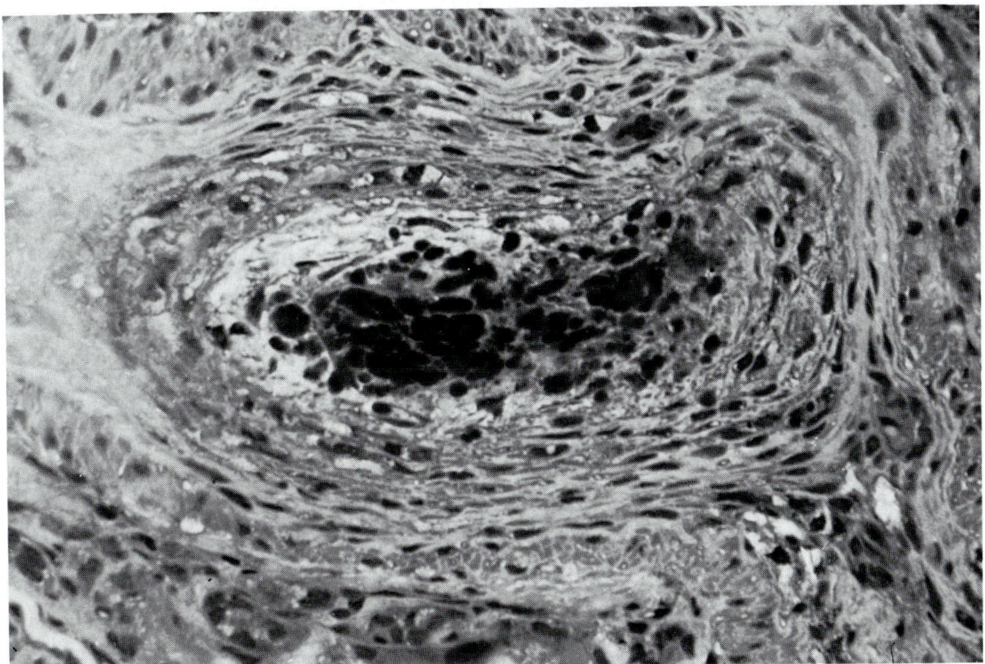

Figure 1–46. Media, hypercellularity. The medial layer of this artery is widened and contains an increased number of smooth muscle cell nuclei. (Masson's trichrome, ×150.)

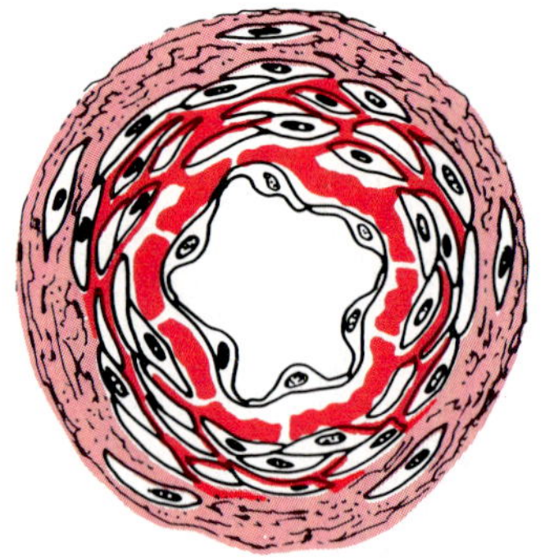

Figure 1–47. Media, sclerosis. Diagram of an increase in the amount of extracellular matrix in the media of an artery.

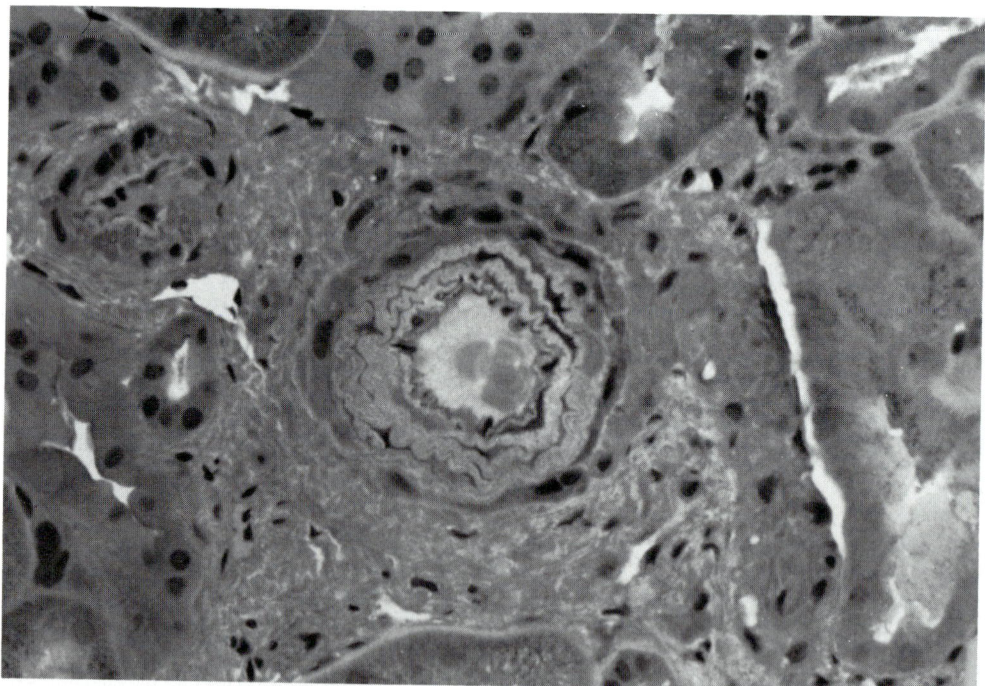

Figure 1–48. Media, sclerosis. There is an increase in the number of elastic laminae and in the amount of other types of extracellular matrix. Although the change primarily affects the media, the intima is also involved. (H&E, ×100.)

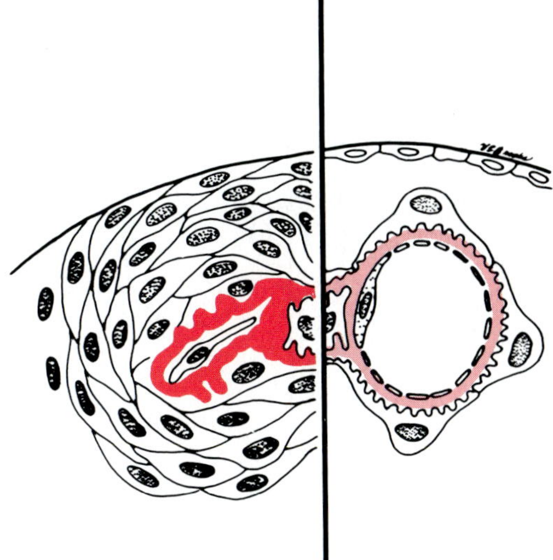

Figure 1–49. Deposits, linear. Diagram of a crescentic glomerulonephritis.

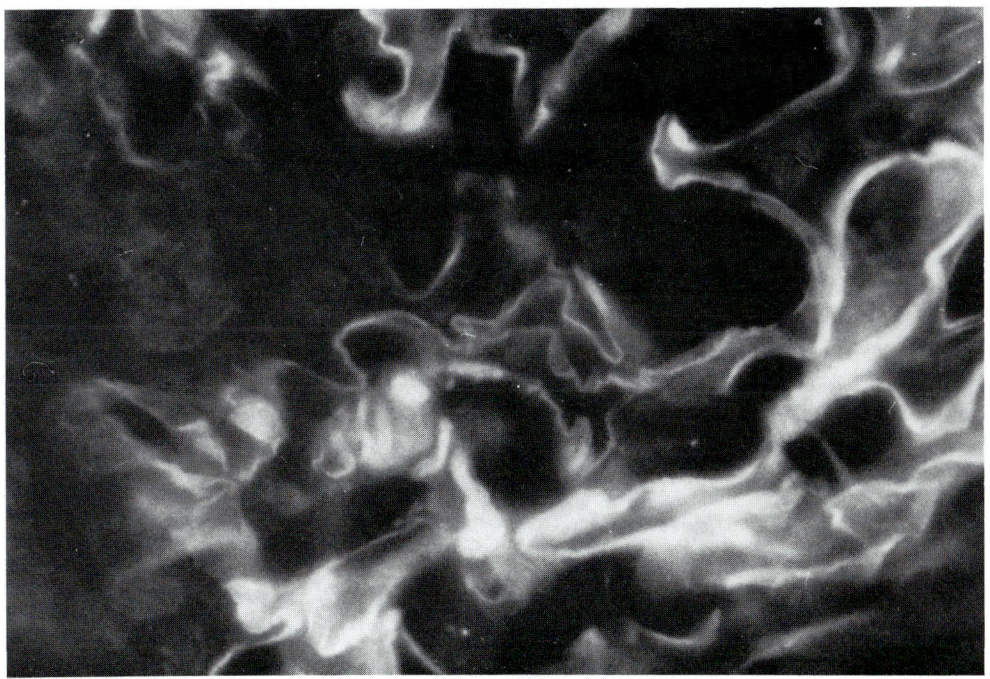

Figure 1–50. Deposits, linear. Immunofluorescence micrograph, anti-IgG. There are linear deposits outlining the glomerular basement membranes. The mesangial matrix is unstained. (×300.)

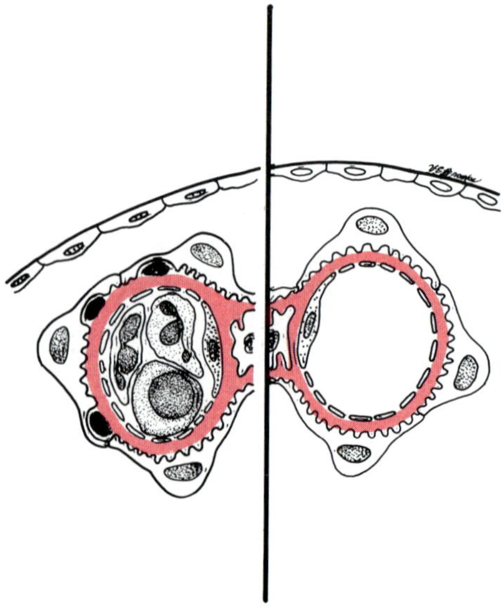

Figure 1–51. Deposits, subepithelial, granular. Diagram of irregular, subepithelial deposits in postinfectious glomerulonephritis.

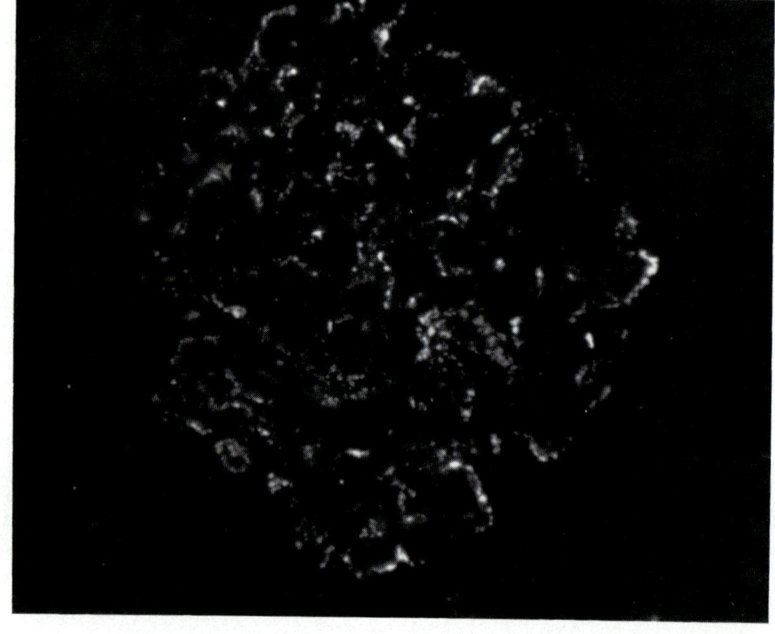

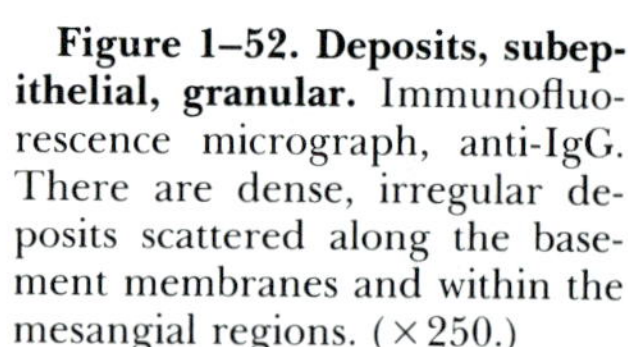

Figure 1–52. Deposits, subepithelial, granular. Immunofluorescence micrograph, anti-IgG. There are dense, irregular deposits scattered along the basement membranes and within the mesangial regions. (×250.)

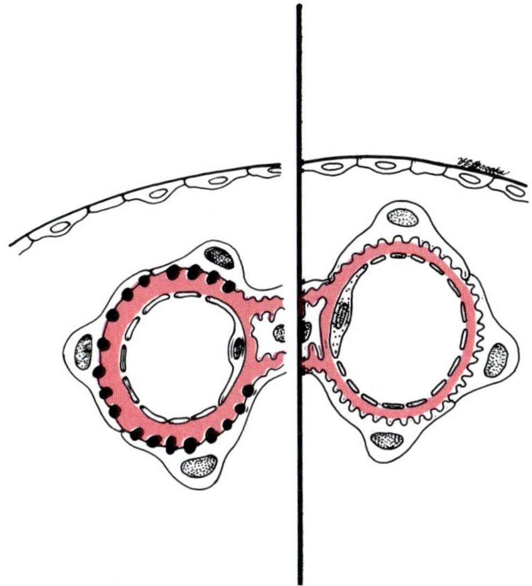

Figure 1–53. Deposits, subepithelial, regular. Diagram of subepithelial deposits in a regular, subepithelial distribution. This pattern is characteristic of membranous glomerulonephritis.

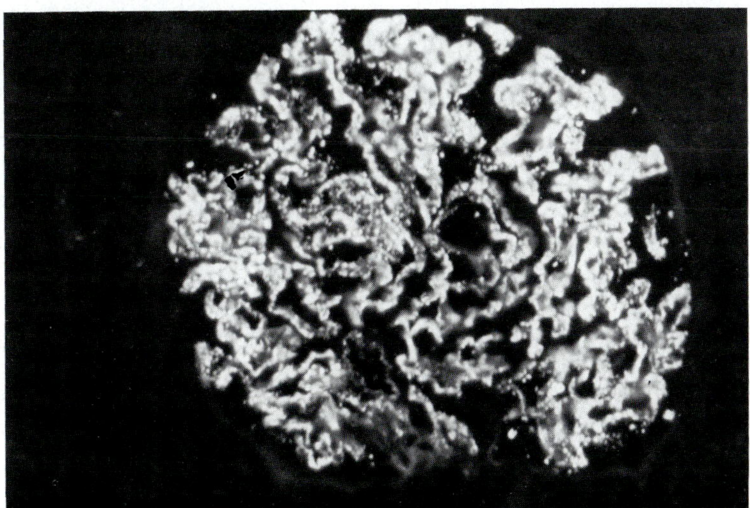

Figure 1–54. Deposits, subepithelial, regular. Immunofluorescence micrograph, anti-IgG. There are fine, subepithelial deposits scattered along the subepithelial aspects of the entire surface of the glomerular basement membranes. The mesangial regions do not contain deposits. (×250.)

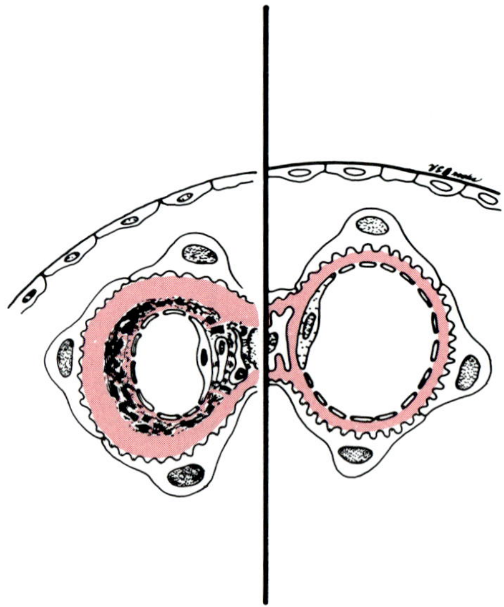

Figure 1–55. Deposits, subendothelial, membranoproliferative glomerulonephritis, type I. Diagram of large, subendothelial deposits with thickened basement membranes.

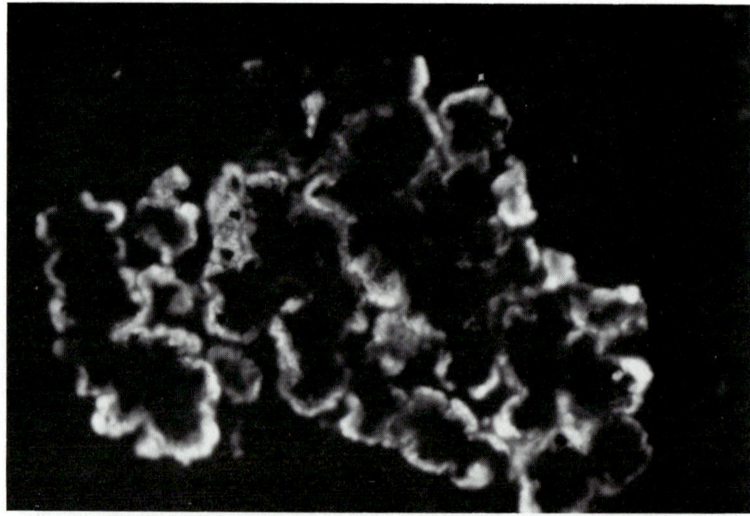

Figure 1–56. Deposits, subendothelial, membranoproliferative glomerulonephritis, type I. Immunofluorescence micrograph, anti-C3. Subendothelial deposits outline the glomerular basement membranes. (×250.)

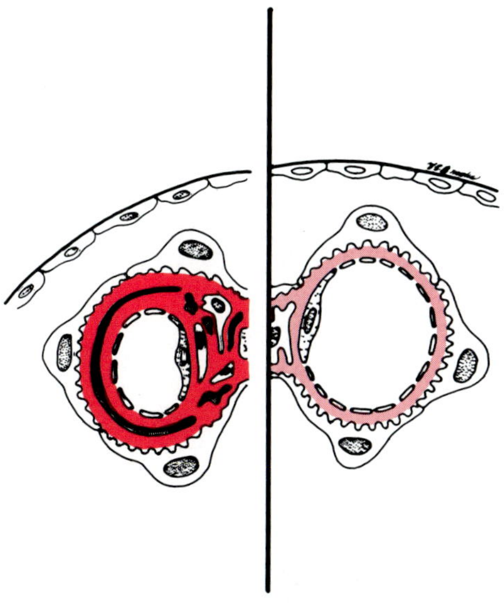

Figure 1–57. Deposits, intramembranous, membranoproliferative glomerulonephritis, type II. Diagram of deposits within a very thickened glomerular basement membrane.

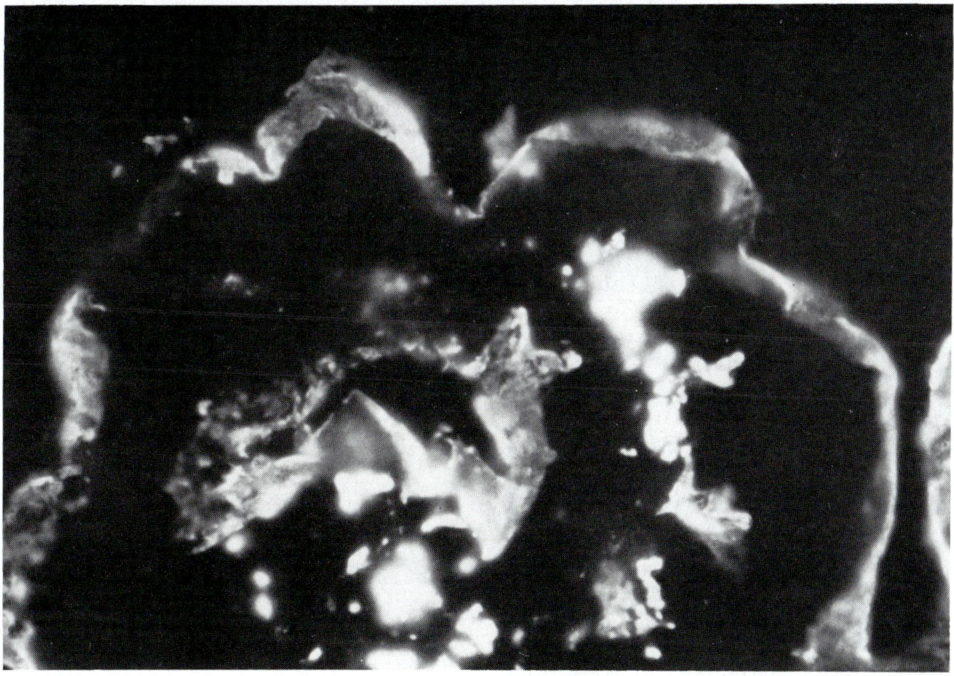

Figure 1–58. Deposits, intramembranous, membranoproliferative glomerulonephritis, type II. Immunofluorescence micrograph, anti-C3. The glomerular basement membranes contain large intramembranous deposits. The mesangial regions contain irregular punctate deposits.

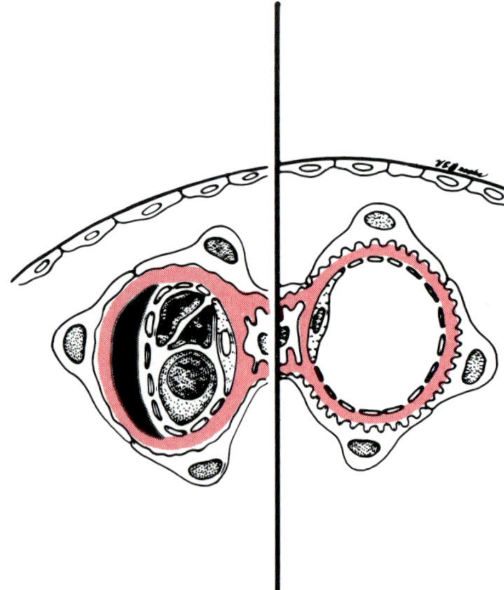

Figure 1–59. Deposits, subendothelial (SLE). Diagram of diffuse, large subendothelial deposits.

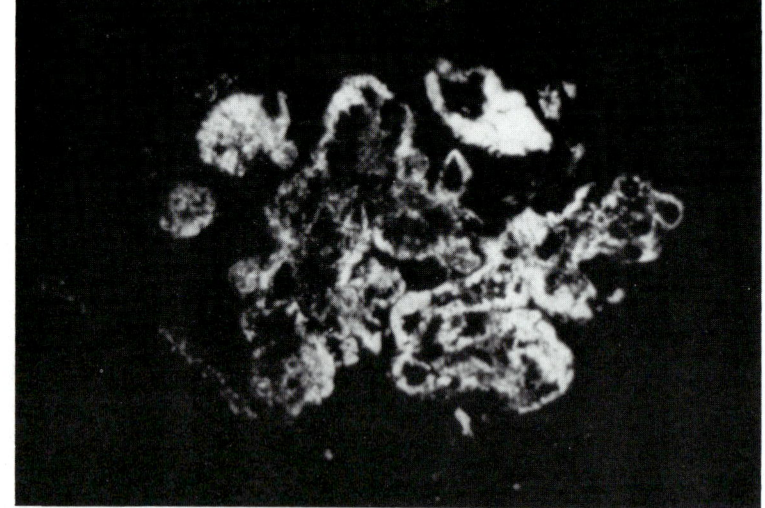

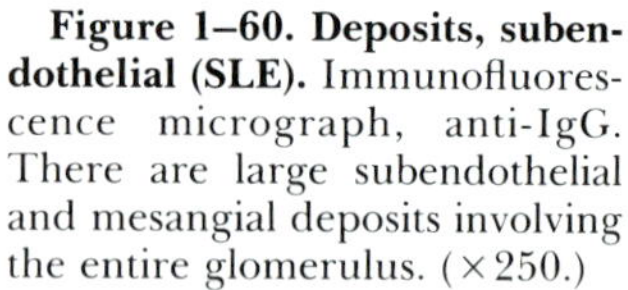

Figure 1–60. Deposits, subendothelial (SLE). Immunofluorescence micrograph, anti-IgG. There are large subendothelial and mesangial deposits involving the entire glomerulus. (×250.)

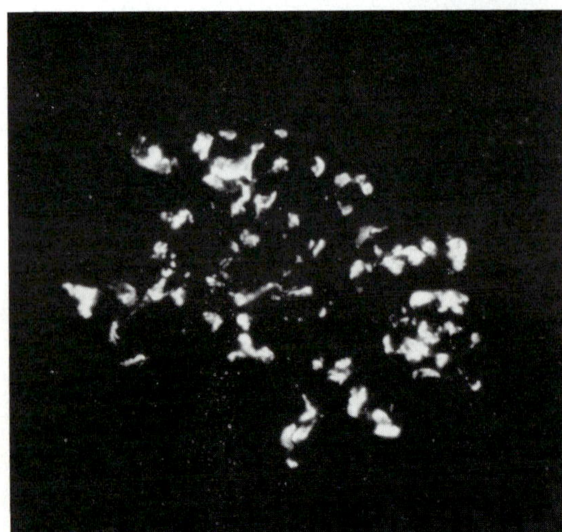

Figure 1–61. Deposits, mesangial. Immunofluorescence micrograph, anti-IgA. There are heavy, irregular deposits in each mesangial region. All glomeruli are affected. (×250.)

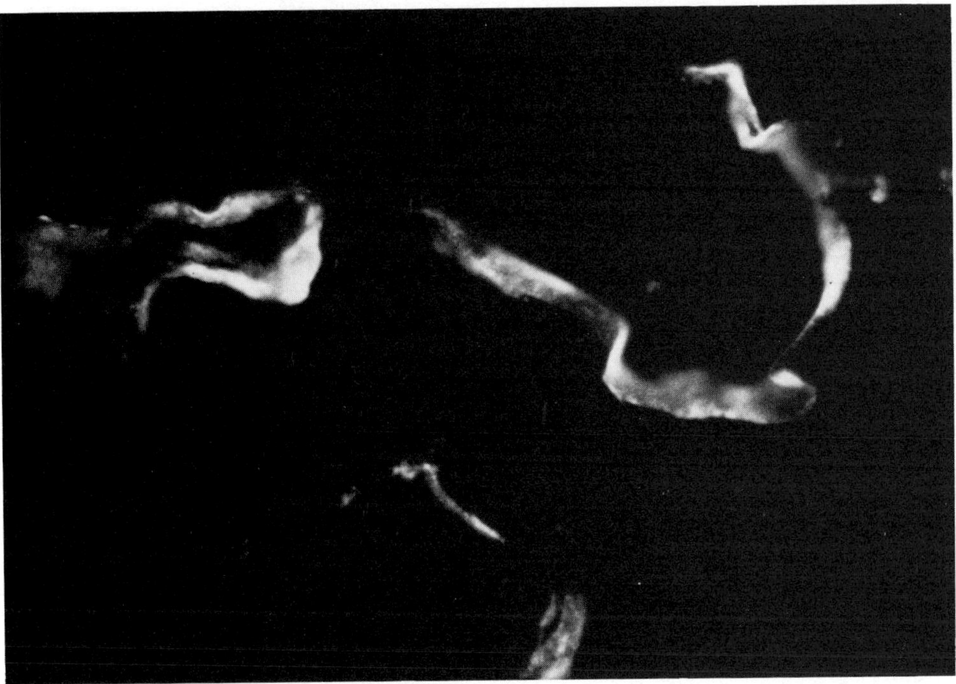

Figure 1–62. Deposits, tubular basement membranes, linear. Immunofluorescence micrograph, anti-IgG. There are deposits outlining the tubular basement membranes. (×300.)

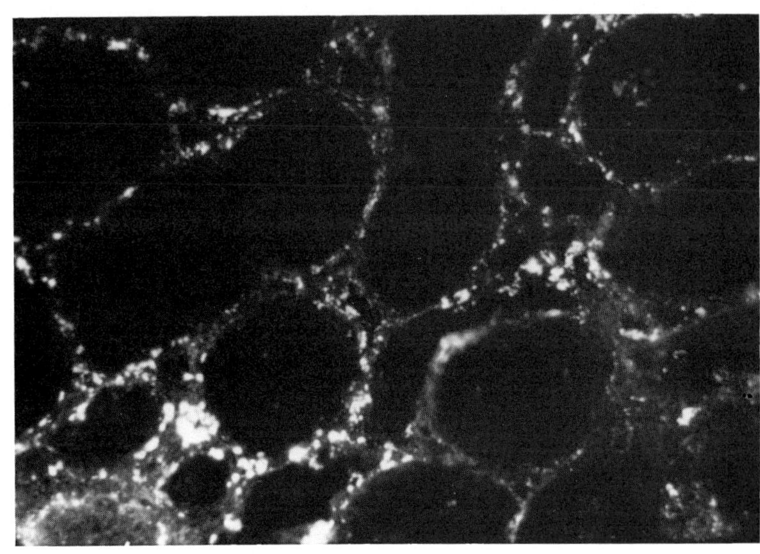

Figure 1–63. Deposits, tubular basement membranes, granular. Immunofluorescence micrograph, anti-IgG. Granular deposits are diffusely spread along the tubular and interstitial capillary basement membranes. (×250.)

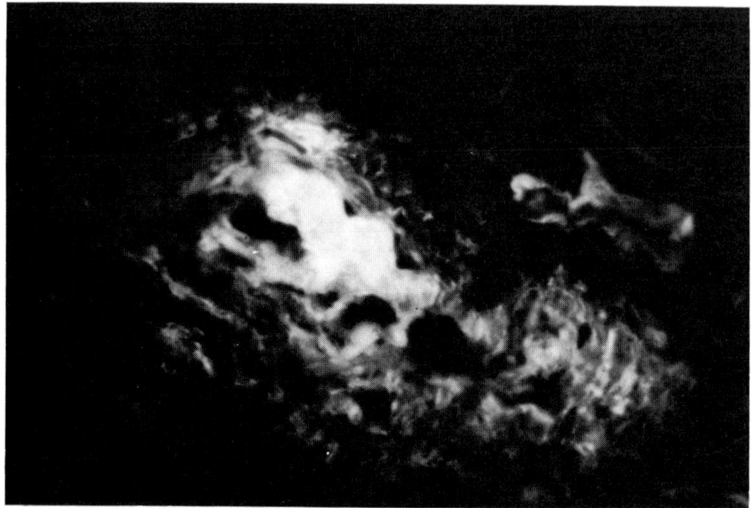

Figure 1–64. Deposits, artery. Immunofluorescence micrograph, antifibrin/fibrinogen antigens. The vascular wall contains large aggregates of deposits without clear margins. (×250.)

Hyalinosis. Acellular material that stains red with eosin and PAS but is unstained by PASM. Contents include serum proteins, other glycoproteins, and lipids.

Necrosis. Loss of structure with disruption of local cells and extracellular matrix, often associated with fibrin deposition.

Mesangiolysis. Disruption of mesangium. May be present in intravascular thrombosis.

Terms Relating to Proliferation

Endocapillary. Within vascular (capillary) loops.

Mesangial. Within the mesangium.

Crescent. Cellular proliferation and/or infiltration composed of glomerular epithelial cells, macrophages, and interstitial cells. If Bowman's capsule has been disrupted, crescents rapidly become sclerotic, resulting in glomerular obsolescence.

Terms Relating to Deposits

Subepithelial or epimembranous. Located between the glomerular basement membrane and the podocytes.

Intramembranous. Within the basement membrane.

Subendothelial. Between the glomerular basement membrane and the endothelium.

Mesangial. Within the mesangium.

Adhesions or synechiae. Localized crescents or bridges of connective tissue that are found between the glomerular vascular loops and Bowman's capsule.

Use of these terms and guidelines will allow categorization of a lesion as glomerular, tubulo-interstitial, or vascular. Glomerular diseases are observed more commonly in renal biopsy specimens than are lesions in the tubulo-interstitial or vascular regions. This distribution reflects both the biopsy policies of the nephrology community and the ability of clinicians and pathologists to suspect and recognize lesions in these other renal compartments.

INITIAL APPROACH TO THE RENAL BIOPSY

The interpretation should be approached systematically, logically, and practically. The first consideration is the nature of the questions that can and should be addressed:

1. What is the nature of the injury—that is, is it inflammatory, proliferative, sclerotic, deposition of foreign material, or a mixture?
2. What is the site of the lesion?
    a. Nephron segment
        Glomeruli
        Tubules
    b. Interstitium
    c. Blood vessels
3. What is its distribution—that is, focal or diffuse?
4. What is the severity—that is, mild or severe?
    a. mild—no disruption of the architecture
    b. moderate—disruption, but basement membranes intact
    c. severe—disruption, basement membranes interrupted

5. Is there evidence/possibility of repair?

After completing this analysis, the next step is to put these observations in context with the disease process and the patient. A summation, diagnosis, and interpretation can then be constructed.

RELATIONSHIP BETWEEN STRUCTURE AND FUNCTION

We and others have found that the measurement of the glomerular filtration rate did not provide a good indication of the underlying renal disease. In our studies, sequential patients from a renal consultation clinic were evaluated without regard to the underlying type or stage of renal disease. We found that there was no correlation between glomerular changes and the glomerular filtration rate, as determined by the clearance of inulin (Fig. 1–65). The best correlation was between the glomerular filtration rate and interstitial disease (Fig. 1–66). This finding remained an enigma until it was recently shown that one of the most important determinants of glomerular filtration rate is the filtration surface area. The filtration surface area can be accurately determined only by renal biopsy, using morphometric techniques. The measurements must be made by electron microscopy. Because it is the only means to determine the residual glomerular surface area available for filtration, electron microscopy may be an important variable in future studies on the progression of glomerular diseases. It now appears that as long as the filtration surface area can be increased, the glomerular filtration rate will remain at or near normal levels in the presence of increasing glomerular damage. These data help explain the lack of correlation between renal structure and function obtained in the past.

Therefore, the renal biopsy not only reveals the type and the extent of renal injury, but it allows their detection and quantification long before they can be measured by other methods.

CONCLUSION

The use of the renal biopsy as a research and clinical tool remains a largely untapped resource. The advent of immunofluorescence and electron microscopy added to its usefulness almost two decades ago. It remains for interested renal physicians to accept the challenge of applying modern biologic techniques to the direct assessment of renal biopsy specimens.

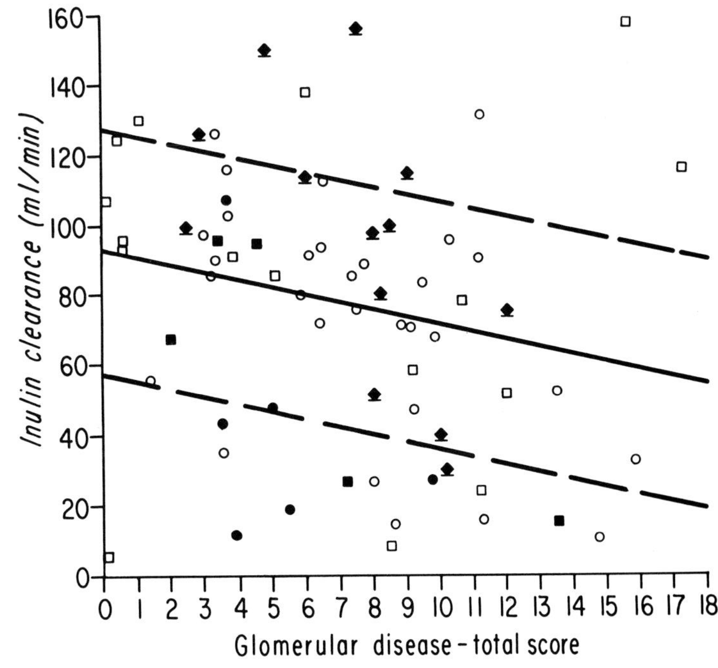

Figure 1–65. Relationship between inulin clearance and glomerular disease. Regression line (solid line) is $y = 92 - 0.02x$ and SEE (dashed line) is 39. The poor correlation is apparent. Symbols refer to cases belonging to conventional diagnostic groups: ▲, acute glomerulonephritis; ○, chronic glomerulonephritis; ●, interstitial nephritis; ■, nephrosclerosis; □, miscellaneous.

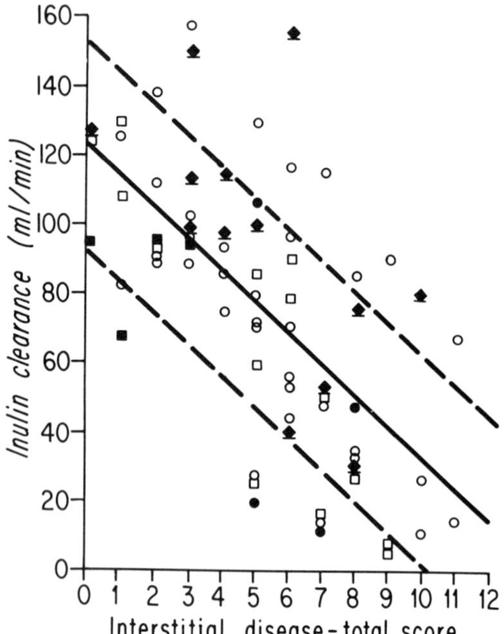

Figure 1–66. Relationship between inulin clearance and interstitial disease. The regression line (solid line) is y = 122 − 8.8x and SEE (dashed line) is 31. The symbols are the same as in Figure 1–65.

SELECTED READINGS

1. Bohle A, MacKensen-Haen S, Gise HV: Significance of tubulointerstitial changes in the renal cortex for the excretory function and concentration ability of the kidney: A morphometric contribution. Am J Nephrol 7:421, 1987.
2. Corwin HL, Schwartz MM, Lewis EJ: The importance of sample size in the interpretation of the renal biopsy. Am J Nephrol 8:85, 1988.
3. Kashgarian M, Hayslett JP, Spargo BH: Teaching monograph. Am J Pathol 89:187, 1977.
4. Morel-Maroger L: The value of renal biopsy. Am J Kidney Dis 1:244, 1982.
5. Morel-Maroger L, Leathem A, Richet G: Glomerular abnormalities in nonsystemic diseases. Relationship between findings by light microscopy and immunofluorescence in 433 renal biopsy specimens. Am J Med 53:170, 1972.
6. Nolasco F, Cameron J, Hartley B, et al: Intraglomerular T cells and monocytes in nephritis: Study with monoclonal antibodies. Kidney Int 31:1160, 1987.
7. Pirani CL, Salinas-Madrigal L, Koss M: Evaluation of percutaneous renal biopsy. *In* Sommer SC (ed): Kidney Pathology Decennial. Appleton-Century-Crofts, New York, 1975, pp. 109–163.
8. Risdon RA, Sloper JC, De Wardener HE: Relationship between renal function and histologic changes found in renal biopsy specimens from patients with persistent glomerulonephritis. Lancet 2:363, 1968.
9. Schainuck LI, Striker GE, Cutler RE, et al: Structural-functional correlations in renal disease. II. The correlations. Hum Pathol 1:631, 1970.
10. Schwartz MM, Bidani AK, Lewis EJ: Glomerular epithelial cell structure and function in chronic proteinuria induced by homologous protein load. Lab Invest 55:673, 1986.
11. Striker GE, Schainuck LI, Cutler RE, et al: Structural-functional correlations in renal disease. I. A method for assaying and classifying histopathologic changes in renal disease. Hum Pathol 1:615, 1970.

Chapter

2

HANDLING AND PREPARATION OF SPECIMENS

The ability to recognize and correctly interpret a renal biopsy specimen requires proper handling of the tissue at all stages of its preparation. Immunofluorescence microscopy is essentially always necessary as an adjunct to light microscopy. Electron microscopy is required in many instances, but this technique may only be available in selected centers. Other special methods may also be required.

The nephrologist (and pathologist) referring specimens must confer with the receiving pathologist regarding the locally preferred methods of transport. In addition, an adequate clinical and laboratory work-up is always required for interpretation of the biopsy findings.

The pathologist may be given two kinds of renal biopsy specimens: wedge and needle samples. Wedge biopsy specimens always include cortex as well as a greater sample of renal tissue than needle biopsy specimens, but they are the exception in the usual pathology practice. In most instances, renal tissue is obtained with a needle and the amount of tissue available is fairly limited.

HANDLING THE GROSS SPECIMEN

Ideally, the pathologist or a histology technician should attend the biopsy procedure to ensure that the tissue is handled properly. If this is not the case, several guidelines will help in obtaining the tissue in the most appropriate state for processing. It is critical to handle the tissue delicately to avoid crushing or tearing the specimen. The cores must be cut with a sharp blade on dental wax using a slicing rather than a crushing motion. Wide mouth pipettes or wooden sticks may be used to place the tissue fragments into appropriate containers. Forceps should never be used. Two separate cores of tissue should be obtained whenever possible. If a small dissecting microscope is available, the first core should be examined for the presence of glomeruli and directly immersed in a bottle of the fixative chosen for light microscopy. Glomeruli are recognizable with a hand lens as tiny reddish structures of less than 1 mm diameter. The second core may be partitioned for immunofluorescence and electron microscopy.

If only one core of tissue is available, it should be gently bisected longitudinally. One-half can then be processed for light microscopy. The second fragment is transected vertically, one-half being used for immunofluorescence microscopy and one-half for electron microscopy. The tissue for electron microscopy can be immediately fixed in the fixative of choice.

The tissue for immunofluorescence microscopy may be stored in a Petri dish and covered with a sterile gauze moistened with sterile TRIS buffer or phosphate-buffered saline (PBS). The tissue should not be carried on ice because it may become partially frozen.

Freezing should be accomplished by snap-freezing in liquid nitrogen or on dry ice. The tissue must not be cut in a cryostat or placed in a freezer before proper snap-freezing. If the tissue cannot be frozen within 2 hours, special transport media allow adequate, if not ideal, preservation of samples for longer periods (up to 36 hours).

In the case of wedge biopsies, ten 1 × 1 × 1 mm pieces of tissue should be placed in fixative for electron miscoscopy. One slice measuring 3 × 3 × 2 mm should be set aside for immunofluorescence microscopy, and the remainder should be placed in a fixative appropriate for light microscopy.

PREPARATION FOR SECTIONING

Light Microscopy

Fixation

Several fixatives have been proposed for light microscopy. The critical point is to choose a fixative that allows the preparation of thin (3 μm) sections and to use multiple stains. The most frequently used fixatives include Duboscq-Brazil or alcoholic Bouin's solution, 10% neutral-buffered formalin, Zenker-formol, Carnoy's solution, or paraformaldehyde. Paraformaldehyde has the advantage of being a reasonable fixative for both light and electron microscopy.

A needle biopsy specimen requires a minimum of 1 hour fixation, whereas wedge biopsies require several hours. The tissue is then processed overnight. The exact sequence of washes may vary and is best determined in the individual laboratory.

Embedding Medium

Paraffin

Paraffin is the most commonly used embedding medium. Paraffins with a high melting point allow the technician to reproducibly obtain thin sections.

Glycol Methacrylate

Glycol methacrylate is used by several laboratories for light microscopy. The exact procedure depends on the manufacturing source. The blocks are quite hard, allowing one to routinely obtain sections of 1 to 2 μm thickness using a JB-4 microtome and a glass knife. The chief advantages of this method are that shrinkage of the tissue is less than in paraffin-embedded specimens and resolution is better because of the thinness of the section. The three main disadvantages are the hygroscopic tendency of the plastic (which results in variation in ease of sectioning because of variations in the ambient humidity), difficulty in storage of the blocks in a condition suitable for future resectioning, and an increased staining time. Most of the standard stains have been altered for use in this medium, and the results are quite satisfactory.

If sections less than 2 μm are obtained, the stains may be too pale for viewing easily and satisfactory photographs may be difficult to obtain.

Cutting

Multiple sections should be cut, and they should be numbered, a useful precaution in the event of focal lesions. We prefer to place three to four sections on each glass slide.

Staining

A battery of stains is used. From paraffin blocks we obtain 12 slides cut at 2 to 3 μm and one at 8 μm. Slide numbers 1, 3, 6, and 12 are stained with hematoxylin and eosin (H&E). Slide 5 is stained with phosphotungstic acid-hematoxylin (PTAH) for fibrin. Slide 7 is stained with periodic acid-Schiff (PAS), which accentuates basement membranes, mesangial matrix, and the brush border of proximal tubular epithelial cells. Various pathologic alterations are also emphasized with this stain, including hyalinosis, cryoglobulin precipitates, and Tamm-Horsfall protein. Slide 8 is stained with a combination of methenamine silver and PAS with an H&E counterstain. This combination aids in the evaluation of lesions involving basement membranes. It is especially useful for photomicrography. Section 9 is stained with a Masson's trichrome, which accentuates fibrosis. It is often possible to detect subepithelial deposits with this stain. The thickest section, number 13, is used for Congo red staining in those biopsies in which there is a suspicion of amyloid deposits. A thick section is required to provide sufficient dye binding for visualization by polarizing microscopy.

The intervening unstained slides can be used for other stains such as those for reticulin or elastin.

Immunofluorescence Microscopy

After it has been properly snap-frozen, the tissue may be stored. However, storage for periods exceeding 4 to 6 weeks results in desiccation, rendering the tissue uninterpretable. The tissue is then cut in a cryostat at a temperature between −25 and −20°C. The sections may not exceed 6 μm and ideally should be 3 to 4 μm in thickness. The slides are fixed for 5 to 10 minutes in acetone, dried at room temperature, washed in buffered saline, and covered for 30 minutes with a drop of fluorescein-labeled antiserum in a moist chamber that is light shielded. After several washes with buffer, the slides are mounted using buffered glycerol. It is possible to delay fading by adding phenylenediamine to the mounting medium.

The sections are then examined using a fluorescence microscope equipped with appropriate excitation and barrier filters. The sections should be photographed because the fluorescence fades on exposure to both ultraviolet and incident light. They also fade on storage, within a few weeks, even without exposure.

Immunoperoxidase

The application of this technique to renal biopsy specimens for the identification of proteins in extracellular deposits has not met with as much success as it has in the identification of cell surface markers. Nonetheless, some use it on fixed and embedded specimens when frozen tissue is not available for immunofluorescence microscopy or when glomeruli are not present in the material obtained for frozen sectioning. Many authors have discussed the vagaries of the technique, including the requirement that the section must be glued to the slides and that the tissue sections require trypsin digestion before exposure to the antibodies. Digestion is used in an attempt to expose antigenic sites. The advantages of this method compared with immunofluorescence microscopy are that frozen tissue is not necessary and that slides are available as a permanent record. The disadvantage is that the technique still gives inconsistent results in many laboratories because of the presence of a high background.

Electron Microscopy

Fixation and Embedding

Many fixatives do not readily penetrate renal tissue. Thus, it is important that the fragments be no larger than 1 × 1 × 1 mm. The most widely used fixative is 3% phosphate-buffered glutaraldehyde. This solution is diluted from a stock solution of 25% glutaraldehyde. The diluted solution has a shelf life of no more than 2 months, even when refrigerated. At room temperature, 3% glutaraldehyde deteriorates within a few hours. Carson's fixative (4% formaldehyde and 1% glutaraldehyde) is an alternate fixative that is available commercially. Fixatives containing glutaraldehyde are not appropriate for light microscopy unless the free aldehyde groups are blocked. Otherwise, the staining patterns are altered and the tissue becomes brittle and difficult to cut in a paraffin-embedded block.

After fixation for a minimum of 2 hours, the tissue is rinsed in buffer, post-fixed in 1% osmium tetroxide, dehydrated, and embedded.

If no glomeruli are present in the material prepared for electron microscopy, the tissue remaining in the light microscopy block can be used. The area of the light microscopy block containing glomeruli is identified and cut from the block. The fragment is rinsed several times in xylene to remove the paraffin. The tissue can then be processed for electron microscopy. The preservation of morphology is less than optimal, but it is often satisfactory for the recognition of significant alterations.

Sectioning and Staining

Thick sections (1 μm) are cut with glass knives and stained with toluidine blue to choose appropriate areas for thin sectioning. In the presence of a diffuse, uniform renal lesion, any region of the cortex that contains all of the representative elements may be suitable. When the lesions are focal or irregular in severity, several representative areas should be chosen. Thin sections (60 to 90 Å) are then cut and stained with uranyl acetate and lead citrate.

Examination

Evaluation of the thin section should include an assessment of all compartments. The section should first be examined at low power. It is helpful to develop a systematic method of assessing the elements of each compartment. For instance, an examination of the glomerulus might include the peripheral vascular wall, all three glomerular cell types (endothelial, epithelial, and mesangial), and the extracellular matrix (glomerular basement membrane and mesangial matrix). An increase in mesangial cell number and matrix is best evaluated with the light microscope because of the small sample size and propensity for sampling errors by electron microscopy. However, the presence and location of immune deposits or amyloid may be best detected and documented by electron microscopy. The several tubular segments should be examined for alterations of either the epithelial cells or tubular basement membranes. The blood vessels, often overlooked, should be carefully evaluated for both cellular and extracellular matrix changes, including the presence of hyalin or other changes related to hypertension. The distribution of interstitial changes is best documented using the light microscope.

Other Specialized Techniques

One new technique is in situ hybridization. This technique still belongs in the category of a research tool, thus applications to clinical problems remain for the future.

Needle aspiration of the kidney is being used in evaluating renal transplants for the presence of rejection in some centers (see Chapter 11). This technique does not have a place in the evaluation of most renal diseases, because the specimen consists of isolated cells.

SELECTED READINGS

1. Agodoa LY, Striker GE, Chi E: Glycomethacrylate embedding of renal biopsy specimens for light microscopy. Am J Clin Pathol 64:655, 1975.
2. Koehler JK: Advanced Techniques in Biological Electron Microscopy. Berlin, Springer-Verlag, 1973.

Chapter

3

CLASSIFICATION OF RENAL DISEASE

The classification of a renal disease depends on recognition and quantification of the predominant lesion. In most cases, careful assessment of a renal biopsy specimen allows its categorization into one of the known disease processes. This does not necessarily mean that each biopsy sample can be neatly placed into a specific disease category that has a clinical counterpart, but certain useful generalizations can be made.

Lesions may affect one, all, or several aspects of the different renal compartments (i.e., the glomeruli, tubules, interstitium, or blood vessels). For the most part, each renal disease affects more than one compartment, even though one site may be more affected than the others. The role of the pathologist is to recognize the site, type, and distribution of lesions and then integrate the information in such a manner that a diagnosis can be reached.

The following list of glomerular, tubulointerstitial, and vascular diseases is not exhaustive but reflects the most common problems encountered in a renal biopsy practice. We have excluded some diseases that are very unusual and those encountered only in tropical countries. Finally, the kidneys are affected by many drugs, toxins, viruses, bacteria, and parasites. We have chosen to list only those that have been reasonably well established.

GLOMERULAR DISEASES

I. GLOMERULAR DISEASE: WITHOUT KNOWN ETIOLOGY
   A. Minimal lesion (or "lipoid nephrosis" or minimal lesion nephrotic syndrome)
      1. Diffuse spreading of pedicels
   B. Diffuse lesions
      1. Diffuse proliferative glomerulonephritis
      2. Membranous glomerulonephritis
      3. Membranoproliferative glomerulonephritis (type I)
      4. Dense-deposit disease (membranoproliferative glomerulonephritis (type II)
      5. Crescentic glomerulonephritis
         a. With immune deposits (granular)
         b. With immune deposits (linear)
         c. Without immune deposits
      6. End-stage sclerosing glomerulonephritis
   C. Focal lesions
      1. Focal proliferative
         a. Without IgA
         b. With IgA
      2. Focal sclerosis or focal and segmental glomerulosclerosis

II. GLOMERULAR DISEASES ASSOCIATED WITH INFECTION
   A. Bacterial
      1. Proliferative glomerulonephritis
         a. Diffuse proliferative and exudative glomerulonephritis (post-streptococcal)

b. Diffuse proliferative glomerulonephritis (other bacteria)
2. Membranoproliferative glomerulonephritis (chronic bacterial diseases)
3. Crescentic glomerulonephritis
a. Post-streptococcal glomerulonephritis
b. Subacute bacterial endocarditis
c. Visceral abscesses
B. Parasitic
1. Membranous glomerulonephritis
a. Filiariasis *(Loa loa)*
2. Membranoproliferative glomerulonephritis
a. *Schistosoma mansoni* (focal proliferative glomerulonephritis)
3. Diffuse basement membrane change
a. Quartan malaria
C. Viral
1. Focal and segmental glomerulosclerosis
a. Acquired immunodeficiency syndrome (AIDS)
2. Membranous and membranoproliferative glomerulonephritis
a. Hepatitis

III. GLOMERULAR LESIONS IN SYSTEMIC DISORDERS
A. Amyloidosis
1. Amyloid AA (secondary)
2. Amyloid AL (primary)
B. Goodpasture's syndrome
C. Hemolytic-uremic syndrome
D. Henoch-Schönlein syndrome
E. Mixed essential cryoglobulinemia
F. Scleroderma
G. Sickle cell disease
H. Systemic lupus erythematosus
I. Systemic vasculitis
J. Myeloma and light-chain systemic deposition disease
K. Carcinoma and lymphoma

IV. GLOMERULAR CHANGES ASSOCIATED WITH MAJOR ORGAN FAILURE
A. Hepatic cirrhosis
B. Cyanotic heart disease
C. Diabetes mellitus

V. GLOMERULAR LESIONS DUE TO TOXINS AND DRUGS
A. Heroin
B. Heavy metals
C. Pharmaceuticals containing a free sulfhydryl group
1. Penicillamine
2. Captopril
D. Immunosuppressive and antineoplastic agents
1. Cyclosporine A
2. Mitomycin C

VI. GLOMERULAR LESIONS IN METABOLIC DISORDERS
A. Diabetes mellitus
B. Lecithin-cholesterol acyltransferase (LCAT) deficiency
C. Cystinosis
D. Fabry's disease
E. Glycogenosis type I

VII. GLOMERULAR LESIONS IN CONGENITAL DISEASES
A. Alport's syndrome
B. Nail-patella syndrome
C. Benign familial hematuria

VIII. TOXEMIA OF PREGNANCY

IX. TRANSPLANTATION

TUBULO-INTERSTITIAL LESIONS

I. TUBULAR
A. Necrosis
1. Acute
2. Regeneration
B. Cellular changes
1. Inclusions (vacuoles)
2. Crystals
C. Atrophy

II. INTERSTITIAL
A. Acute
1. Infectious (bacteria, spirochetes, Hantaan virus)
2. Drug-induced (non-steroidal anti-inflammatory agents and beta-lactam antibiotics)

3. Immune-mediated (uveitis)
4. Granulomatous (tuberculosis, sarcoid, drug-induced)

B. Chronic
1. Infectious
2. Drug-induced (phenacetin)
3. Heavy metals

DISEASES OF THE BLOOD VESSELS

I. ARTERIOSCLEROSIS
II. SCLERODERMA
III. CHOLESTEROL EMBOLI
IV. VASCULITIS

Chapter

4

PRIMARY GLOMERULAR DISEASE OF UNKNOWN ETIOLOGY

MINIMAL LESION

The terms *minimal change nephrotic syndrome, minimal change disease, minimal change,* and *lipoid nephrosis* encompass a clinicopathologic entity that consists of the nephrotic syndrome in association with a specific configurational change that is limited to the visceral epithelial cells of the glomerulus. For the sake of brevity and consistency, we will refer to this syndrome as minimal lesion. This syndrome is defined by the presence of normal-appearing glomeruli by light and immunofluorescence microscopy, with an electron microscopic lesion consisting only of effacement of the pedicels. The result is that the urinary side of the glomerular basement membrane is covered by a homogeneous layer of epithelial cell cytoplasm rather than the complex interdigitation of pedicels from adjacent cells.

Pathogenesis

The pathogenesis of minimal lesion is unknown, but one of the current beliefs is that one mediator of the disease is a low-molecular-weight substance derived from T-lymphocytes. The effect of this substance could be to alter the podocytes so that the charge and size-selective characteristics of the glomerular vascular wall are altered. The net result of this change is the development of proteinuria. This hypothesis is strengthened by the rapid response of the proteinuria and pedicel effacement to steroid therapy and the presence of this clinical and morphologic entity in patients with certain malignancies of T-lymphocytes.

Patient Presentation

Minimal lesion is the most common underlying disease in nephrotic children. It is most frequently seen after 2 years of age, with a peak incidence at age 3. It is much more common in boys than in girls. Curiously, adults of both sexes are affected equally often.

The syndrome is characterized by multiple exacerbations and remissions, sometimes over a period of years, with long intervals between incidents. The precipitating events are not known, but minimal lesion has been associated with allergic reactions, including bee stings. The onset is heralded by the development of progressive edema and selective proteinuria (i.e., albuminuria). Hypertension and hematuria are rare and when present should lead to the suspicion of some other renal disease than minimal lesion.

Few children now undergo biopsy unless they do not respond to steroids, and few pathologists have the opportunity to see this disease by renal biopsy. The sole exceptions are those few patients with this syndrome who do not show a prompt response to steroid therapy and in whom the nephrotic syndrome is severe enough to prompt the question of treatment with more aggressive therapeutic agents.

Although the overwhelming majority of children with the nephrotic syndrome have this renal picture, it is much less frequent in adults, in whom it accounts for approximately 20% of patients presenting with the idiopathic nephrotic syndrome. Therefore, adults are much more likely to undergo renal biopsy before a trial of steroid therapy is undertaken.

Histology

Light Microscopy

Because the diagnosis of minimal lesion depends on the absence of obvious glomerular changes by light microscopy, it is imperative that multiple sections of each biopsy sample be prepared and examined thoroughly (Figs. 4–1 and 4–2). The glomeruli of children are smaller than those of adults and may appear to be hypercellular to pathologists who do not often examine pediatric renal tissue. If there is any question about cellularity or extracellular matrix changes by light microscopy, normal tissue from a child of similar age should be used for comparison.

The peripheral vascular loops may occasionally appear to be dilated but are otherwise normal. The podocyte cytoplasm appears swollen or vacuolated. The pedicel abnormalities (i.e., effacement) may be apparent in sections of methacrylate-embedded tissue (Fig. 4–3).

No cellular proliferation or mesangial matrix change is seen.

There is some controversy in the current literature about whether minimal change, mesangial proliferative glomerulonephritis, and focal or segmental glomerulonephritis all are part of a continuum. It has been said that patients are encountered in whom one can demonstrate a transition between these different diseases. We are of the strong opinion that minimal lesion belongs in a separate category based on its morphologic appearance and clinical behavior. In our combined experience, we are not aware of any patient who has progressed from minimal lesion to any sclerosing or proliferative disease. However, it should be carefully stated that this conclusion is based on the study of biopsies in which multiple sections have been examined by light, immunofluorescence, and electron microscopy and includes only those cases in which an adequate sample of renal tissue has been available for study. In the absence of this type of detailed search, focal lesions may be missed.

Only very minor changes are ordinarily present in the extraglomerular regions. They consist mainly of slight interstitial widening, apparently due to edema, and the presence of hyalin droplets in the cytoplasm of the proximal tubules. In biopsies of older patients, lesions in the tubulo-interstitial or vascular compartments may be associated with arteriosclerosis.

Immunofluorescence Microscopy

The characteristic feature of this disease is the complete absence of immune reactants, fibrin, and other foreign materials. Some have suggested that small amounts of IgM and C3 may be found, but most agree that the hallmark of minimal change is the lack of such substances.

Electron Microscopy

The electron microscopic changes are so restricted to the glomerular visceral epithelial cells that some have dubbed minimal lesion the "epithelial cell disease." The characteristic podocyte abnormality is the complete effacement of the pedicels, resulting in a smooth and homogenous layer of epithelial cell cy-

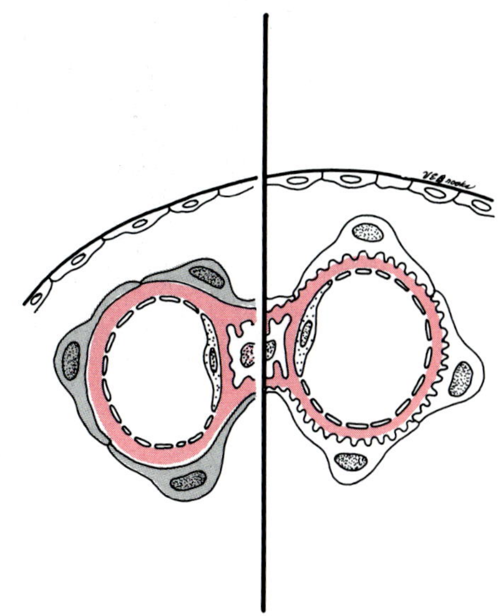

Figure 4–1. Diagram of diffuse podocyte spreading.

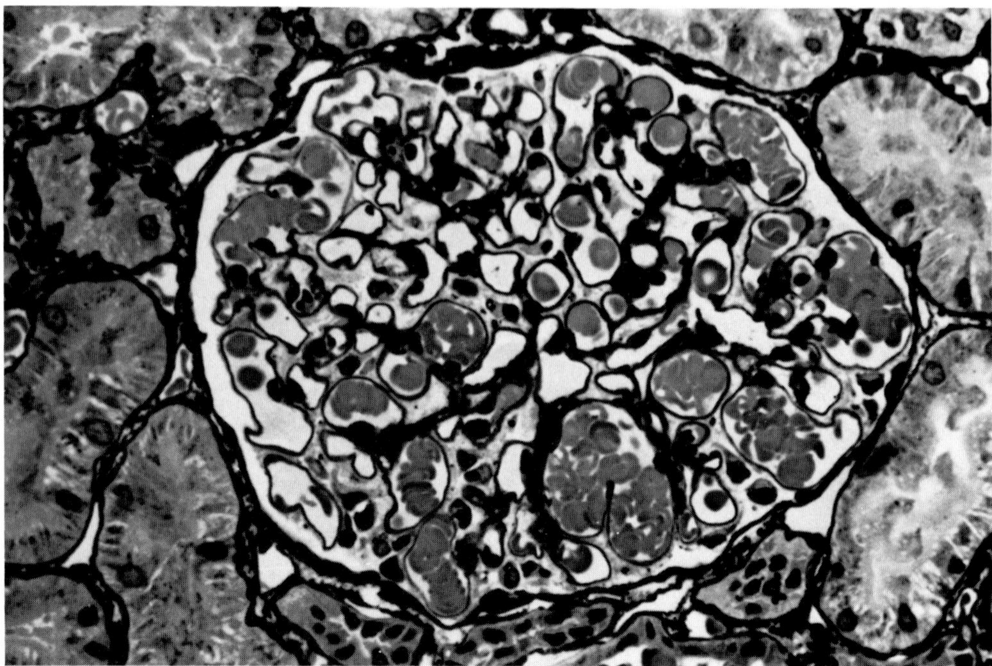

Figure 4–2. The basement membrane and mesangial regions are unremarkable. The vascular spaces are widely patent. (PASM, ×300.)

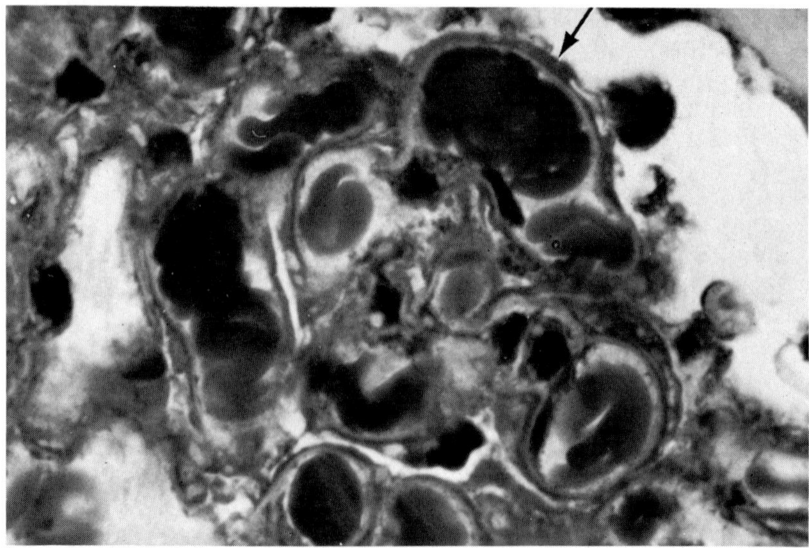

Figure 4–3. High-power light micrograph of a methacrylate-embedded specimen. Podocyte spreading can be seen over most of the peripheral glomerular basement membranes. (H&E, ×1200.)

toplasm that lacks interdigitations (Fig. 4–4). In the past, this change in the architecture of the visceral epithelial cells was called fusion. However, it would more likely seem to represent loss of the normal fingerlike interdigitations (pedicels) between adjacent visceral epithelial cells, rather than fusion of cell membranes. The epithelial cell processes, adjacent to and covering the peripheral basement membrane, are thickened but otherwise appear normal. The cytoplasm in the body of the epithelial cells may contain many large, clear vacuoles as well and an apparent increase in the number of other cell organelles. The urinary surface of the epithelial cells may also contain an increased number of microvilli; this change has been called microvillous transformation.

One clue to the presence of a focal lesion is that the pedicel spreading is less diffuse and regular. This stands in sharp contrast to that in the minimal lesion, where pedicel spreading is almost monotonous in its regularity and diffuseness.

The lamina rara externa, the lamina densa, and the lamina rara interna all appear normal.

The endothelial cell cytoplasm may also appear somewhat more prominent than normal, but quantitative studies of pore size have not been performed.

The mesangial cells and matrix appear normal.

No deposits are seen.

Prognosis

The outcome in children has been extensively studied, and a few long-term studies in adults have been reported. The outcome in children is complete remission of the nephrotic syndrome after steroid therapy. Although there may be multiple exacerbations of the disease, each seems to be steroid sensitive. The podocyte changes rapidly revert to normal after steroid therapy, coincident with the loss of proteinuria. More than 70% of children have only one or a small number of episodes of the nephrotic syndrome. In our experience, when there has been a course other than that just described, careful reassessment of the original biopsy material has revealed a lesion previously overlooked. In these cases, control of the nephrotic syndrome often requires the continuous administration of steroids (so-called steroid dependence) or addition of a cytotoxic agent.

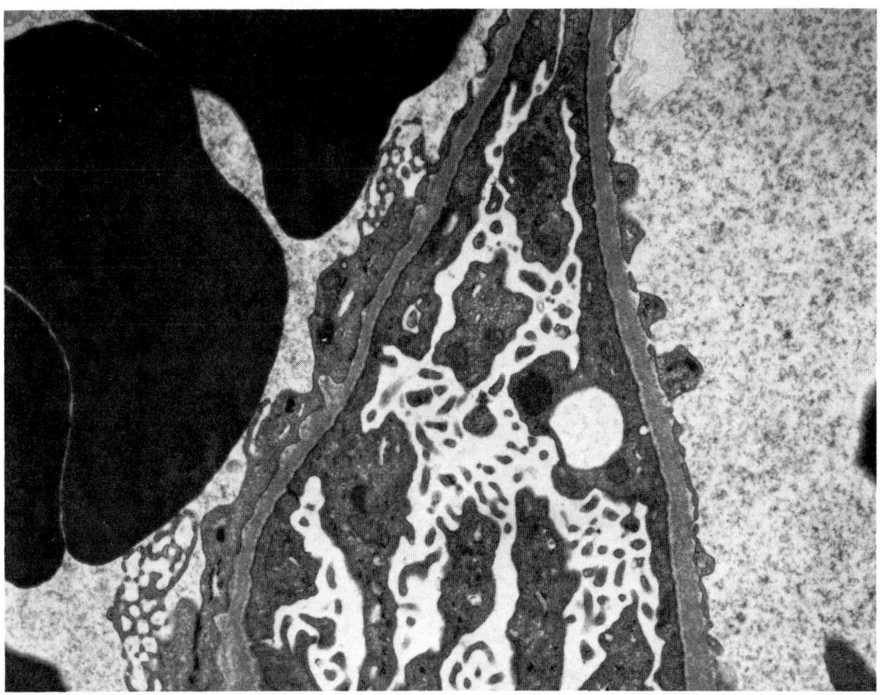

Figure 4–4. The epithelial cells form a continuous sheet of cytoplasm. Note that the cell junctions are widely spaced. The basement membrane and the endothelial cell cytoplasm are not affected. (×5000.)

Although the disorder is much less common in adults, several studies suggest that the prognosis in adults appears to be similar to that in children.

It remains to be firmly established whether or not a relationship exists between the various forms of nephrotic syndrome, but in our opinion it serves no useful purpose to draw parallels without clear reasons to do so. Thus, IgM disease, mesangial proliferative glomerulonephritis, and like categories with demonstrable morphologic abnormalities should be considered as separate entities. The fact that they all are idiopathic, all are associated with the nephrotic syndrome, and may have at least a temporary response to steroid administration does not provide sufficient justification to place them into a category entitled minimal lesion, in our opinion.

SELECTED READINGS

1. Black DAK, Rose G, Brewer DB: Controlled trial of prednisone in adult patients with the nephrotic syndrome. Br Med J 3:421, 1970.
2. Cameron JS: Histology, protein clearances, and response to treatment of nephrotic syndrome. Br Med J 4:352, 1968.
3. Churg J, Habib R, White RHR: Pathology of the nephrotic syndrome in children. Lancet 1:1299, 1970.
4. Hayslett JP, Kashgarian M, Bensch KG, et al: Clinicopathological correlations in the nephrotic syndrome due to primary renal disease. Medicine 52:93, 1973.
5. Trompeter RS, Hicks J, Lloyd BW, et al: Long-term outcome for children with minimal-change nephrotic syndrome. Lancet 1:368, 1985.

FOCAL AND SEGMENTAL GLOMERULOSCLEROSIS

Focal and segmental glomerulosclerosis has many synonyms, including *focal sclerosis, focal hyalinosis,* and *focal glomerulosclerosis.* It is defined by the presence of localized areas of sclerosis or solidification within the glomerular tufts (Table 4–1).

Table 4–1. Conditions that May Be Associated with Focal/Segmental Glomerulosclerosis*

Clinical Conditions	Hyalinosis
Idiopathic nephrotic syndrome	+
Asymptomatic proteinuria	+
Obesity	–
Unilateral renal agenesis	+
Obstructive or reflux nephropathy	+
Heroin-associated nephropathy	+
AIDS-associated nephropathy	+
Post-infectious glomerulonephritis (resolving glomerulonephritis)	–
Systemic lupus erythematosus (treated)	–
Vasculitis (treated)	–
Glycogenosis	+
Sickle cell disease	–
Alport's syndrome	–
Familial deficiency of lecithin-cholesterol acyltransferase	+

*Excluding congenital disorders appearing before 1 year.

Focal and segmental glomerulosclerosis is one of the common histologic lesions in the idiopathic nephrotic syndrome in adults but is much less common in children. For this reason and also because many of the patients with this disease initially respond to steroid treatment, this entity was initially considered to be part of the group of diseases or syndromes collectively referred to as lipoid nephrosis. This term should now be considered to have only historic significance, because most investigators now believe that minimal change nephrotic syndrome, focal sclerosis, and IgM mesangial nephropathy are separate disorders. Others consider them as a continuous spectrum of lesions with a common pathogenesis. It is not our purpose to resolve this controversy, but pathologists and clinicians alike should be aware that the presence of areas of sclerosis and hyalinosis, or of synechiae, in a patient with an idiopathic nephrotic syndrome portends a different clinical course than in a patient with no lesions in the renal biopsy. Namely, patients with light microscopic histologic lesions respond poorly to (or remain dependent on) steroids, and they have an increased risk of recurrent disease as well as a propensity to progress to end-stage renal disease. The exact risk of end-stage renal disease awaits appropriate study.

Patients who have these histologic lesions but who do not have the nephrotic syndrome do not seem to have such a worrisome prognosis. Some focal and segmental sclerotic lesions, usually in the absence of hyalin material, may result from preexisting acute lesions (e.g., infectious glomerulonephritis). Thus these lesions may represent a benign outcome of an acute, severe glomerulonephritis and must be clearly distinguished from the progressive conditions just described. In these cases of "resolved glomerulonephritis," the patients seldom have significant proteinuria. In fact, if the nephrotic syndrome is present, this sequence of events and the diagnosis of post-infectious glomerulonephritis must be questioned.

Segmental and focal sclerosis may be seen in other diseases such as acquired immunodeficiency syndrome and heroin nephropathy (see Chapter 5).

Pathogenesis

There is increasing evidence that proteinuria in these disorders is secondary to a loss in the permselectivity of the glomerular filtration barrier. There is some controversy about the nature of the physiopathology—that is, whether the change is a loss in the size selectivity, the charge, or some combination. The most current evidence suggests that a loss in size selectivity is the most significant change. A loss in charge selectivity also occurs; it can be recognized by the loss of the glomerular polyanion layer by light microscopic stains. The loss of glomerular polyanion could be either the cause or the result of the visceral epithelial cell lesions. The effect of changes in basement membrane charge has been clearly demonstrated in experimental models using infusions of polycationized substances. The infused polycations localize to the glomerular basement membrane. The animals develop proteinuria, which has been linked to neutralization of the normal anionic nature of the glomerular basement membrane. The administration of the aminonucleoside of puromycin to rats also results in a loss of anionic charge and is associated with the concomitant development of effacement of the pedicels and massive albuminuria. There is agreement that both the glomerular basement membrane and the visceral epithelial lesions have a critical role in the development and expression of the disease.

In experimental models, glomerulosclerosis seems to progress relentlessly, even though the initial stimulus is no longer present. This also seems to be the case in humans. Micropuncture studies in rats suggest that glomerular hyperfiltration, mediated by increased intravascular hydrostatic pressure, is the initiating agent and was responsible for the progression of the lesions. Recent studies indicate that many other factors may also influence this process, including dietary intake, growth factors, and arachidonic acid metabolites.

Whether focal and segmental glomerulosclerosis in humans is associated with hyperfiltration, perhaps aggravated by a high-protein diet, or whether elevated glomerular hydrostatic pressure plays a part in human disease is the subject of current investigation.

The disorder is more common in children, in whom it represents a significant percentage of all nephrotic syndrome patients, with a clear-cut predominance of boys being affected. There is no apparent difference in predominance between adult men and women. We found focal glomerulosclerosis in 57 nephrotic adults out of a total of 250 patients who presented with the nephrotic syndrome at Tenon Hospital, Paris, between 1965 and 1974.

Immunologic causes of this disease have also been proposed. In the case of the minimal change disease, various mediators released by lymphocytes have been incriminated. These, of course, include the various lymphokines. The strongest case for a role of circulating factors in focal sclerosis comes from observations on recipients of renal allografts, who develop proteinuria very shortly after graft function commences. Because cadaveric grafts are genetically different from the recipient, the best interpretation of this observation is that the appearance of proteinuria is related to some factor in the recipient. Another group of observations that suggest a role for immunologic factors are reports that certain clinical events, including atopy, bee stings, and upper respiratory tract infections, may precede the onset of proteinuria. Various immune disturbances characterized by depression of immune responses have been described as being associated with focal glomerulosclerosis, although there is no consensus on the role that they might have in triggering the disorder.

There may be a familial propensity to develop the nephrotic syndrome. Although the genetic basis of these disorders has not been clearly established, patients with minimal change or focal and segmental glomerulosclerosis are more likely to have an affected family member than can be explained on the basis of chance alone.

Patient Presentation

As in minimal change nephrotic syndrome, focal and segmented glomerulosclerosis is characterized by the rapid development of edema; however, in this case the proteinuria is non-selective. Patients with focal sclerosis tend to have microscopic hematuria more commonly than those with minimal changes. Hypoalbuminemia is prominent, as is hypercholesterolemia. Complement levels are normal.

Histology

Light Microscopy

The lesion of focal glomerulosclerosis is not specific and should always be interpreted along with the clinical and laboratory data. Table 4–1 lists the various clinicopathologic syndromes associated with focal sclerosing lesions, and this lengthy list is by no means complete.

In general, many glomeruli appear normal, contrasting with those in which segmental glomerulosclerosis is found. In the early stages, limited areas of glomerulosclerosis are seen, with solidification of the tuft and disorganization of the normal architecture (Fig. 4–5). These areas often contain large, eosinophilic deposits that stain bright red by periodic acid-Schiff (PAS) or trichrome stains, are located on the endothelial aspect of the glomerular basement membrane, and are often referred to as hyalin. This material is not positive with silver stains and may resemble fibrin in hematoxylin and eosin (H&E) preparations. In the vicinity of the hyalin lesions, foam cells or vacuoles containing lipid may be encountered. In the early stages, the mesangial spaces contain large accumulations of matrix. The mesangial spaces may later become obliterated by the confluence of segmental lesions, resulting in masses of eosinophilic material occupying the area of several lobules. In this latter case, the hyalinized masses may be connected to Bowman's capsule via a connective tissue bridge that occludes a part of the urinary space (Fig. 4–6). Occasionally, synechiae are outlined by visceral epithelial cells, and the adjacent Bowman's capsule cells are prominent, giving the false impression that this is a localized crescent. Bowman's capsule is usually multilaminated in the immediate vicinity of the bridge between the glomerular vascular loops and the capsule. The rest of the capsule may be normal. This finding is so characteristic that the presence of localized multilaminations in a section suggests that a synechia exists in the glomerulus, even though it may not be seen in the section under examination. In the affected glomeruli, there appears to be a clear-cut line of demarcation between the affected segment and the rest of the glomer-

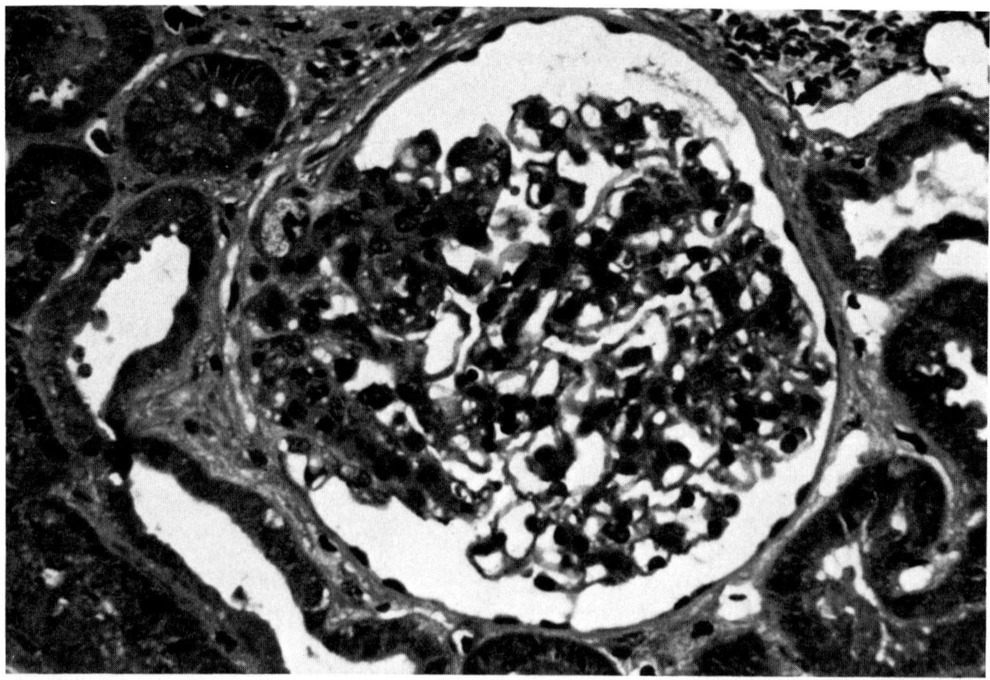

Figure 4–5. A well-organized synechia is present. Synechiae are most commonly seen in the region of the urinary pole. In this case there is mesangial hypercellularity and sclerosis. (H&E, ×300.)

ulus, which is usually either normal or shows few lesions. Whether the rest of the "normal" glomerulus contains normal cells and matrix awaits the development of more sensitive methods of analysis, although some researchers believe that there are subtle abnormalities in these adjacent areas. The segmental lesions may affect the vascular pole, but they are otherwise randomly distributed throughout the glomerular tufts. It is our impression that synechiae, when present, are often located in the vicinity of the urinary pole. Finally, the proportion of affected glomeruli and the extension of the lesions within the individual glomeruli require an adequate sample. The lesion preferentially affects the juxtamedullary glomeruli. This pattern has not been established as a necessary condition, but it is often difficult to state precisely the anatomic localization of glomeruli in biopsy specimens.

The presence of obsolescent glomeruli has led some to call this lesion "global sclerosis." Whether this represents a subset of focal glomerular sclerosis is open to question. When patients have advanced renal failure, most glomeruli may appear obsolescent, but even in those only partly affected there is clear evidence of the underlying focal sclerosing process. The areas of hyalinosis tend to persist even when the basic architecture of the tufts has been extensively modified.

The interstitium shows irregular areas of fibrosis, which may contain mononuclear inflammatory cells. Very commonly, one finds aggregates of foam cells in association with these interstitial lesions. Foam cells, once thought to be a marker of hereditary nephritis, seem rather to be simply an indication of proteinuria.

The tubules show focal atrophy with localized thickening of their basement membranes. These changes coincide with the interstitial lesions. In some instances, these foci are more obvious than the glomerular lesions, which may be so minimal as to have been overlooked. When present, this change is of sufficient consequence that one can be suspicious that the patient does not have minimal lesion nephrotic syndrome, and one should examine multiple additional sections to search for a focal and segmental glomerular lesion. Protein, granular, and red blood cells casts in the tubules are common. As in other glomerular lesions, the state of the interstitial change is the compartment most closely correlated with the glomerular filtration rate.

The blood vessel lesions parallel the glomerular changes. The arterioles and the juxtaglomerular vasculature often show hyalinosis or so-called fibrinoid material resembling that in the glomeruli. Duplication and thickening of the elastic laminae of the middle-sized arteries is common, as is smooth cell hyperplasia. These changes often herald hypertension.

Immunofluorescence Microscopy

The glomeruli do not contain significant amounts of immunoglobulin, complement components, or fibrin except for the areas of sclerosis. In the sclerotic areas, one finds large aggregates of IgM that are often in combination with C3 (Fig. 4–7). C1q is also common in these areas. Bowman's capsule and tubular basement membranes may also contain irregular aggregates of C3. The arterioles often contain IgM and C3 (a common finding in many sclerosing diseases). The membrane attack complex antigens of the complement proteins are invariably present in the areas of sclerosis, and some report that these areas also contain IgG.

Some patients also have minute, comma-like IgM deposits in the mesangial areas. It is difficult to delineate the difference between these minimal deposits and the larger deposits present in the so-called IgM mesangial nephropathy. Small granular deposits of C3 may codistribute with the IgM, but they are also very discrete.

Electron Microscopy

In the non-sclerotic areas, there may be some degree of epithelial change characterized by irregular flattening and widening of the pedicels. The cytoplasm of the podocytes has an increased number of organelles of various types and frequently has large empty vacuoles, leading some to say that there are "pseudocysts" in the cells. The peripheral areas of sclerosis are characterized by an increase in the amount of extracellular material that seems to envelop and encase the peripheral basement membrane. One is often able to recognize the original glomerular basement membrane as a wrinkled, dark structure within the sclerotic zone. In the area of a synechia, this matrix meets and fuses with the thickened Bowman's capsule (Fig. 4–8). Thus, the new mass of extracel-

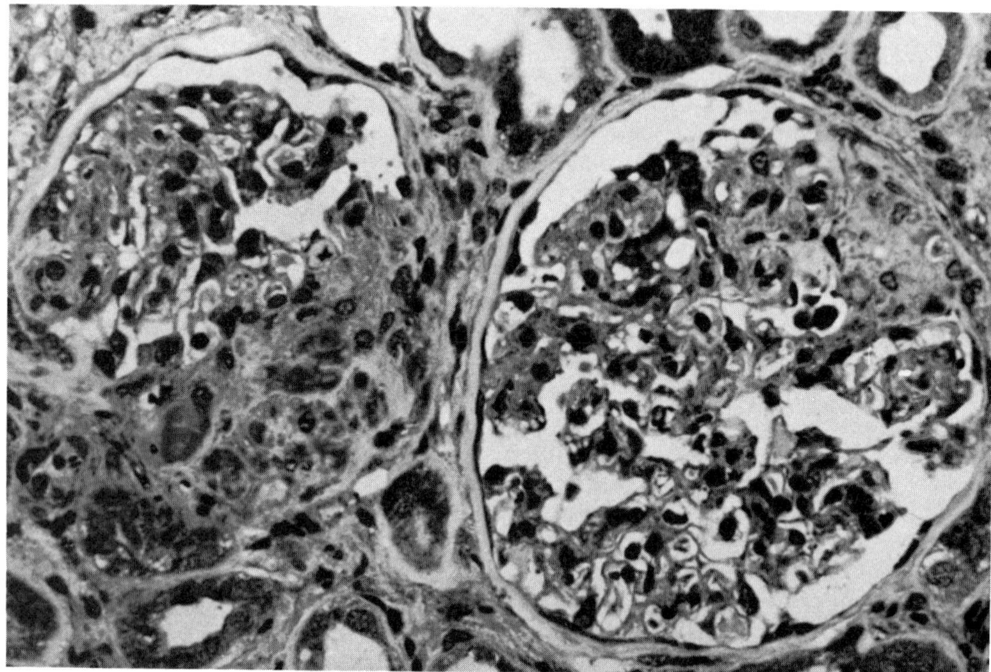

Figure 4–6. The two glomeruli demonstrate various degrees of sclerosis, with approximately 20 to 50% of the structures remaining relatively normal. All mesangial regions are abnormal, ranging from mild sclerosis to almost complete effacement. (H&E, ×300.)

lular material forms the bridge between the glomerular tuft and the capsule, rather than the original basement membrane of either structure. The glomerular basement membranes near the mesangial regions are frequently wrinkled and present a corrugated, thickened, and contracted appearance. The sclerotic zones in the mesangium are generally hypocellular and contain cellular debris resembling fragments of double-layered cell membranes (Fig. 4–9). The vascular spaces in these regions are compromised by this sclerotic process. The endothelial cell cytoplasm adjacent to the sclerotic zones is thickened, contains many cytoplasmic organelles, and frequently lacks fenestrae.

Prognosis

The prognosis of focal sclerosis, unassociated with the nephrotic syndrome, is vir-

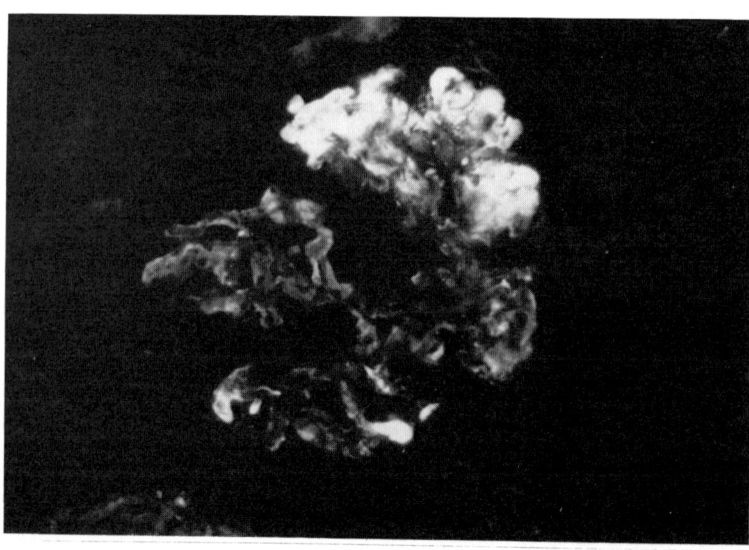

Figure 4–7. Immunofluorescence micrograph, anti-IgM. There are large, local aggregates in the sclerotic areas. (×250.)

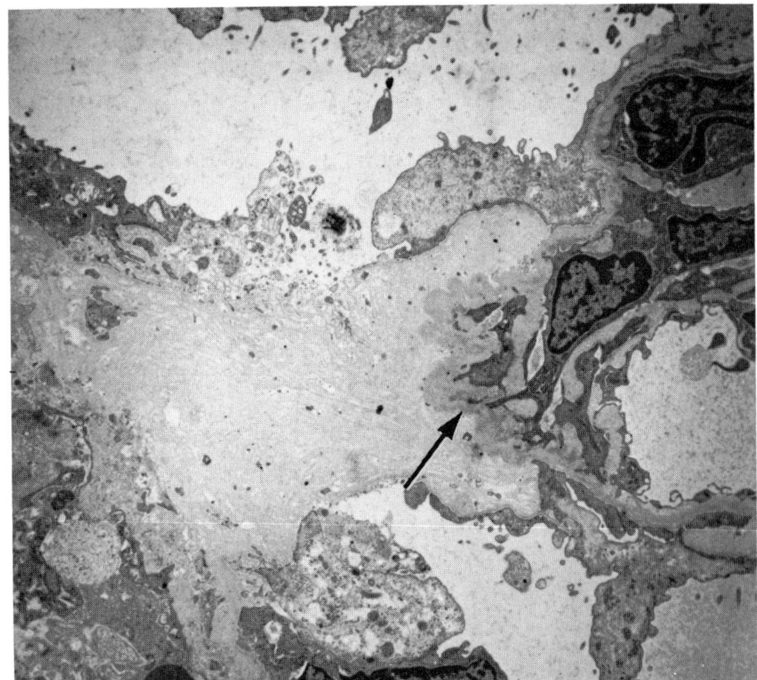

Figure 4–8. In the areas of sclerosis, the basement membranes (arrow) are either collapsed or extended around masses of lightly stained extracellular material. In this case, the sclerosis forms a bridging connection between the basement membranes of the glomerulus and Bowman's capsule. (×1500.)

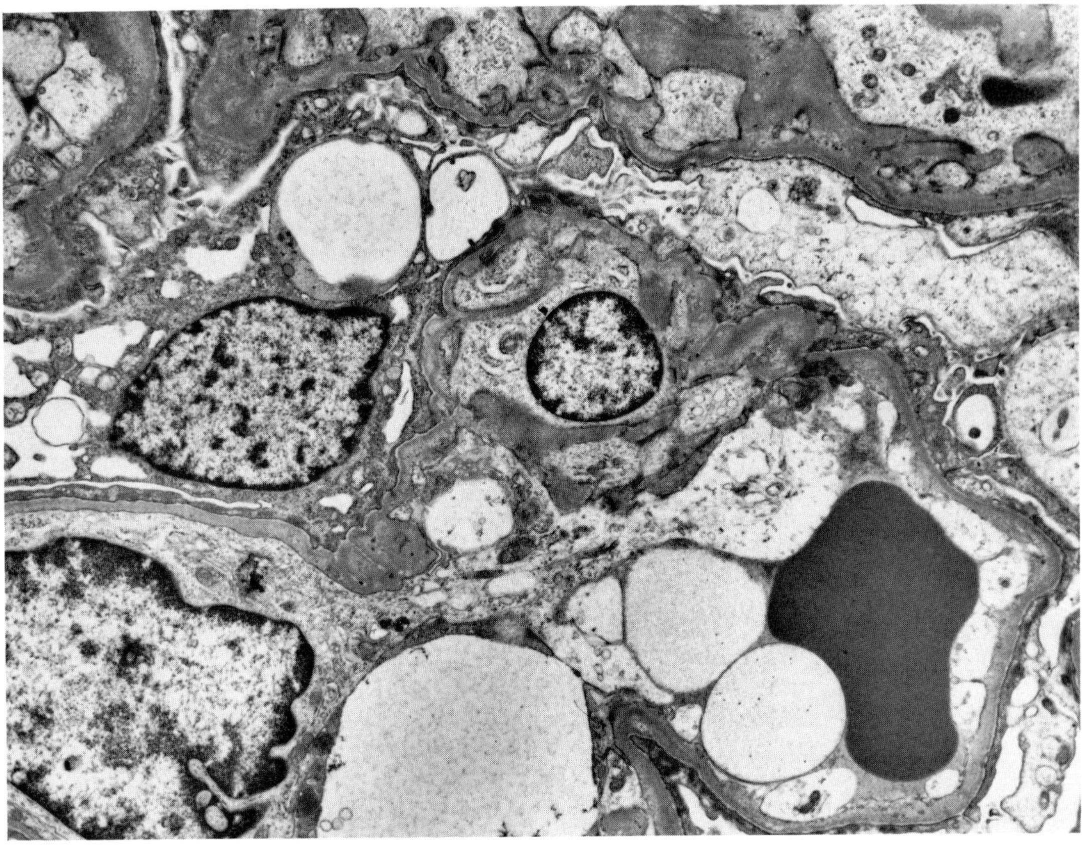

Figure 4–9. The mesangial matrix is increased. The glomerular basement membrane is collapsed, forming a wrinkled mass near the mesangium. (×1600.)

tually unknown. In the presence of the nephrotic syndrome, the prognosis can best be determined by the response to corticosteroids. In children, who have a prompt response, the outcome approaches that in the minimal lesion group. Those who are steroid resistant or steroid dependent may develop progressively worsening renal function. In adults, Cameron has reported that approximately one-half of patients will develop chronic glomerulonephritis within 10 years. Some investigators have identified a subgroup of these patients who pursue a course of rapid progression to end stage. The glomerular lesions in this group are quite severe, and it may be difficult to be sure that the underlying lesion was focal.

SELECTED READINGS

1. Border WA: Distinguishing minimal change disease from mesangial disorders (nephrology forum). Kidney Int 34:419, 1988.
2. Churg J, Habib R, White RMR: Pathology of the nephrotic syndrome in children. A report of the international study of kidney disease in children. Lancet 1:1299, 1970.
3. Habib R: Focal glomerular sclerosis. Kidney Int 4:355, 1973.
4. Jao W, Pollak VE, Noraris SH, et al: Lipoid nephrosis: An approach to the clinicopathologic analysis and dismemberment of idiopathic nephrotic syndrome with minimal glomerular changes. Medicine 52:445, 1973.
5. Olson JL, De Urdaneta AG, Heptinstall RH: Glomerular hyalinosis and its relation to hyperfiltration. Lab Invest 52:387, 1985.
6. Schwartz MM, Lewis EJ: Focal segmental glomerular sclerosis. The cellular lesion. Kidney Int 28:968, 1985.
7. Velosa J, Glasser RJ, Nevins TE, Michael AF: Experimental model of focal sclerosis: II. Correlation with immunopathologic changes, macromolecular kinetics and polyanion loss. Lab Invest 36:527, 1977.
8. Whitworth JA, Turner DR, Leibowitz S, et al: Focal segmental sclerosis or scarred focal proliferative glomerulonephritis. Clin Nephrol 9:229, 1978.

MESANGIAL PROLIFERATIVE DISEASE

This category of renal disease is clinically indistinguishable from minimal change. The age, sex, and prior history of this group of patients are identical to those in patients with minimal lesion. The only feature that may be useful in making a distinction is that these patients may, at onset or soon thereafter, become dependent on continuous steroid therapy to remain free from the stigmata of the nephrotic syndrome.

This category represents a mixed group of diseases sharing the common features of mild mesangial proliferation, often coexisting with IgM deposits. Some researchers do not believe that this is a separate diagnostic entity and would group it with minimal change nephrotic syndrome.

Histology

Light Microscopy

The mesangial regions are uniformly but moderately more prominent than normal. This change appears to be principally the result of an increase in the number of cells (Fig. 4–10). Mesangial nodules are not seen, and the glomerular extracellular matrix appears normal in both the mesangial and peripheral basement membrane zones.

Immunofluorescence Microscopy

In contrast to minimal change, in this disease, immune deposits are clearly evident. As seen by light microscopy, the lesions are limited to the mesangial regions. Deposits of IgM and C3 are present in each mesangial region, and all glomeruli are affected. In fact, were it not for the immunofluorescence findings, it would be possible to overlook the light microscopic changes and conclude that the disease belongs to the minimal change category.

Electron Microscopy

The visceral epithelial cell pedicels are widened and in many areas are effaced in a manner approaching that seen in minimal change. Nonetheless, the pattern of the alterations of the pedicels is not as uniform and diffuse as in minimal change (Fig. 4–11). The epithelial cell cytoplasm contains many vacuoles, as well as an increased number of other intracellular organelles. The plasma membranes on the urinary surface show villous transformation.

The mesangial regions contain easily detectable electron-dense deposits within the extracellular matrix. No other changes are visible.

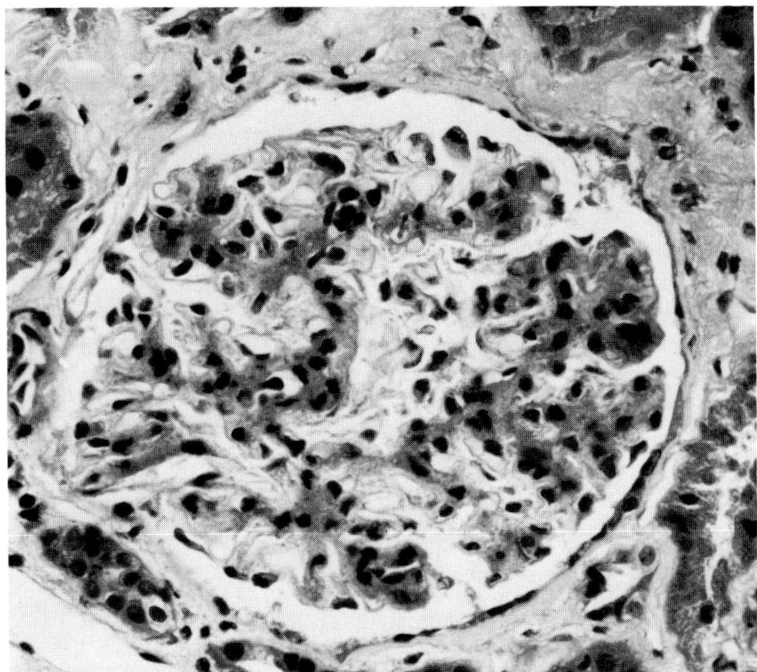

Figure 4–10. There is a diffuse increase in the number of intraglomerular cells. (H&E, ×250.)

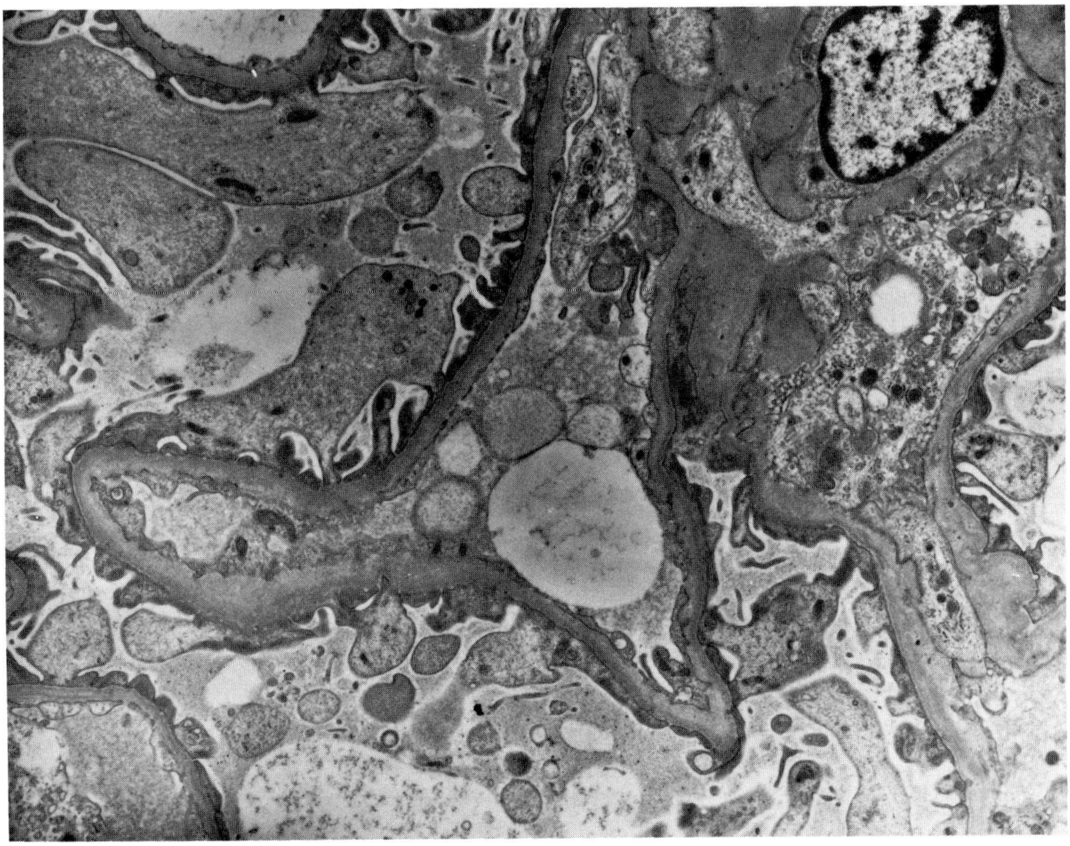

Figure 4–11. The pedicels are locally spread, and the mesangial matrix is increased in amount. (×6700.)

Prognosis

The outcome in this disease is not well established. A number of reports lump these patients together with those who have minimal change. However, in the many series that separate the patients by category, only 30 to 50% of patients with mesangial changes achieve complete remission with steroid therapy. In addition, most investigators agree that this group of patients has an increased risk of developing focal and segmental glomerulosclerosis and subsequent renal functional deterioration.

SELECTED READINGS

1. Border WA: Distinguishing minimal-change disease from mesangial disorders. Kidney Int 34:419, 1988.
2. Brown EA, Upadhyaya K, Hayslett JP: The clinical course of mesangial proliferative glomerulonephritis. Medicine 58:295, 1979.
3. Cohen AH, Border WA, Glassock RJ: Nephrotic syndrome with glomerular mesangial IgM deposits. Lab Invest 38:610, 1978.
4. International Study of Kidney Disease in Children: Primary nephrotic syndrome in children: Clinical significance of histopathologic variants of minimal change and of diffuse mesangial hypercellularity. Kidney Int 20:765, 1981.
5. Southwest Pediatric Nephrology Study Group: Childhood nephrotic syndrome associated with diffuse mesangial hypercellularity. Kidney Int 24:87, 1983.
6. Trompeter RS, Lloyd BW, Hicks J, et al: Long-term outcome for children with minimal change nephrotic syndrome. Lancet 1:368, 1985.
7. Waldherr R, Gubler MC, Levy M, et al: The significance of pure diffuse mesangial proliferation in idiopathic nephrotic syndrome. Clin Nephrol 10:171, 1978.

MEMBRANOUS GLOMERULONEPHRITIS

The term *membranous nephropathy* (also called membranous, epimembranous, or extramembranous glomerulonephritis) designates a morphologic entity characterized by the presence of immune deposits distributed uniformly along the outer aspects of the glomerular basement membranes. This lesion, the most common glomerular pattern observed in adult patients with the nephrotic syndrome, may also be found in association with systemic diseases (e.g., systemic lupus erythematosus), uptake of toxins such as heavy metals, and exposure to certain drugs such as penicillamine and gold salts (Table 4–2).

Table 4–2. Membranous Glomerulonephritis

Idiopathic
Secondary to toxins
Gold
Bismuth
Mercury
Silver
Drug-induced
Penicillamine
Non-steroidal anti-inflammatory agents
Captopril
Associated with other diseases
Systemic lupus erythematosus (and mixed connective tissue disease)
Autoimmune thyroiditis
Sickle cell disease
Sarcoidosis
Myasthenia gravis
Carcinoma
Infections
Syphilis
Schistosomiasis
Filariasis
Hepatitis B

Pathogenesis

It is now thought that this glomerular disease results from the formation of immune deposits locally on the epithelial aspects of the glomerular basement membrane. It has been postulated that antibodies, mostly of the IgG class, react with an antigen present on the podocytes. This conclusion is based on studies of a rat model (Heymann's nephritis), which is considered to be a satisfactory experimental counterpart of the human disease. The immune deposits in this model consist of IgG antibodies that have been shown to react with an antigen present on the pedicels of the rat podocyte. The presence and nature of a locally synthesized glomerular antigen have not been demonstrated in humans.

The localization of antibodies to the subepithelial space might be predisposed to by antigens that arrive passively and become fixed or "planted" because of the physical characteristics of the antigen. For instance, materials could be localized to the subepithelial space on the basis of charge selectivity. It has been shown that a number of substances, including cationized proteins of the appropriate size, localize to the subepithelial spaces and act as "planted antigens" in experimental animals. These antigens are responsible for the in situ formation of immune complexes. A potential role for complement in the induction of proteinuria has been demonstrated in several animal models but remains unproved in humans.

Thus the experimental models have shown that membranous glomerulonephritis can occur as the consequence of immune complexes formed locally along the glomerular walls. The antigen has been shown to derive either from the circulation or is a biosynthetic product of the cells abutting the glomerular basement membrane. The antigens derived from the circulation arrive at the subepithelial site either because of the hemodynamic forces operative within the glomerulus or as a consequence of the size and charge of the antigen, or both. The result is that the number of antigens that can lead to this anatomic localization is quite diverse, and the morphologic pattern is representative but not diagnostic of a particular etiology. For instance, several putative antigens have been suggested to play a pathogenetic role. These include glycoproteins derived from rat podocytes (Heymann's nephritis) and DNA in systemic lupus erythematosus. Other antigens have been demonstrated in a few clinical syndromes: thyroid antigens in patients with autoimmune thyroiditis, hepatitis virus-associated antigens (HBsAg, HBe antigen), tumor antigens (carcinoembryonic antigen), parasite or fungal antigens (*Treponema, Schistosoma,* and *Echinococcus*), and antigens belonging to the coagulation cascade.

The exact role that each antigen might play and the frequency of their association with either the underlying disease or with the syndrome of membranous glomerulonephritis remains to be proved, and the etiologic factors remain largely undetermined. Thus, this syndrome remains in the category of idiopathic diseases.

Patient Presentation

Membranous glomerulonephritis is the most common entity in adult patients who present with the nephrotic syndrome. It is also present in children but is less common as a cause of the nephrotic syndrome. Interestingly, this lesion may spontaneously regress in children, but this outcome is less common in adults.

The proportion of patients with idiopathic membranous glomerulonephritis in a group of nephrotic adults seems to vary with the geographic location of the survey and with the clinical use of renal biopsy in the evaluation of the nephrotic syndrome. It should be remembered that a significant percentage of patients with membranous glomerulonephritis have an underlying extrarenal disease or have been exposed to toxins. Thus the clinical manifestations of the primary process may overshadow or mask the renal lesion.

Membranous glomerulonephritis is most frequently found after the third decade of life. Proteinuria is more or less constantly present in membranous glomerulonephritis and is often associated with the nephrotic syndrome. Microscopic hematuria and hypertension are also common. Renal failure may occur as the disease progresses but is seldom found as the presenting problem, and this lesion is not a common cause of chronic renal failure. Serum complement levels are normal, and cryoglobulin levels remain at normal levels in the serum unless there is an associated disease.

Histology

Light Microscopy

The glomeruli are large, and the lesions are homogeneous and diffuse. There is no cellular proliferation. The principal finding is uniform, diffuse thickening of the peripheral glomerular vascular wall. For this reason, the lesion was initially given the name *membranous* glomerulonephritis. It appears as if the lesion is restricted to the glomerular basement membranes. Examination of the basement membranes by PAS or silver stains reveals that there are regular subepithelial spikelike projections of the glomerular basement membrane, between which are deposits of proteinaceous material (Fig. 4–12). The overlying visceral epithelial cells are not conspicuous, except for the occasional presence of cytoplasmic protein-containing droplets. As the lesion evolves, the "spikes" progress from being just detectable, to becoming progressively more conspicuous, and eventually occupying the entire subepithelial space as a broad band of extracellular matrix with sub-

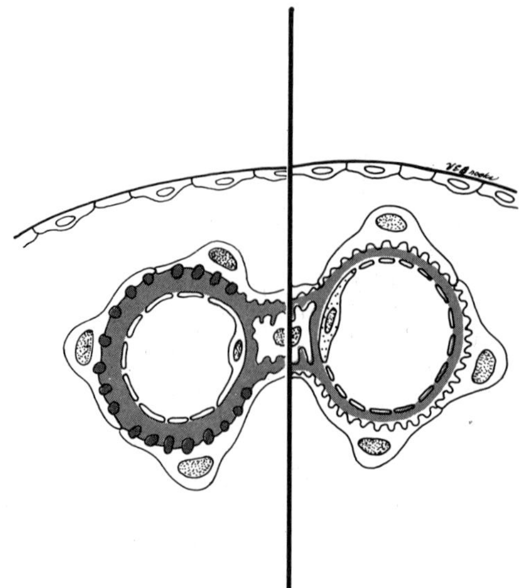

Figure 4–12. Diagram showing multiple small subepithelial deposits. The epithelial cells cover both the deposits and the "spikes" of glomerular basement membrane that lie between the deposits. The endothelial cells, the mesangium, and the lumen are not affected.

stantial distortion of the glomerular architecture. This transition has been arbitrarily divided into four stages:

Stage 1. The vascular walls may appear normal by H&E and PAS stains, but fine stippling of a widened subepithelial space may be appreciated by silver stains because the subepithelial deposits are not stained and thus appear as negative images. This change does not affect all vascular loops uniformly, and the change may be missed by light microscopy. However, at this stage, the changes are easily detectable by immunofluorescence microscopy.

Stage 2. Diffuse, uniform thickening of the peripheral vascular wall is present in every glomerulus (Fig. 4–13). Note that the mesangial regions are unaffected.

Stage 3. The peripheral glomerular vascular walls are uniformly and diffusely thickened. At this stage, the spikes are thickened and in many regions may have fused. The end result is that there may be an irregularly thickened peripheral basement membrane without clear spike formation (Fig. 4–14). In some of the thickened walls, deposits may be seen to be incorporated within the matrix.

Stage 4. Many glomeruli are obsolescent in this stage. The glomeruli remain large even when obsolescent, and the underlying thickened basement membranes may still be appreciated by PAS or silver stains. The nonobsolescent glomeruli are very sclerotic, and it may be difficult to determine the nature of the disease except for the fact that the pe-

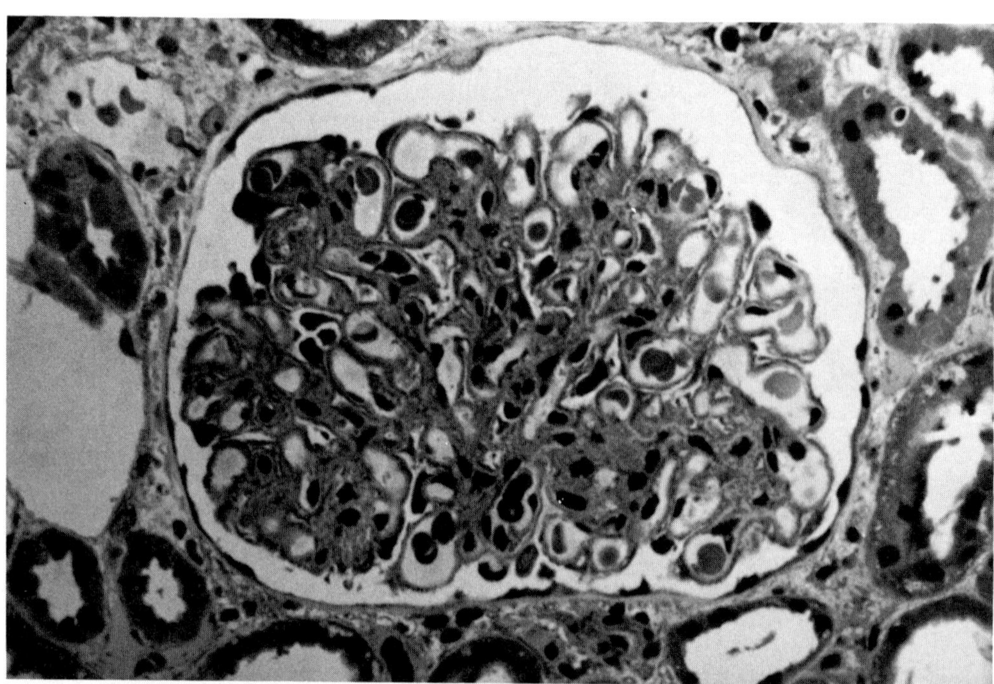

Figure 4–13. The major histologic change is diffuse thickening of the basement membranes. Silver staining is necessary to reveal the spikes and deposits. (H&E, ×300.)

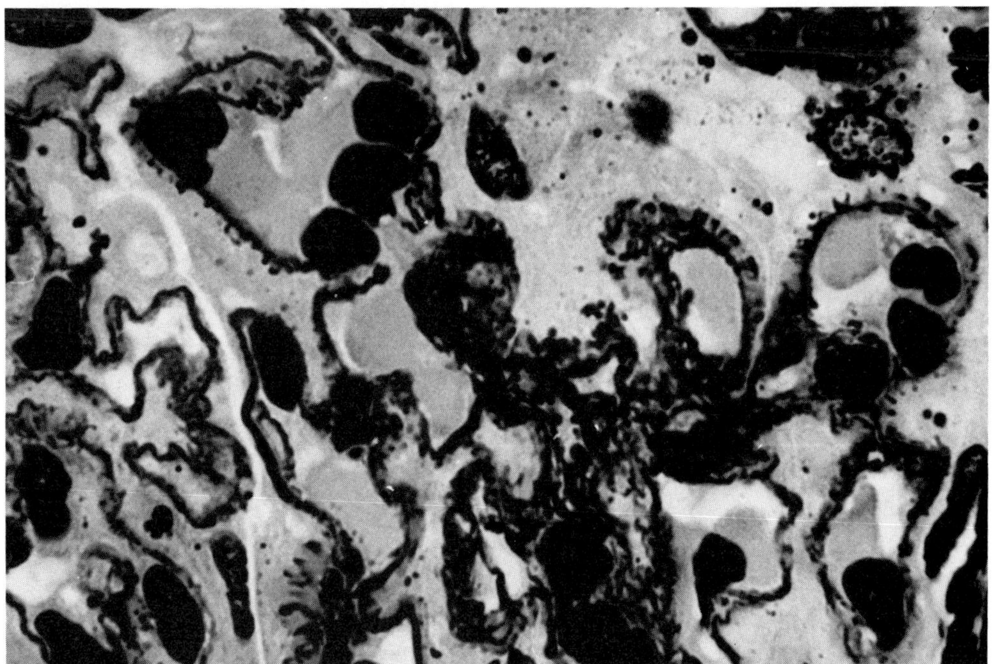

Figure 4–14. Silver methenamine stain demonstrating an advanced lesion in which the large subepithelial spikes are regular in distribution. (PASM, ×1200.)

ripheral basement membranes are quite thickened.

The tubules and the interstitium are not affected early in the disease except for evidence of a large glomerular protein leak. Later, as the number of obsolescent glomeruli increases, nephron loss becomes evident because of tubular atrophy and interstitial fibrosis.

Vascular lesions are not a primary feature of this disease but instead parallel the stage of the disease or the age of the patient.

Immunofluorescence Microscopy

The deposits are readily apparent, even in stage 1. They consist of IgG (C3 is present in 20 to 40%) distributed in a regular, granular pattern over the epithelial aspects of the glomerular basement membrane. The mesangial regions are unaffected, unless there is an associated systemic disease, such as systemic lupus erythematosus (Fig. 4–15). Granular deposits of IgA and IgM are occasionally found, but they are always in lesser amounts than IgG.

The deposits become progressively larger and more sparsely distributed as they are displaced and incorporated into the increasing quantities of basement membrane (Fig. 4–16). The deposits may persist in the obsolescent glomeruli.

C4 and C1q are not usually present in idiopathic membranous glomerulonephritis and if present should suggest that a search for systemic lupus erythematosus is warranted.

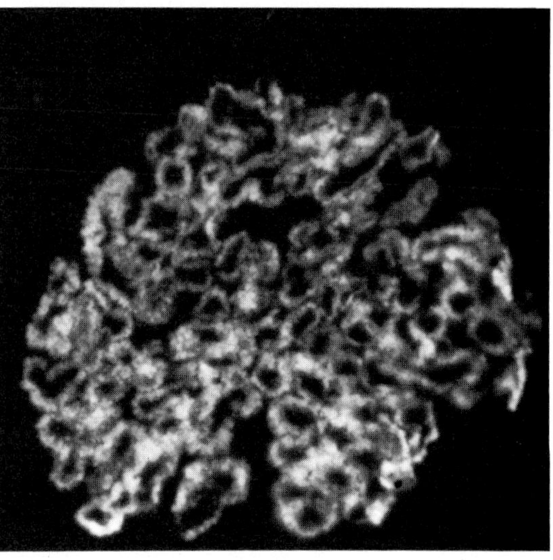

Figure 4–15. Immunofluorescence micrograph, anti-IgG. There are multiple granular deposits covering the urinary side of the glomerular basement membranes. (×250.)

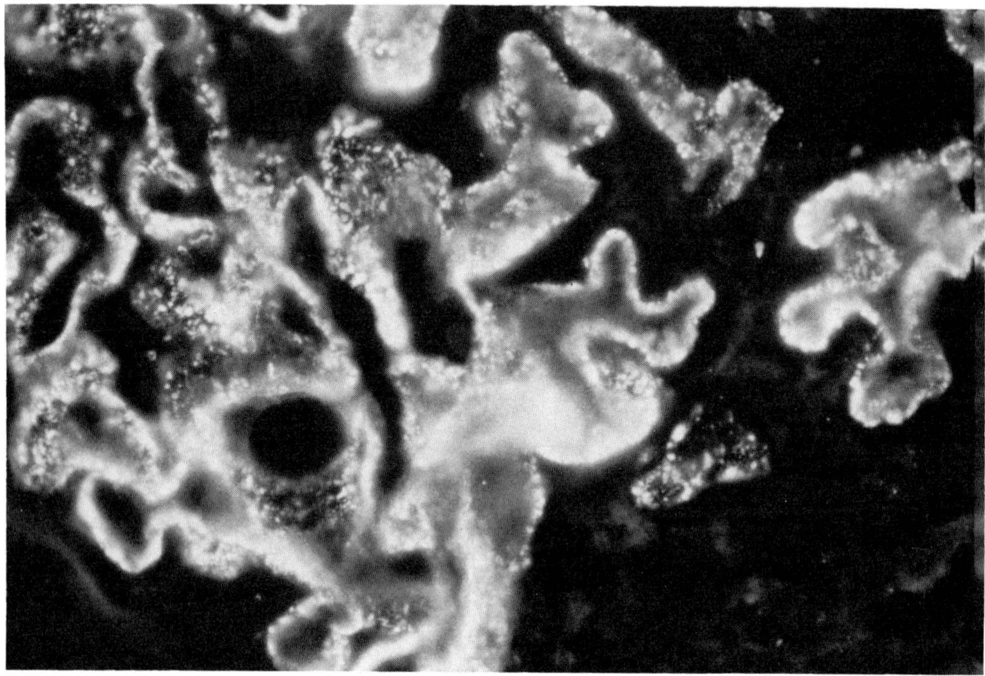

Figure 4–16. Immunofluorescence micrograph, anti-IgG. At high power the deposits appear nearly confluent. (×400.)

Electron Microscopy

Stage 1. The subepithelial deposits are small and indistinct and may appear to be concentrated under the slit diaphragms. The basement membranes often appear normal, and the spikes are not conspicuous. The epithelial cell cytoplasm changes are often quite prominent, with an increased number of cytoplasmic organelles and broadened pedicels containing an accumulation of microfilaments near the deposits (Fig. 4–17).

Stage 2. The subepithelial deposits and the subepithelial spikes are regularly spaced as well as relatively uniform in size and shape (Figs. 4–18 and 4–19). The cytoplasm of the visceral epithelial cells is prominent and contains many organelles. The pedicels are broadened and irregular in width. The mesangial regions remain unremarkable.

Stage 3. The peripheral basement membranes are markedly thickened and irregular in contour. Electron-dense deposits are found within the thickened basement membranes as well as on the epithelial aspects. The visceral epithelial cells are similar in appearance to stage 2, but the pedicels are even more irregular (Fig. 4–20).

Stage 4. The basement membranes are diffusely and markedly thickened (Fig. 4–21). Electron-dense deposits are much less frequently encountered than in stage 3; they are instead thought to largely disappear, leaving lucent areas within the basement membranes (Fig. 4–22).

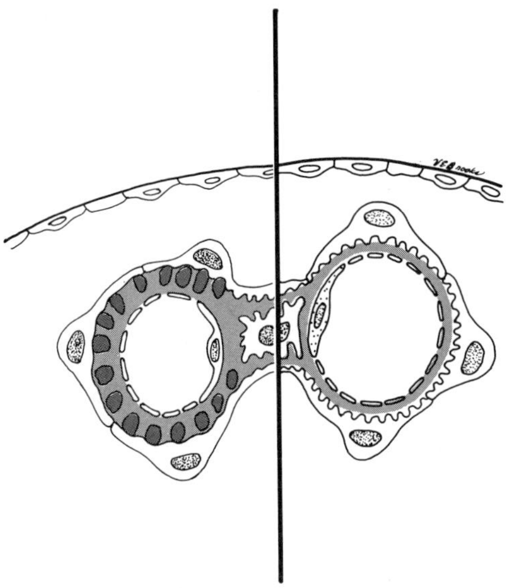

Figure 4–17. Diagram demonstrating larger subepithelial deposits, which have been partially incorporated within the substance of the thickened glomerular basement membranes.

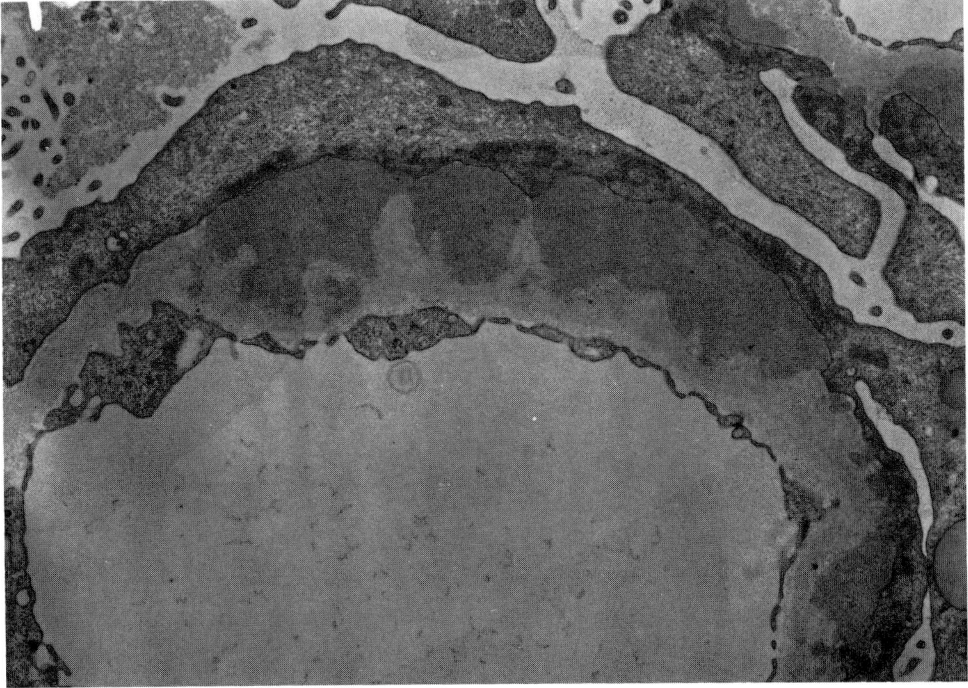

Figure 4–18. On the subepithelial aspects of the lamina densa, irregularly shaped deposits are found. Between the deposits are extensions of the lamina densa. (×6000.)

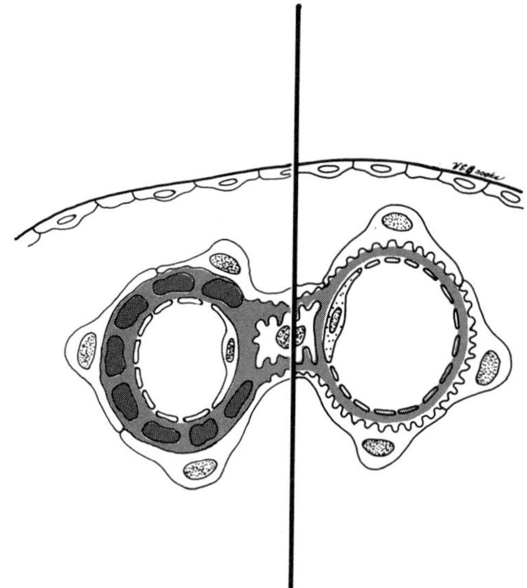

Figure 4–19. Diagram of the stage 3 lesion. The deposits are surrounded and partially incorporated within the glomerular basement membranes. The mesangial regions are normal.

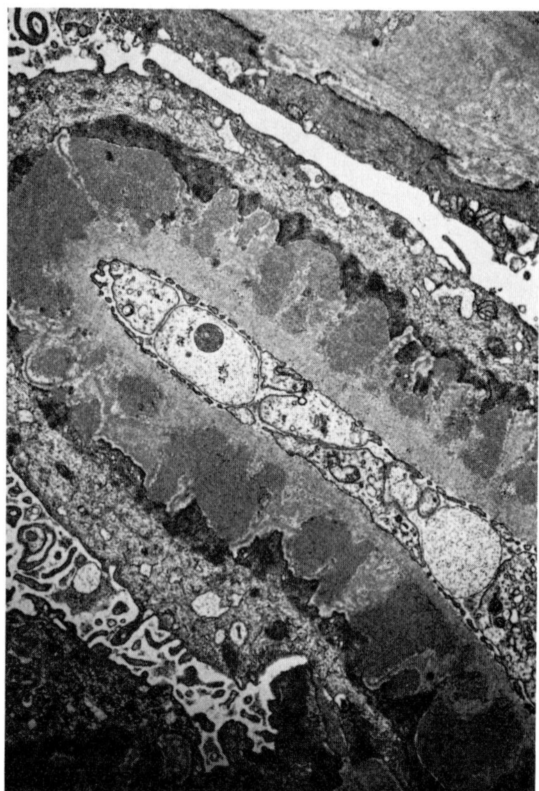

Figure 4–20. The deposits are larger and much more uniform. The lamina densa forms large subepithelial spikes. (×7500.)

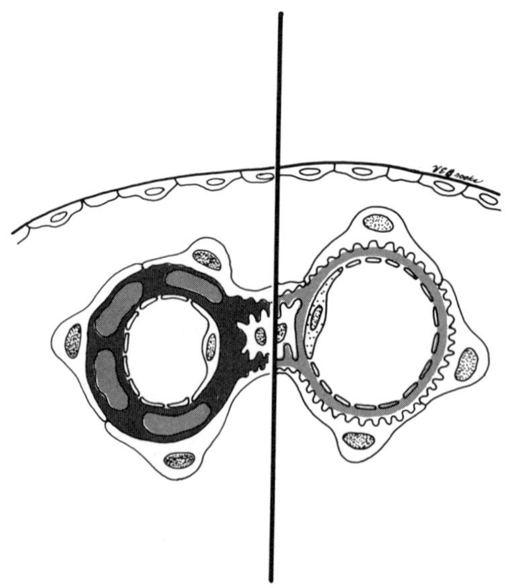

Figure 4–21. Diagram of a stage 4 lesion. The basement membranes are massively thickened. The deposits are almost completely incorporated within the lamina densa.

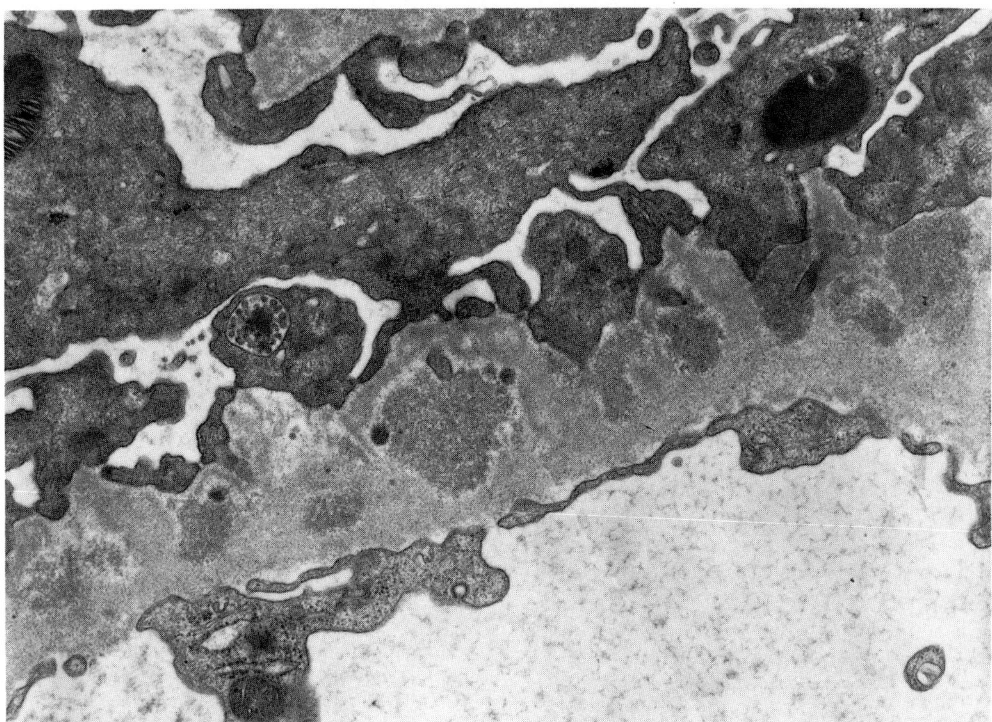

Figure 4–22. The basement membranes are markedly, but irregularly, thickened. The electron-dense deposits are surrounded by lamina densa. (×7500.)

Associations with Other Diseases, Drugs and Toxins

Systemic Lupus Erythematosus

Membranous glomerulonephritis is present in less than 10% of systemic lupus erythematosus-associated glomerular disease. The epimembranous deposits are most often found in association with deposits in the subendothelial or mesangial spaces or with mesangial hypercellularity. In these latter cases, the presence of other glomerular lesions should lead one to suspect the presence of systemic lupus erythematosus in a biopsy sample thought to represent membranous glomerulonephritis.

Immunofluorescence microscopic examination reveals diffuse, regular, and granular deposits of IgG along the peripheral aspects of the glomerular basement membranes. Deposits may also be found in the mesangial areas, along tubular basement membranes, and along the intertubular capillaries. Complement components are invariably found, and C1q and C4 often codistribute with IgG. Other immunoglobulins, IgA and IgM, may be conspicuous components of the glomerular deposits.

Rheumatoid Arthritis

The association between rheumatoid arthritis and membranous glomerulonephritis is very tenuous. We, along with others, believe that when membranous glomerulonephritis is found in patients with rheumatoid arthritis, the renal disease is secondary to drug therapy. The drugs most commonly associated with membranous glomerulonephritis in these patients are penicillamine and gold salts.

Infectious and Parasitic Diseases

Membranous glomerulonephritis has been associated with certain infectious and parasitic diseases. This association is uncommon in the United States and Western Europe. The diseases most often implicated include syphilis, schistosomiasis, hydatidosis, and filiariasis.

Drugs

The occurrence of membranous glomerulonephritis as an adverse reaction to drug therapy is well documented. In general, the clinical course is benign, because the glomerulonephritis most often reverses when the drug is withdrawn. The presence of a free sulfhydryl group is the most common chemical structural correlate (e.g., in antihypertensive agents, penicillamines, and so on), but non-steroidal anti-inflammatory agents have also been reported as causal agents.

Heavy metals associated with membranous glomerulonephritis include gold, lead, and mercury. Silver and bismuth have only rarely been reported.

Renal Vein Thrombosis

The occurrence of renal vein thrombosis in patients with membranous glomerulonephritis has been reported to be more common than can be attributed to chance alone. Several findings should lead one to suspect this diagnosis: interstitial edema, dilation of the peritubular capillaries, and the presence of leukocytes in distended glomerular capillaries. These morphologic features are far from specific and should be regarded as nothing more than suggestive unless there are strong clinical reasons to suggest an association.

Prognosis

Two factors make it difficult to predict prognosis in membranous glomerulonephritis. First, complete remission of the nephrotic syndrome and, less commonly, of proteinuria may spontaneously occur. In addition, the causes may be multifactorial, and the underlying condition may be difficult to diagnose or treat. Thus, interpretation of therapeutic interventions is fraught with difficulty in the absence of prospective, long-term studies with an adequate number of well-studied patients. It is thought that membranous glomerulonephritis, in common with other forms of chronic glomerulonephritis, leads to an inexorable downhill course. However, few long-term studies are available for documenting this event. In those studies that are published, the course has been said to follow an irregular and somewhat unpredictable course. There have been reports that therapy with corticosteroids results in amelioration of the nephrotic syndrome, and some groups now use them routinely. Recent reports bring this practice into sharp question. The use of azathioprine has been reported as primary therapy or for its "steroid-sparing" effect, but its use is not currently widespread. For these reasons, there is no currently agreed on therapy, except for removal of the causal agent when it can be identified and remedied.

Attempts to find histologic predictors of subsequent outcome or of treatment efficacy have thus far been unsuccessful, but quantitative (morphometric) studies of renal biopsies have not been reported. The presence of interstitial fibrosis remains the best indicator of severe, irreversible disease. However, this would seem to represent simply the residuum of nephron loss and thus may not be useful to predict other than the stage of the disease. The ability to find predictors that will be useful in the prevention of nephron loss remains an unsolved problem.

SELECTED READINGS

1. Agodoa LCY, Striker GE, George CRP, et al: The appearance of nonlinear deposits of immunoglobulins in Goodpasture's syndrome. Am J Med 61:407, 1976.
2. Doi TM, Mayumi K, Kanatsu F, et al: Distribution of IgG subclasses in membranous nephropathy. Clin Exp Immunol 58:57, 1984.
3. Forland M, Spargo BH: Clinicopathological correlations in idiopathic nephrotic syndrome with membranous nephropathy. Nephron 6:498, 1969.
4. Jennette J, Iskandar S, Dalldorf FG: Pathologic differentiation between lupus and non lupus membranous glomerulopathy. Kidney Int 24:377, 1983.
5. Rosen SL: Membranous glomerulonephritis: Current status. Hum Pathol 2:209, 1971.
6. Southwest Pediatric Nephrology Study Group: Comparison of idiopathic and systemic lupus erythematosus-associated membranous glomerulonephropathy in children. Am J Kidney Dis 7:115, 1986.
7. Wehrman M, Bohle A, Bogenschutz O, et al: Long-term prognosis of chronic idiopathic membranous glomerulonephritis. Clin Nephrol 31:67, 1989.

MEMBRANOPROLIFERATIVE GLOMERULONEPHRITIS AND DENSE DEPOSIT DISEASE

The term *membranoproliferative glomerulonephritis* refers to a histologic pattern characterized principally by an increased number of intraglomerular cells and thickening of the peripheral glomerular vascular walls (Table 4–3). This term, widely used throughout the world, includes both diseases of unknown cause and some associated with systemic and infectious disorders. Membranoproliferative glomerulonephritis therefore designates a

Table 4–3. Membranoproliferative Glomerulonephritis: Histologic Patterns

Idiopathic
Membranoproliferative glomerulonephritis type I (subendothelial deposits)
Membranoproliferative glomerulonephritis type II (dense deposits, intramembranous deposits)

Infectious/parasitic
- Subacute bacterial endocarditis
- Shunt nephritis
- Other deep infections
- Schistosomiasis *(S. mansoni)*

Other diseases
- Systemic lupus erythematosus
- Liver cirrhosis, $alpha_1$-antitrypsin deficiency
- Drash's syndrome: nephroblastoma
- Mixed cryoglobulinemia
- Chronic lymphocytic leukemia
- Complement deficiency (C3)
- Chronic active hepatitis
- Benign monoclonal gammopathy

morphologic pattern that should be integrated within an etiologic context when possible.

This chapter reviews the idiopathic forms of membranoproliferative glomerulonephritis. Another term commonly applied to this disease is *mesangiocapillary glomerulonephritis.* This name reflects the belief that abnormalities in and of the mesangium are the crucial determinants in the development of the disease process.

Pathogenesis

There are two major and distinct categories of idiopathic membranoproliferative glomerulonephritis, often referred to as types I and II. These two types are histologically separable, but their clinical features and subsequent course are identical. In the past few years, other histologic subcategories have been proposed, based on minor variants of the two major categories. We believe that further designations are unnecessary and that there is no need to add further complexity to an already confusing disease in which the histologic nuances do not have etiologic, therapeutic, or clinical outcome correlates. In other texts, these lesions have been referred to as lobular glomerulonephritis, but this term has been replaced by the descriptor membranoproliferative glomerulonephritis in most recent communications. We therefore describe only two categories: type I, which is associated with duplication of the peripheral glomerular basement membranes (so-called tram tracks) and glomerular immune deposits; and type II, which is associated with dense, homogeneous deposits of material occupying and expanding the lamina densa of many renal basement membranes. Complement abnormalities are frequent in both conditions but are of different types. Patients with dense deposits (type II) often show persistent C3 activation because of the presence of a circulating IgG autoantibody known as C3 nephritic factor. Patients with this factor have marked depression of C3 plasma levels, whereas the early complement components are at normal levels. The nephritic factor is rarely found in patients with type I membranoproliferative glomerulonephritis. The exact role of the complement abnormalities in these diseases is unknown, but some investigators believe that these patients have a complement deficiency that becomes clinically manifest as a glomerulonephritis.

Clarification of the pathogenesis of type II membranoproliferative glomerulonephritis has been further complicated by the fact that the biochemical composition of the dense deposits remains unknown.

Both types I and II were initially described in children and, although not restricted to this age-group, are much more common therein.

Finally, both types are rare, and their incidence seems to have markedly decreased in the Western world over the past two decades.

Patient Presentation

As noted earlier, children or adolescents are more frequently affected than adults. The nephrotic syndrome is the most common clinical presentation and is usually accompanied by changes in the urine sediment (red blood cells and red blood cell casts). Occasional patients present with macroscopic hematuria or the nephritic syndrome.

At the time of diagnosis, approximately one-half of the patients have a low CH50 and C3 plasma level; C1q and C4 are also depressed in type I membranoproliferative glomerulonephritis. In families with a hereditary deficiency of complement, type I membranoproliferative glomerulonephritis has been reported in the absence of other signs of systemic disease. Finally, some patients with lipodystrophy have been reported to

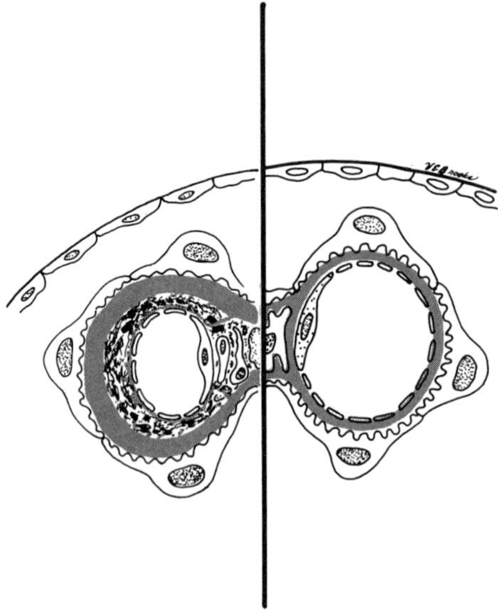

Figure 4–23. Diagram of type I membranoproliferative glomerulonephritis with a markedly widened subendothelium that contains deposits, cytoplasmic extensions of adjacent cells, and a second layer of basement membrane beneath the endothelial cell layer. This has been called mesangial interposition, but the exact nature of the cells has not been established. The mesangium contains an increased number of cells as well as deposits.

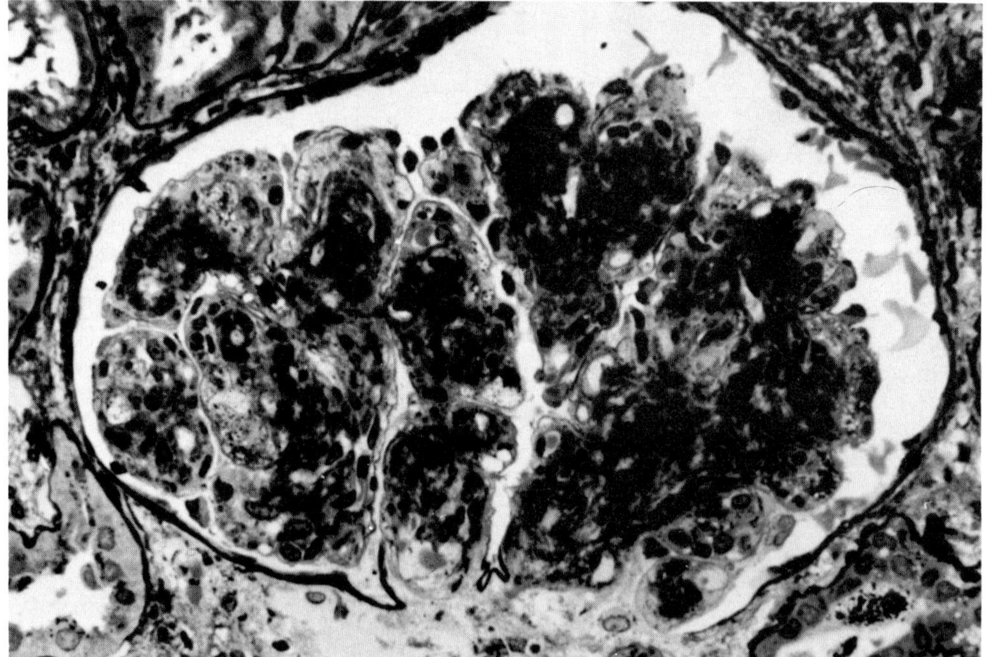

Figure 4–24. The architecture of the glomerulus is distorted by the large masses of mesangial matrix, the diminution of the vascular lumen, and the large increase in overall size. (PASM, ×300.)

have type II membranoproliferative glomerulonephritis (dense deposit disease).

Histology

Light Microscopy

Type I Membranoproliferative Glomerulonephritis

The most common type of membranoproliferative glomerulonephritis is type I, which is characterized by enlarged, hypercellular glomeruli with a marked increase in extracellular matrix (Figs. 4–23 and 4–24). There often is an infiltrate of neutrophils and mononuclear inflammatory cells, although this is seldom as marked as in acute postinfectious glomerulonephritis.

The mesangial regions are the site of the most intense hypercellularity, as well as a marked increase in matrix (Fig. 4–25). This mesangial change is diffuse and uniform and may have an almost nodular appearance. The mesangial regions are thus quite enlarged and impinge on the vascular spaces. This encroachment on the vascular spaces gives the appearance that the mesangium is growing out into the subendothelial region. The term given to this change is *mesangial interposition*. It represents marked expansion of the mesangium, both cells and matrix, with concomitant compression of the vascular lumen.

The peripheral glomerular basement membranes are diffusely and irregularly thickened. They have a double contour configuration (the so-called tram tracks). The width of the zone between the two laminae of the glomerular basement membrane varies widely, and irregular profiles of basement membrane may be seen bridging the space, giving it a honeycomb appearance (Fig. 4–26). There may be cytoplasmic elements between the two layers of the glomerular basement membrane, but it is not clear whether this cytoplasm represents mesangial or endothelial cells.

Endothelial cells are difficult to see, but they may have a swollen cytoplasm. Subendothelial or intramembranous deposits may occasionally be recognizable.

As this lesion progresses, the hypercellularity becomes less prominent and the matrix increases. The lesion thus becomes more nodular in appearance. It is this stage that was previously given the name lobular glomerulonephritis.

The tubules show no specific lesions but rather reflect the presence of a glomerular

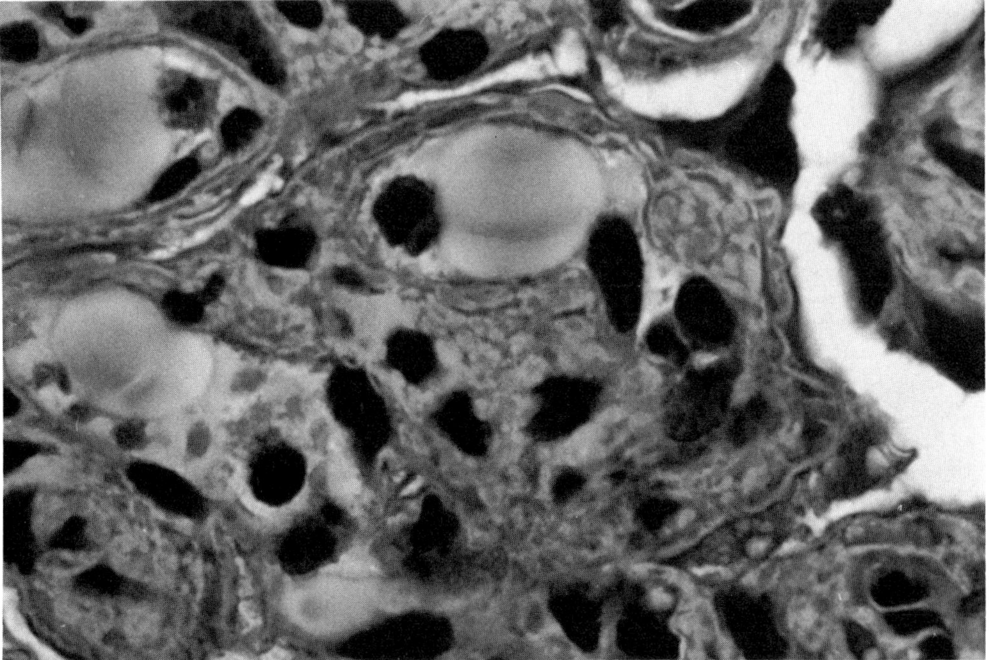

Figure 4–25. At high power the spreading of the podocytes and duplication of the glomerular basement membranes are evident. There is a prominent increase in the number of mesangial cells and in the amount of mesangial matrix. (H&E, ×1200.)

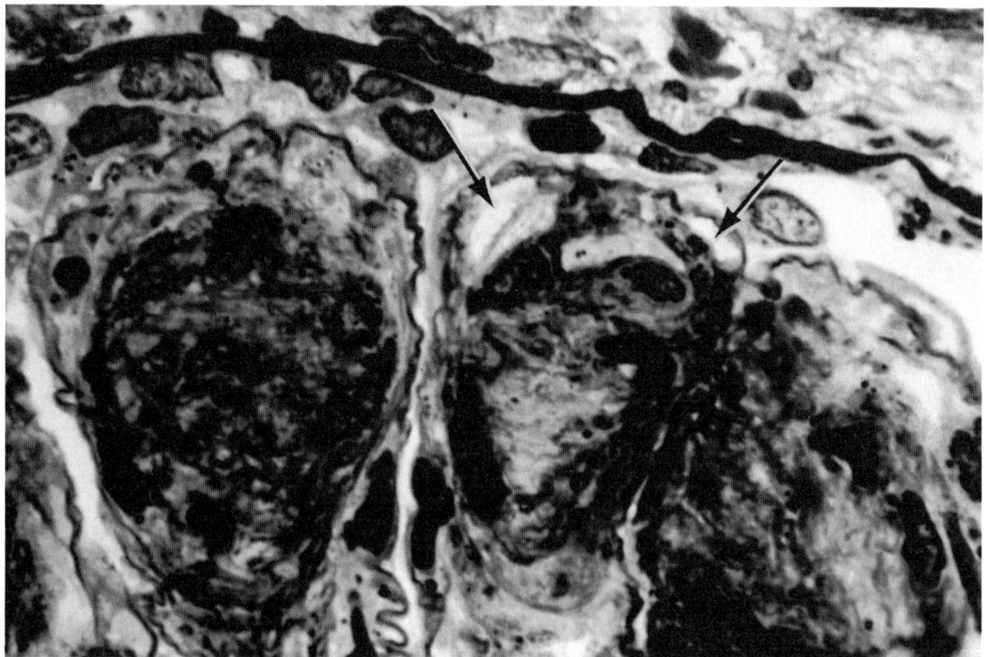

Figure 4–26. The marked mesangial sclerosis and narrowing of the vascular spaces (arrows) are highlighted. (PASM, ×1200.)

protein leak. Thus, there are cytoplasmic hyalin droplets and occasional red blood cells.

The interstitium does not appear to be a primary site of involvement, and lesions in this compartment follow and mirror those in the glomeruli.

The blood vessels are only involved in late stages of the disease.

Type II Membranoproliferative Glomerulonephritis: Dense Deposit Disease

Type II membranoproliferative glomerulonephritis is a unique histologic lesion that should not be confused with type I. We and others prefer the term *dense deposit disease.* The glomeruli are enlarged and may be hypercellular, as in type I, but the glomerular basement membrane changes are very specific by each histologic method (Fig. 4–27). The changes are diffuse, regular thickening of the glomerular basement membranes that outline the glomerulus, even over the mesangial regions (Fig. 4–28). They are easily seen on H&E sections because they are densely eosinophilic. The deposits may be interrupted or may exist as strings of deposits connected by a thin thread of material, giving them a sausage-shaped contour. These lesions are PAS positive and stain brownish with periodic acid-silver methenamine (PASM).

The mesangial cellularity is not as marked as in type I, but the mesangial sclerosis may be prominent in its late stages. Thus, this lesion may be as lobular in appearance as type I.

Epithelial hypercellularity is not often present early in the disease, but crescents are frequently seen late in the disease as it progresses rapidly to renal failure.

Similar deposits are found in tubular basement membranes and Bowman's capsule, where they have the same shape and tinctorial characteristics as those in the glomerular basement membranes.

Immunofluorescence Microscopy

Type I Membranoproliferative Glomerulonephritis

Deposits are found in the subendothelial and mesangial areas in a coarse, granular pattern along peripheral glomerular basement membranes and in the mesangium. C3 is always present and is usually accompanied by lesser amounts of C1q, C4, and properdin (Figs. 4–29 and 4–30). In some cases, C3 is the only immune reactant found in the mesangial areas. However, IgG and IgM usually

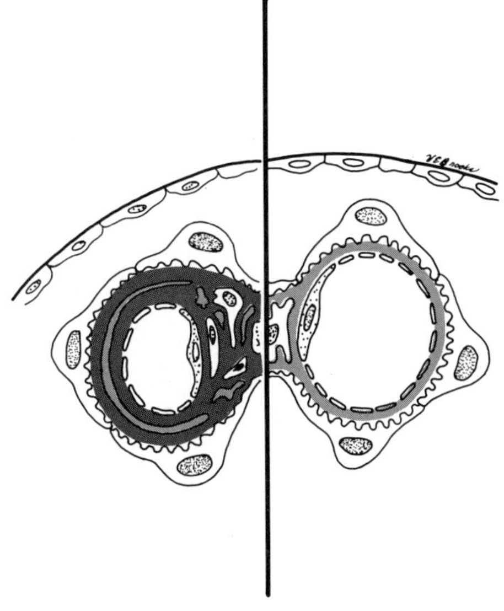

Figure 4–27. Diagram of type II membranoproliferative glomerulonephritis. The glomerular basement membrane contains a dense, continuous deposit. There is an increase in the number of mesangial cells and in the amount of mesangial matrix.

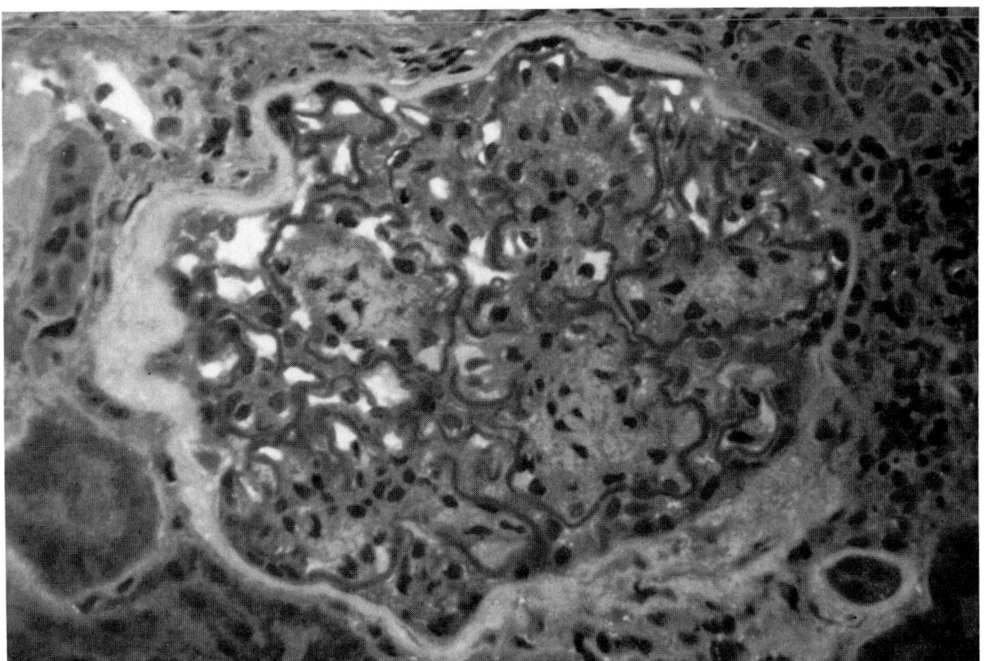

Figure 4–28. The glomerular basement membranes are outlined by a continuous dense deposit. Note that the mesangium is covered by the deposit but does not contain the densely staining material. Bowman's capsule is thickened. (H&E, ×200.)

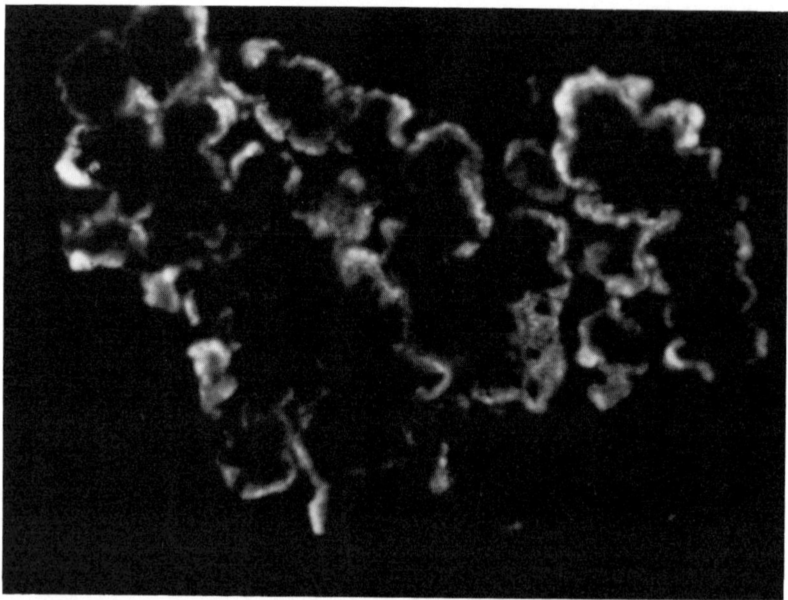

Figure 4–29. Immunofluorescence micrograph, anti-C3. There are nearly continuous, bulky deposits outlining the glomerular basement membranes. The mesangial regions are not affected. (×250.)

are also present as heavy, coarse granular deposits in both subendothelial and mesangial areas (Figs. 4–29 and 4–30). IgA deposits are unusual.

The deposits are found in all glomeruli. C3 may also be detected in Bowman's capsule and tubular basement membranes. Fibrin is often present in the glomeruli in a distribution identical to that of the immunoglobulins. In the absence of C3 deposits, the diagnosis of membranoproliferative glomerulonephritis should be questioned.

Type II Membranoproliferative Glomerulonephritis: Dense Deposit Disease

The immunofluorescence microscopic pattern in membranoproliferative glomerulonephritis type II, or dense deposit disease, is unique in both the composition and the distribution of the immunoreactants. Smooth, linear deposits of C3 outline the basement membranes. Importantly, C3 is the only immunoreactant found in these deposits. The deposits are often quite faint and may not be

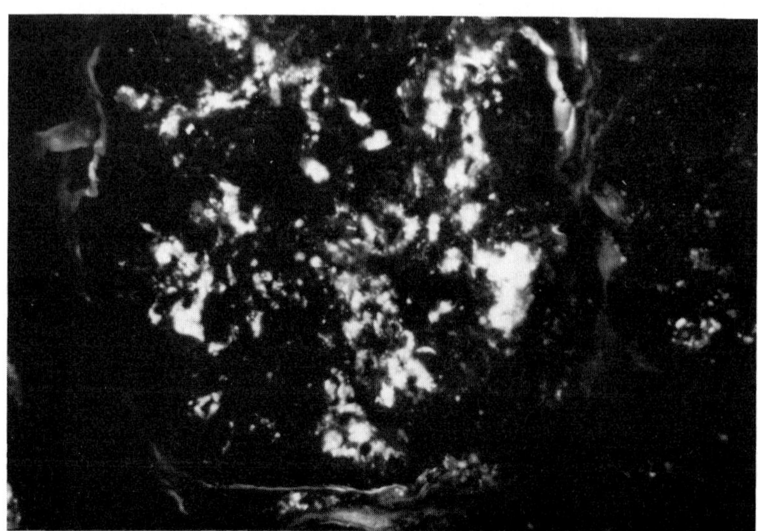

Figure 4–30. Immunofluorescence micrograph, anti-IgG. The mesangium contains large aggregates in this case. The peripheral basement membranes of the glomerulus and that of Bowman's capsule contain few deposits. (×250.)

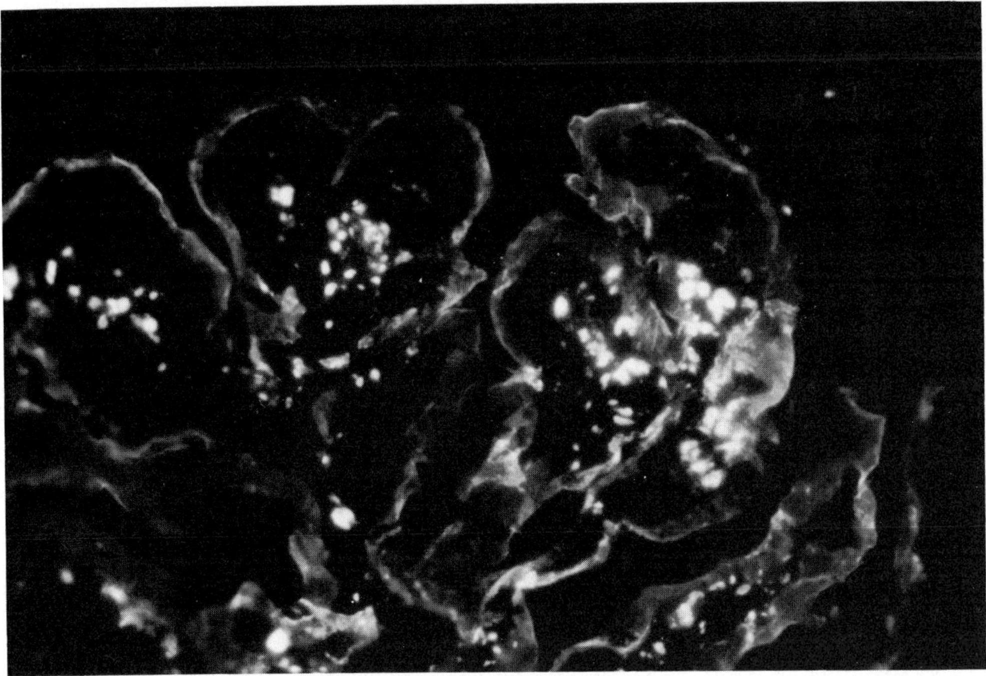

Figure 4–31. Immunofluorescence micrograph, anti-C3. The glomerular basement membranes are faintly stained, and the mesangium contains brightly staining punctate deposits. (×500.)

apparent except with the appropriate antibody and fluorescence light source. In addition to this linear basement distribution of C3, there are also scattered brightly staining granules of C3 throughout the glomerulus (Fig. 4–31).

Electron Microscopy

Type I Membranoproliferative Glomerulonephritis

The characteristic features at the ultrastructural level are deposits and marked distortion of the glomerular basement membranes (Fig. 4–32). The deposits are located in both the mesangial and subendothelial regions. The subendothelial deposits are present in one-third to one-half of the patients and vary considerably in size from loop to loop and between individual patients.

The peripheral basement membrane "duplication" is seen to consist of retention of the normal, or native, basement membrane adjacent to the epithelial cells and the addition of new segments of basement membrane beneath the endothelial cell layer. The subendothelial layer is not as regular in thickness as the native glomerular basement membrane, and it is quite often discontinuous. Lying between these two layers of basement membrane is a space containing cytoplasmic elements, scattered deposits, and a large amount of flocculent material without definite substructure, often referred to as mesangial interposition.

Fibrin tactoids may be found in the vascular regions.

Type II Membranoproliferative Glomerulonephritis: Dense Deposit Disease

As noted by light and immunofluorescence microscopy, the glomerular basement membrane deposits are the most prominent feature (Fig. 4–33). They are strongly electron dense, and distort the vascular wall architecture. The deposits underlie the native glomerular basement membrane, and segments of the glomerular basement membrane are often formed between the endothelial cells and the adjacent deposits. Deposits may also be found in Bowman's capsule basement membranes, as well as in those of the tubules. In these regions, the deposits are most often segmental and discontinuous. The mesangial regions are expanded principally by an increase in the amount of extracellular matrix. There are few deposits, and the number of cells is not often increased. Mesangial "interposition" is not a common finding.

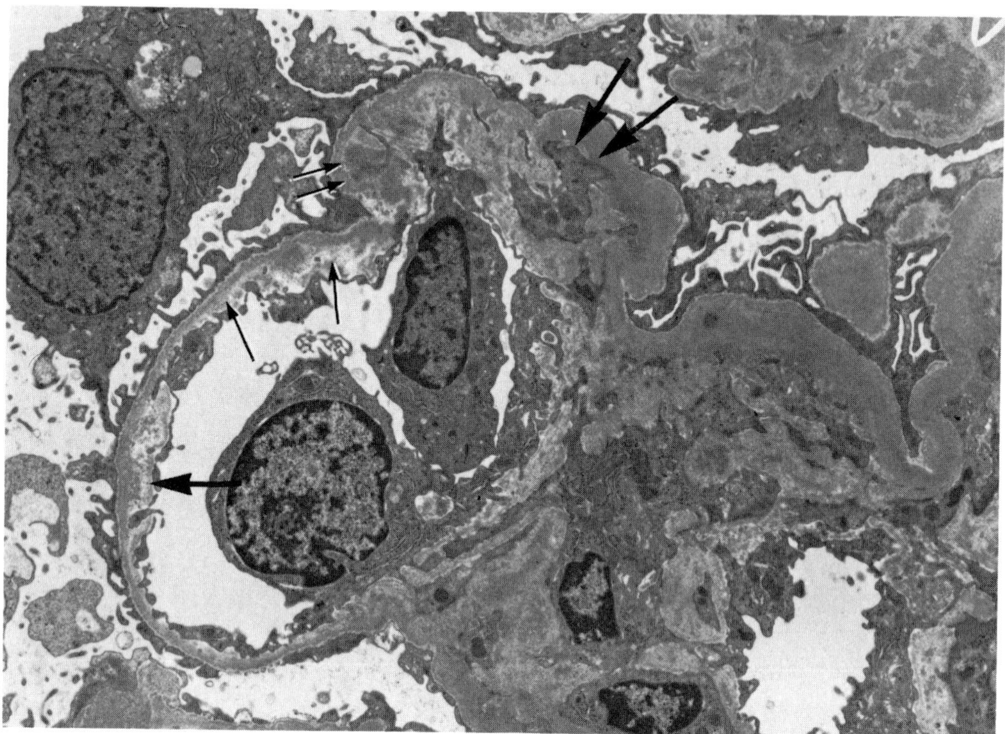

Figure 4–32. The lamina densa is intact. The subendothelial spaces contain large, irregular deposits of flocculent material (single light arrows) and irregular segments of a second layer of basement membrane (heavy arrow). In other areas there are deposits (double light arrows) and cell cytoplasm extensions (double heavy arrows). The mesangium contains deposits and an increased amount of extracellular matrix. The endothelial cell cytoplasm is thickened and contains few fenestrae. (×2500.)

There may be occasional subepithelial deposits, but they are usually scattered and are not a prominent feature. Visceral epithelial cells show spreading of the pedicels and microvillus formation.

Other Diseases

Type I membranoproliferative glomerulonephritis occurs in widely disparate clinical disorders (Table 4–3). Lesions that mimic the idiopathic forms have been associated with hereditary complement deficiencies, are occasionally seen in patients with systemic lupus erythematosus, and have been reported in patients with mixed cryoglobulinemia and in some patients with light-chain systemic disease (see Chapter 9). In addition, this is a common form of glomerular disease in patients with chronic bacterial infections or parasitic infections (see Chapter 5). It has also been reported in patients with various forms of liver disease, including hepatitis and alcoholic cirrhosis. In the latter, the glomerular immunoglobulin deposits consist mainly of IgA.

Interestingly, the glomerular lesion in patients with hepatitis appears to be age dependent. In children, the principal lesion is membranous glomerulonephritis, whereas in adults, type I membranoproliferative glomerulonephritis is more typical. The latter may be differentiated from the usual case of type I membranoproliferative glomerulonephritis by the presence of hepatitis B viral antigens in the deposits of some patients.

Prognosis

The clinical course appears to be comparable in both types of membranoproliferative glomerulonephritis. They both are thought to be relatively slowly progressive, although it should be noted that 50 to 60% of the patients are in renal failure 10 years after clinical onset. Some believe that patients with type II membranoproliferative glomerulonephritis (or dense deposit disease) have a

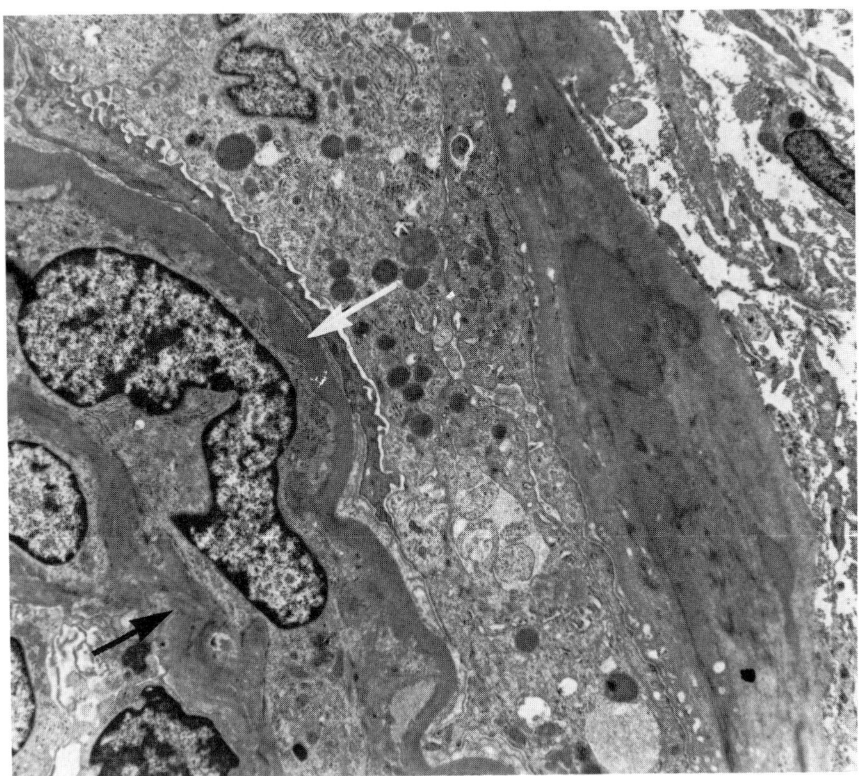

Figure 4–33. The peripheral glomerular basement membrane is almost completely replaced by a dense deposit (light arrow). The vascular space is separated from the external lamina by a zone containing cell cytoplasmic extensions and a second layer of basement membrane (heavy arrow). Bowman's capsule basement membrane also contains deposits. (×1500.)

more protracted course than those with type I. In both types I and II progression to renal failure is heralded by the appearance of crescentic glomerulonephritis.

It has also been stated that the so-called lobular forms progress more rapidly to renal failure, but these suggestions have not been rigorously tested, and it is likely that cases in this category represent late stages of membranoproliferative glomerulonephritis.

The presence of crescents and of extensive tubulo-interstitial lesions is the most reliable predictor of a poor short-term outcome.

Clinical remission independent of therapeutic measures may occur in both types of membranoproliferative glomerulonephritis. This fact, coupled with its declining incidence in the Western world, has made it difficult to evaluate the effectiveness of therapy. However, the use of inhibitors of platelet aggregation combined with aspirin and steroids has been stated to be effective in ameliorating the disease process.

Finally, type II membranoproliferative glomerulonephritis very frequently recurs in patients with a renal allograft, whereas this is an infrequent occurrence in patients with type I.

SELECTED READINGS

1. Donadio JV, Slack TK, Holley KE, et al: Idiopathic membranoproliferative (mesangiocapillary) glomerulonephritis: A clinicopathological study. Mayo Clin Proc 54:141, 1979.
2. Habib R, Gubler MC, Loirat D, et al: Dense deposit disease: A variant of membranoproliferative glomerulonephritis. Kidney Int 7:204, 1975.
3. Hayslett, JP, Kashgarian M, Bensch KG, et al: Clinicopathological correlations in the nephrotic syndrome due to primary renal disease. Medicine 52:93, 1973.
4. Kim Y, Michael AF, Fish AJ: Idiopathic membranoproliferative glomerulonephritis. Contemp Issues Nephrol 9:2337, 1982.
5. Mandelenakis N, Mendoza N, Pirani CL, et al: Lobular glomerulonephritis and membranoproliferative glomerulonephritis. Medicine 50:319, 1971.
6. Ooi YM, Vallota EH, West CD: Classical complement pathway activation in membranoproliferative glomerulonephritis. Kidney Int 9:46, 1976.

IgA GLOMERULONEPHRITIS

IgA nephropathy has emerged as a defined entity based entirely on the extensive use of immunofluorescence microscopy in renal pathology. It was described by Berger in 1968, and thus its first eponym was Berger's disease. IgA nephropathy was initially recognized because of the unusual finding of large mesangial deposits of IgA in patients whose only evidence of renal disease was macroscopic hematuria. In adult patients, the mesangial deposits frequently contained other immunoglobulins (IgM and IgG), and there were associated focal and segmental glomerular lesions (Table 4–4). This disease, described first in Paris, was initially considered benign and thought to be restricted to Europe. It took several years for it to become apparent that this disease was not only widespread but that, rather than being a benign condition, it represented the most common cause of chronic, progressive glomerulonephritis in the Western world and in Asia. It also became clear that the presence of mesangial IgA deposits as the predominant feature was not restricted to a single disease but that a spectrum of diseases was associated with glomerular deposits of IgA. These included several other diseases: Henoch-Schönlein purpura, systemic lupus erythematosus, and cirrhosis. Because of the diversity of clinical manifestations associated with the presence of mesangial IgA deposits, the use of the term *IgA nephropathy* has remained controversial and tends to obscure the varied types of glomerulonephropathy that share this finding. The other names proposed for this morphologic and clinical entity are *mesangial IgA glomerulonephritis, IgA mesangial disease, IgA-IgG nephropathy,* and *Berger's disease.* None is satisfactory, and we must rely on a combination of clinical, laboratory, and morphologic descriptors to arrive at a clear communication of the underlying process. Perhaps this must suffice until the etiology is clarified.

Pathogenesis

The diagnosis relies entirely on the finding of IgA as the predominant immune reactant in the mesangial areas and occasionally along the glomerular basement membranes. It also depends on the exclusion of Henoch-Schönlein purpura, systemic lupus erythematosus, and liver disease on clinical and laboratory grounds.

IgA glomerulonephritis has received considerable attention through multiple clinical and morphologic studies. The clinicopathologic features and geographic distribution of IgA nephropathy are now well defined, but the etiology and pathogenesis remain undefined. A wide variation exists in the frequency with which different countries report IgA nephropathy in the acute phases, but there now seems to be general agreement that it accounts for approximately 10% of all cases of end-stage renal disease. In Europe, it appears to be more common in France, Italy, and Spain. In Asia, the frequency of the disease is high, especially in Japan, where it represents 30 to 40% of all end-stage glomerular diseases. Countries with large African populations seem to have a low incidence of IgA nephropathy. Taken together, these

Table 4–4. Focal Proliferative Glomerulonephritis

Etiology	Clinical	Deposits
Idiopathic	Focal proliferative glomerulonephritis	IgA
	Other focal proliferative glomerulonephritis	IgG-IgM
	IgM mesangial glomerulonephritis	C_3
		IgM
Infectious	Subacute bacterial endocarditis	IgG-IgM
Systemic	Henoch-Schönlein purpura	IgA
	Systemic lupus erythematosus	IgG
	Mixed connective tissue disease	IgG
	Vasculitis	Fibrinogen
	Cirrhosis	IgA
	Mixed cryoglobulinemia	IgM/IgG
Antiglomerular basement membrane	Goodpasture's syndrome (anti-glomerular basement membrane)	Linear IgG

data suggest a strong genetic component. One must take this information in the context in which it is presented—namely, that few investigators have performed prospective long-term studies based on renal biopsies.

It is not established, therefore, whether this is a single disease or a group of diseases. Nonetheless, the presence of large deposits of IgA in the mesangium provides a useful way to distinguish this group of patients from those with glomerular aggregates composed principally of other immunoglobulins. It is widely accepted that this is an immune complex disease, based on animal studies that demonstrate that glomerular IgA deposits can be induced by oral immunization. This method of immunization results in circulating IgA immune complexes. The animal studies reinforce suspicions of a similar pathogenesis in humans. Many investigators have noted that in some patients the clinical syndrome follows an upper respiratory tract infection or is exacerbated by the presence of such an event. Some patients have been found to have high levels of circulating IgA complexes, and some have high levels of polymeric IgA. Both of these findings remain in the category of interesting observations with uncertain pathogenetic significance, but they leave open the possibility of a role for immunologic factors in the pathogenesis of this disease. Interestingly, some of the circulating complexes contain IgA rheumatoid factor that reacts with autologous IgG. The nature of the antigens present in the circulating immune complexes and the question of whether there is a similar antigen in the mesangial aggregates of IgA remains a question for future research. Possibilities for such antigens include food and viral and microbial antigens. Finally a defect in either the production of IgA or the clearance of macromolecular IgA has recently been proposed.

The question of a genetic predisposition remains unanswered. This latter topic has recently received impetus based on the finding of clustering in families and on the preferential association with some C3 or C4 phenotypes and HLA histocompatibility antigens.

Transplantation has also provided some interesting clues about the pathogenesis of this disease. Several patients have developed recurrent IgA nephropathy in their renal allograft. It is important to observe that many such patients have been monitored for extended periods and none have developed a progressive sclerosing disease in the glomeruli of the graft. This suggests that the disease requires both some circulating substance and a kidney that responds by the development of a sclerosing glomerular lesion. This tentative conclusion has received further support from observations on a cadaver kidney that contained mesangial deposits and that was transplanted into a patient who did not have IgA disease. The IgA deposits disappeared from the mesangial regions of the allograft placed into this patient. These data cause speculation that (1) IgA nephropathy might be treated by removing the source of the mesangial IgA aggregates and (2) that the renal response is the critical factor in the determination of the pathogenicity of the materials that deposit in the mesangium.

Patient Presentation

IgA nephropathy may occur at any age but is more common in young adults. There is a male predominance in the Western world, but this does not appear to be the case in Asia. The majority of patients have asymptomatic microscopic hematuria and mild proteinuria and a protracted clinical course. In one-third of patients, the hematuria is macroscopic, recurrent, and may be associated with flank pain. The hematuric episodes are often immediately preceded (a few hours or days) by an episode of a mild upper respiratory tract viruslike infection. Some patients with mild gastrointestinal flulike symptoms have also been reported. The episodes of hematuria may last for only a few hours and dissipate. Other patients may develop symptoms of an acute nephritic syndrome, including renal failure, hypertension, edema, and heavy proteinuria. Finally, a small number of patients may have short episodes of acute oliguric renal failure that spontaneously remit.

A benign course is typical in children. Unfortunately adults most often show signs of significant renal disease by the time the syndrome is diagnosed. Some patients may present with the nephrotic syndrome, but this is not common.

Histology

Light Microscopy

Although the disease was first classified as a focal proliferative glomerulonephritis, it has been recognized that there are multiple histologic patterns, including the absence of detectable light microscopic abnormalities. The most characteristic histologic lesions are focal and segmental mesangial proliferation. In the mild forms, the lesions are minimal and the glomeruli may appear normal or show minimal increases in the amount of extracellular matrix or the degree of cellularity. In addition, these changes may affect only a small number of glomeruli or a small portion of individual glomeruli.

Proliferative and sclerotic lesions of different ages often coexist in the same biopsy specimen. Localized crescents are also present near the foci of mesangial proliferation. Areas of necrosis, if present, are rare and limited and like cellular crescents are more common in biopsies performed early after an acute episode of hematuria. Large crescents with foci of necrosis have been described during episodes of acute renal failure, in which case the diagnosis of Henoch-Schönlein purpura must be excluded on clinical grounds.

Areas of sclerosis involve segments of the glomerular tuft, and in the presence of synechiae, the immediately adjacent Bowman's capsules are frequently thickened and multilaminated. When glomerular basement membrane thickening occurs, it is usually present as irregular, segmental areas of multilamination, in contrast to the diffusely laminated pattern characteristic of membranoproliferative glomerulonephritis. Many or most peripheral glomerular basement membranes appear normal with silver stains. The presence of obsolescent glomeruli attests to the chronic nature of the disease.

The mesangial matrix occasionally contains eosinophilic mesangial deposits, often called "fibrinoid," which appear red on trichrome-stained sections. This is a misleading term, because newly formed hyalin also has this appearance. The use of the descriptor *fibrinoid* denotes a more acute process than is ordinarily present in these patients. Therefore, we prefer the use of the term *hyalin* to describe this material.

Tubulo-interstitial lesions are often conspicuous and closely parallel the degree of renal functional impairment. Scattered areas of interstitial edema or sclerosis with interstitial inflammatory cell infiltrates predominate around the more severely damaged glomeruli. In adults, there often are obvious chronic vascular lesions.

The World Health Organization working group on classification of glomerular disease has proposed the following categorization:

Class I: Minimal lesion

Class II: Minor changes with small, segmental areas of proliferation (Figs. 4–34 and 4–35)

Class III: Focal and segmental glomerulonephritis with less than 50% of the glomeruli showing obvious changes (Fig. 4–36)

Class IV: Diffuse mesangial lesions with proliferation and sclerosis (Fig. 4–37)

Class V: Diffuse sclerosing glomerulonephritis affecting more than 80% of glomeruli (Fig. 4–38)

Although this classification provides a descriptive framework, many cases cannot be easily categorized using this method.

Immunofluorescence Microscopy

IgA nephropathy, as described earlier, can only be accurately diagnosed by immunochemical methods. Although the light microscopic lesions may be focal, the immunoglobulins are always present in a diffuse pattern by immunofluorescence microscopy.

The single constant finding in this disease is the presence of diffuse deposits of IgA in the mesangium, forming either discrete granules or large aggregates (Figs. 4–39 and 4–40). When large, the deposits may also be found in the subendothelial areas. Uncommonly there are focal, granular subepithelial deposits. IgG codistributes with IgA in more than one-half of the cases, but it is usually present in smaller amounts. The term *IgA-IgG nephropathy* was coined because of the frequent coexistence of these two immunoglobulins in the mesangium. IgM has also been reported in the mesangium of one-half of the patients. C3 is present in most patients and has the same distribution as IgA. C1q and C4 complement components are not commonly present. As in other sclerosing diseases, the membrane attack components may be present.

Fibrinogen deposits, also common, are most often small and inconspicuous. This fact may help in the differentiation of IgA ne-

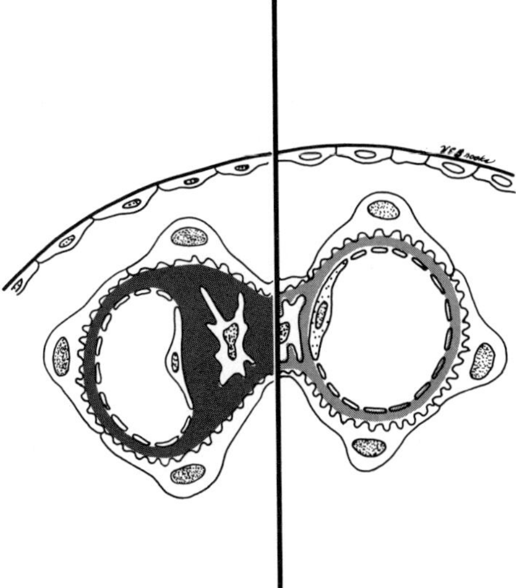

Figure 4–34. Diagram of a glomerulus with an increase in the amount of mesangial matrix.

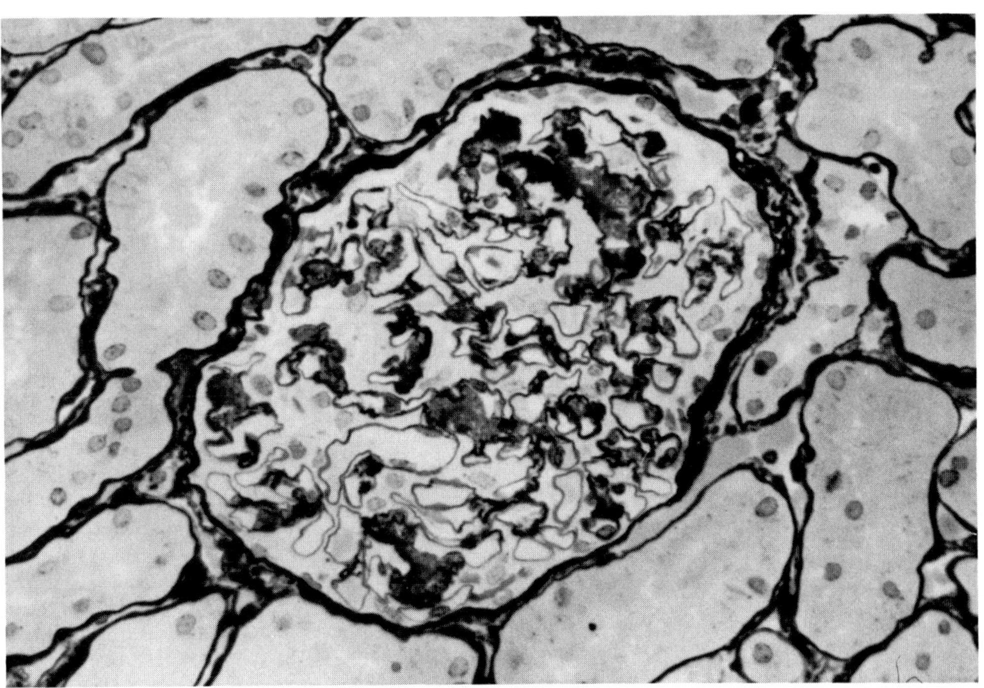

Figure 4–35. All glomeruli have mesangial regions expanded by a PASM-positive material. The number of glomerular cells is normal. Although the glomerular basement membranes are normal, those of Bowman's capsule may be thickened. (PASM, ×300.)

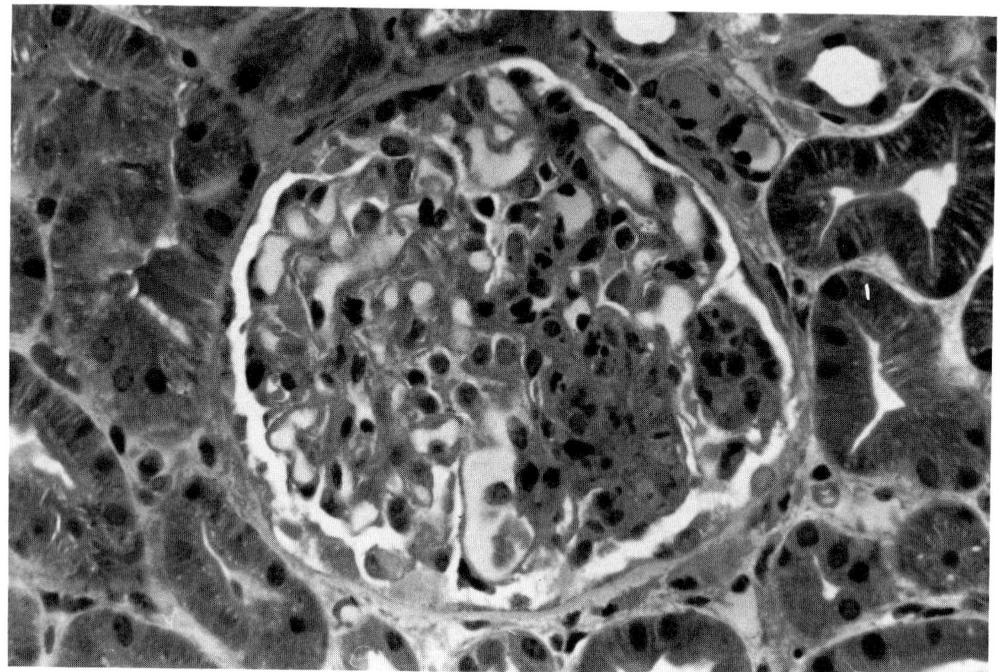

Figure 4–36. The focal area of proliferation contains neutrophils and a small focus of necrosis. (H&E, ×300.)

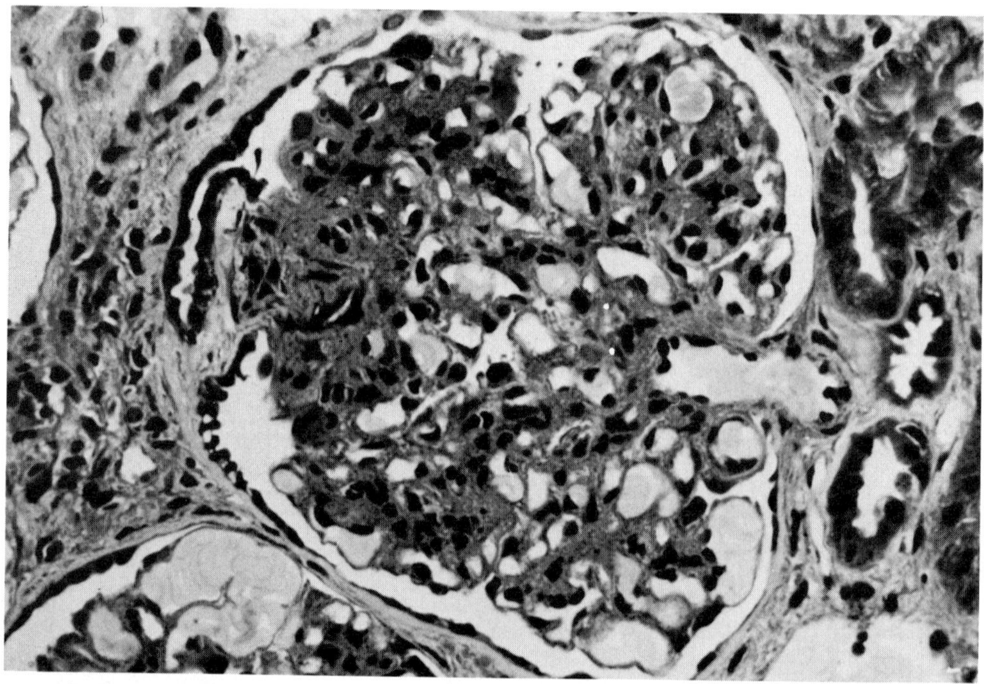

Figure 4–37. There is diffuse mesangial proliferation and sclerosis. An organized synechia is seen near the urinary pole of the glomerulus. (H&E, ×300.)

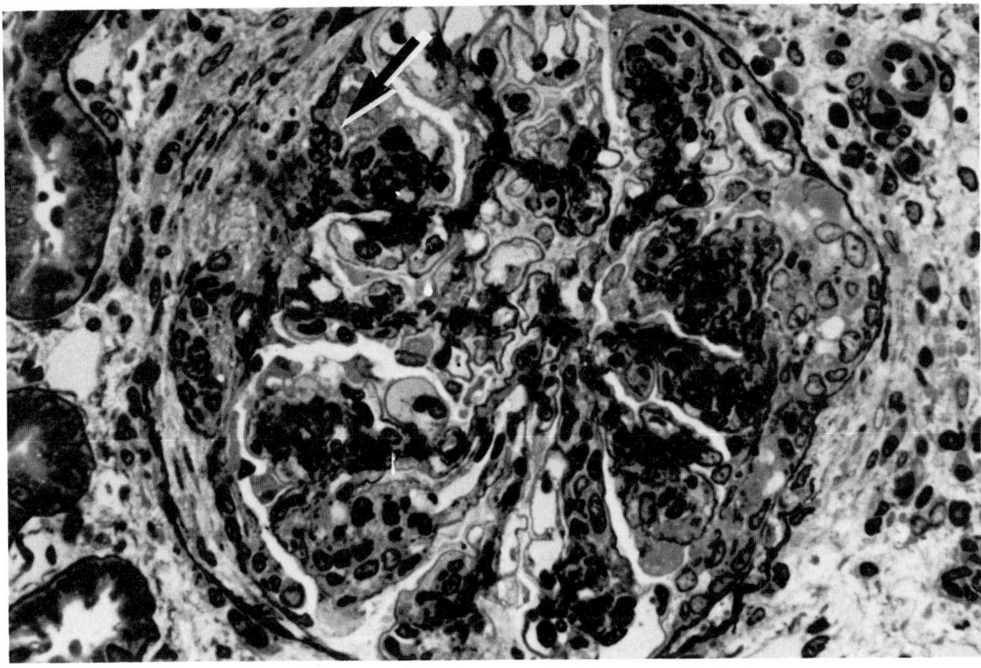

Figure 4–38. There is diffuse mesangial sclerosis and proliferation, as well as localized epithelial cell proliferation with both cellular and organized synechiae. (PASM, ×300.)

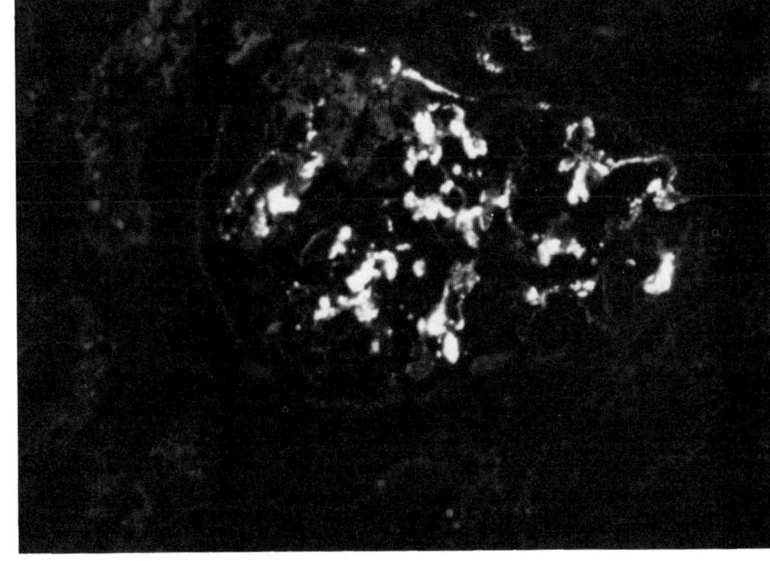

Figure 4–39. Immunofluorescence micrograph, anti-IgA. The mesangial regions of all glomeruli contain deposits. (×100.)

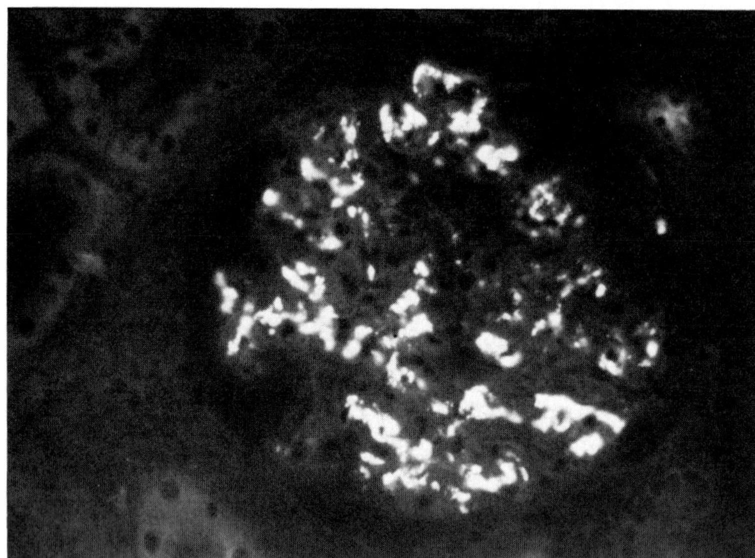

Figure 4–40. Immunofluorescence micrograph, anti-IgA. At higher power, each mesangial space is seen to contain deposits. (×250.)

phropathy from the nephropathy of Henoch-Schönlein purpura because of the prominence of fibrinogen deposits in the latter.

The only other immune complex-mediated glomerular disease in which significant IgA deposits are present is systemic lupus erythematosus. IgA deposits may also be found in patients with chronic liver disease.

Electron Microscopy

The deposits, recognizable as electron-dense granular material, are irregularly spread throughout the mesangial matrix, and some mesangial regions are completely free from recognizable dense deposits. Deposits are rarely found in the cytoplasm of mesangial cells. The associated mesangial matrix may be expanded, and the number of cells in the mesangium may be increased. The deposits are irregular in size and often lie between the mesangial cells and the adjacent paramesangial peripheral basement membrane (Fig. 4–41). Subendothelial deposits are most commonly found adjacent to a mesangial region (Fig. 4–42). Although rare, subepithelial deposits may be noted. They most often are separated from the overlying epithelial cells by a thin layer of electron-dense material resembling basement membrane. The peripheral basement membrane frequently shows thinning and multilamination in patients who have sclerosing lesions by light microscopy. In these areas, there may be localized spreading of the pedicels.

Prognosis

There is no specific treatment for IgA nephropathy, and the natural history is so variable as to make generalizations precarious. As many as 10 to 20% of affected adults develop end-stage renal disease. The most frequent clinical course is thought to be one of slow, progressive deterioration. Various attempts have been made to define the histologic features that predict a poor prognosis. There appear to be none unique to IgA nephropathy, and one must rely on general criteria that are applicable to all other types of severe, progressive glomerular diseases. These include the presence of crescents, abundant sclerosis, severe tubulo-interstitial lesions, and advanced vascular lesions. Thus, no single histologic feature or constellation of features provides assistance to the pathologist in predicting which cases of early disease will deteriorate and which will resolve.

SELECTED READINGS

1. Berger J, Hinglais N: Les depots intercapillaires d'IgA-IgG. J Urol Nephrol 74:694, 1968.
2. Beukhof JR, Kardaun O, Schaafsma W, et al: Toward individual prognosis of IgA nephropathy. Kidney Int 29:549, 1986.
3. Clarkson AR, Woodroffe AJ, Bannister KM, et al: The syndrome of IgA nephropathy. Clin Nephrol 21:7, 1984.
4. D'Amico G, Imbasciati E, diBelgioioso GB, et al: Idiopathic IgA mesangial nephropathy. Medicine 64:49, 1985.

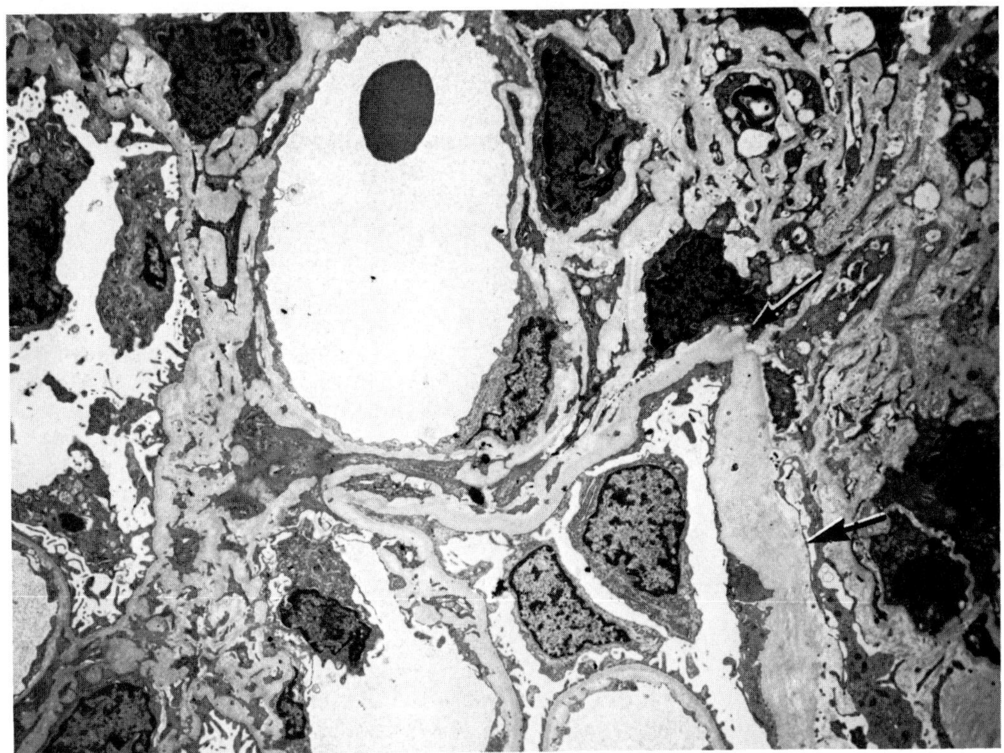

Figure 4–41. The mesangial matrix is diffusely increased in amount in this electron micrograph of the vascular pole region (heavy arrow). Bowman's capsule basement membrane is irregularly thickened (arrows). (×2200.)

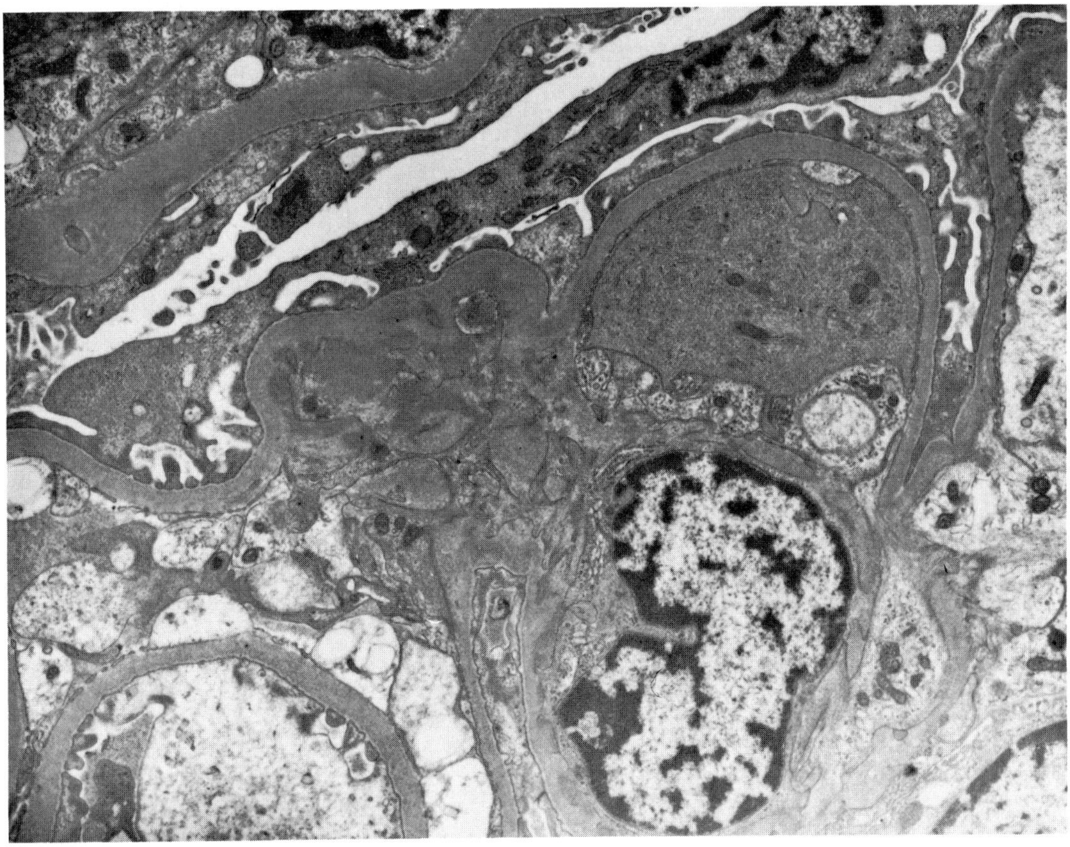

Figure 4–42. Granular deposits lie within the mesangial matrix. (×5400.)

5. Julian BA: Familial IgA nephropathy: Evidence of an inherited mechanism of diseases. N Engl J Med 202:312, 1985.
6. Julian BA, Waldo FB, Rifai A, et al: IgA nephropathy. The most common glomerulonephritis worldwide. Am J Med 84:129, 1988.
7. Morel-Maroger LJ, Verroust PJ: Clinicopathological correlations in glomerular diseases. *In* Jones NF (ed): Advances in Renal Diseases. Churchill Livingstone, Edinburgh, Scotland, 1975, pp 48–79.
8. Yoshikawa N, Iijima K, Maehara K, et al: Mesangial changes in IgA nephropathy in children. Kidney Int 32:585, 1987.
9. Yoshikawa N, Ito H, Yoshiya S, et al: Henoch-Schönlein nephritis and IgA nephropathy in children: A comparison of clinical course. Clin Nephrol 27:233, 1987.

CRESCENTIC GLOMERULONEPHRITIS OR RAPIDLY PROGRESSIVE GLOMERULONEPHRITIS

Crescentic glomerulonephritis is the histopathologic term coined to designate an array of severe glomerular diseases that share the common feature of crescents in a large percentage of the glomeruli. This category of disease is also known as rapidly progressive, subacute, malignant, and extracapillary glomerulonephritis. It is characterized histologically by extensive crescents and clinically by the rapid deterioration of renal function that reaches end stage within a period of days or weeks.

This process was first recognized in the early part of the 20th century. The definition, a purely histologic categorization, encompasses several varieties of glomerular disorders characterized by their light microscopic and immunopathologic features. The classification of this group of disorders rapidly evolved after the application of immunopathologic techniques to renal biopsies. As pointed out in Chapter 3, crescents may occur in a large number of glomerular diseases, but the discussion in this chapter is restricted to those diseases in which they constitute the main histologic feature. Crescentic glomerulonephritis in association with systemic diseases is reviewed in other chapters.

Pathogenesis

In the past few years, there has emerged a working classification of crescentic glomerulonephritis based on immunofluorescence microscopic findings. The categories are as follows:

Glomerulonephritis due to antibodies directed toward glomerular basement antigens (anti-glomerular basement membrane)
Glomerulonephritis due to the deposition or formation of immune complexes in the glomeruli
Glomerulonephritis in which no immunoglobulins are found in the glomeruli (so-called non-immune or idiopathic)

An attempt has been made to relate these findings to a presumptive underlying mechanism, based on animal studies. However, the cause of the disease remains unknown in most patients.

This classification, as will be demonstrated, is of use principally because it provides clinicians with help in determining the treatment approach best suited to each patient.

Crescentic glomerulonephritis (Table 4–5) is an infrequently encountered disease, constituting fewer than 10% of all renal biopsies performed for the diagnosis of glomerulonephritis. Thus, it is difficult for any one group to mount a study of the diagnostic criteria, the pathogenesis and its possible geographic or genetic differences, the best means to treat the various subcategories, and the number of patients in each category. However, the best estimates of the number of patients in each of the categories are as follows:

Antiglomerular basement membrane antibodies, 20%
Immune complex, 40%
Non-immune, 40%

The mechanism of crescent formation has been the subject of considerable investigation. It was initially assumed that the origin of the cells composing the crescent was exclusively epithelial. Further, these epithelial cells were thought to be derived from Bowman's capsule. However, early electron icroscopic studies pointed out the heterogeneity of cells within the crescent, noting that there were both light and dark cells. The application of cell markers revealed that the crescent was indeed a mixed population of cells and that some were derived from macrophages. One of the early events in the development of crescents is the appearance of fibrin in the

Table 4–5. Crescentic Glomerulonephritis

Light Microscopy	Immunofluorescence Microscopy	Possible Pathogenesis	Association
Crescents/necrosis	Linear IgG Fibrinogen	Anti-glomerular basement membrane	Pulmonary hemorrhage
Crescents/proliferation in the tuft	Granular IgG Complement Fibrinogen	Immune complexes	Bacterial infections
Crescents/necrosis	Negative Fibrinogen (?)	Non-immune	Systemic symptoms (rash, arthralgias, fever)

urinary space. An influx of macrophages into the urinary space follows. It was suggested that breaks in the glomerular basement membrane, so-called gaps, allowed the passage of both the high-molecular-weight precursors of fibrin and subsequently the macrophages. These two events presage and are thought to induce the proliferation of the indigenous glomerular cells.

The variable cellular composition of the crescent, the multiplicity and variety of the lesions occurring in the underlying glomerular tuft, and the different patterns of immunologic involvement all point to the conclusion that crescentic glomerulonephritis is a syndrome with diverse causes. The common features that draw this group together into one diagnostic category are the presence of large numbers of crescents and a clinical course characterized by abrupt onset and rapid progression to renal failure.

Patient Presentation

Crescentic glomerulonephritis most commonly affects adults, being very uncommon before the age of 30. There is a male predominance, especially in the anti-glomerular basement membrane variety. This form is also more common in patients with the HLA-Dr2 phenotype.

The presenting symptoms may be vague, and the patients often complain of weakness, nausea, and general fatigue. In most instances, the renal disease is characterized by severe, unremitting oliguric or anuric renal failure, which is occasionally heralded by macroscopic hematuria. Hypertension is uncommon and never prominent unless there is severe volume expansion due to sodium retention.

The cause of the disease is completely unknown, for the most part. However, various antecedents have been observed and reported on. Approximately one-half of the patients have a history of an influenza-like illness preceding the onset of renal symptoms. In this respect, anti-glomerular basement membrane disease has been thought to follow influenza A2 infections, but in most patients, acute and convalescent sera either have not been obtained or have not been informative. Even less well established is a relation between exposure to organic solvents and crescentic glomerulonephritis.

Pulmonary hemorrhage is a complication in almost one-third of patients with anti-glomerular basement membrane crescentic glomerulonephritis, either at presentation or shortly thereafter. This presentation in concert with crescentic glomerulonephritis and circulating anti-glomerular basement membrane antibodies has been called Goodpasture's syndrome. In these patients, there is a strong correlation between the presence of the antibodies, a history of smoking (or other pulmonary injury), and the presence of pulmonary hemorrhage (see Chapter 6).

The autoantibodies react with the NC-1 region of the type IV collagen of the glomerular basement membrane. This region of the molecule is referred to as the Goodpasture's antigen.

Patients with immune complex glomerulonephritis may come to medical attention because of the underlying infectious disease process—for example, with a visceral abscess. Crescentic glomerulonephritis following streptococcal infection is essentially only encountered in children and is very unusual in the United States and Western Europe. Infections such as abdominal abscesses, infected vascular shunts, or sepsis have been associated with crescentic glomerulonephritis and should always be considered because they represent potentially curable causes of crescentic glomerulonephritis.

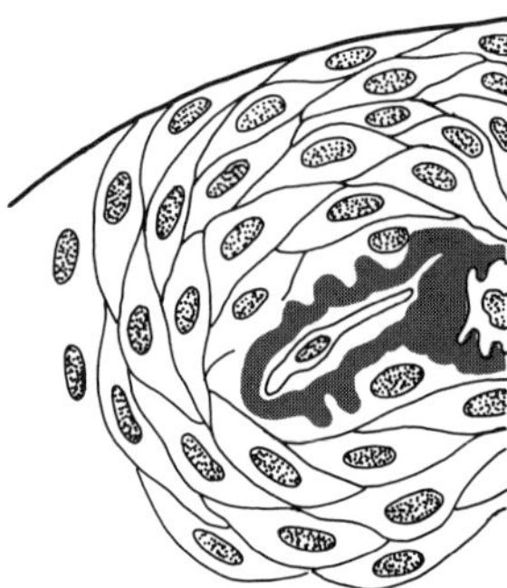

Figure 4–43. Diagram of epithelial cell proliferation and collapse of the glomerulus.

Patients with non-immune crescentic glomerulonephritis often present with rash, arthritis, and fever. This triad may lead to confusion between this syndrome and a vasculitis.

Histology

Crescentic glomerulonephritis is one of the renal disorders in which it is imperative that pathologists examine the renal biopsy by light and immunofluorescence microscopic techniques and report the results in the shortest interval consistent with accurate interpretation.

Light Microscopy

Crescentic glomerulonephritis is characterized by the obliteration of Bowman's space by cells (Figs. 4–43 and 4–44). The underlying glomerular tuft is compressed and often obliterated. Although there is no agreement about the exact number of crescents required for the diagnosis of crescentic glomerulonephritis, most researchers agree that 80% or more of the glomeruli should be affected. Because this diagnosis carries such a poor prognosis, the pathologist must observe an adequate specimen before this diagnosis is rendered.

The size of the crescent may also have prognostic significance, and it is obvious that glomeruli with large circumferential crescents represent more severely affected glomeruli than those with more limited involvement.

The cells that form the crescents are often large. Those that have a pale, swollen cytoplasm and a regular oval nucleus are most likely macrophages. They are identifiable as macrophages with the use of monoclonal antibodies to cell surface markers. Occasional

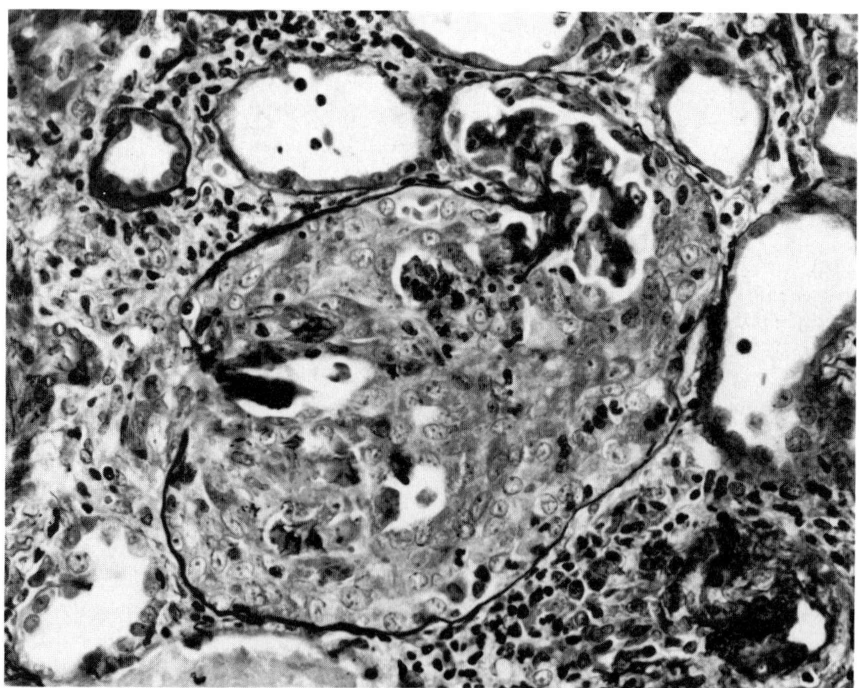

Figure 4–44. There is diffuse proliferation of glomerular epithelial cells, which completely occupy the urinary space. The underlying glomerular tuft is compressed and collapsed. (H&E, ×300.)

mitotic figures may be observed in the smaller, darker cells admixed with the large, clear cells. The latter cells are epithelial in origin. These are the predominant cell type in the crescents when biopsies are performed at a later time. In addition, neutrophils and red blood cells are frequently observed. Fibrin is often found between cells of the crescent. It is recognized as strongly eosinophilic areas that are red with trichrome stains (Fig. 4–45). Fibrin, present in early cases, disappears soon thereafter. The crescents may contain interstitial cells, if the basement membrane of Bowman's capsule has been breached. This is best seen with silver stains (Fig. 4–46). In this instance, there is continuity between the crescent and a rich periglomerular infiltrate. We believe that this feature is most common in non-immune crescentic glomerulonephritis and portends a grave prognosis, because it reflects an aggressive inflammatory lesion that repairs by scarring and destruction of the glomerulus.

It is unusual to find multinucleated cells in the crescent except in patients with Wegener's granulomatosis.

Another unusual pattern is found when the basement membrane of Bowman's capsule has been interrupted. Interstitial cells cross the basement membrane, invading Bowman's space, and form an array of palisading fibroblast-like cells. In this case, as one might expect from the presence of such a large number of collagen-producing cells, the glomerular crescents rapidly organize and the glomeruli become completely and rapidly obsolescent.

One interesting and unexplained finding is the frequent observation of a mixture of cellular and partially or completely fibrotic crescents. This would lead one to suspect that the injury may actually be a much more indolent or perhaps recurrent process than the clinical and laboratory data would suggest.

The evaluation of the underlying tuft may give precious insight into the underlying pathologic process. Focal and segmental areas of necrosis are often prominent. These are more widespread in the non-immune form but may also occur in the anti-glomerular basement membrane and immune complex varieties. The areas of necrosis involve an ill-defined segment of the tuft, usually in direct contact with the overlying crescent. The necrosis, as with the appearance of fibrin in the crescent, is typical of early lesions. These two findings tend to presage an aggressive fibrotic response. When crescents are extensive, the glomerular tuft is compressed

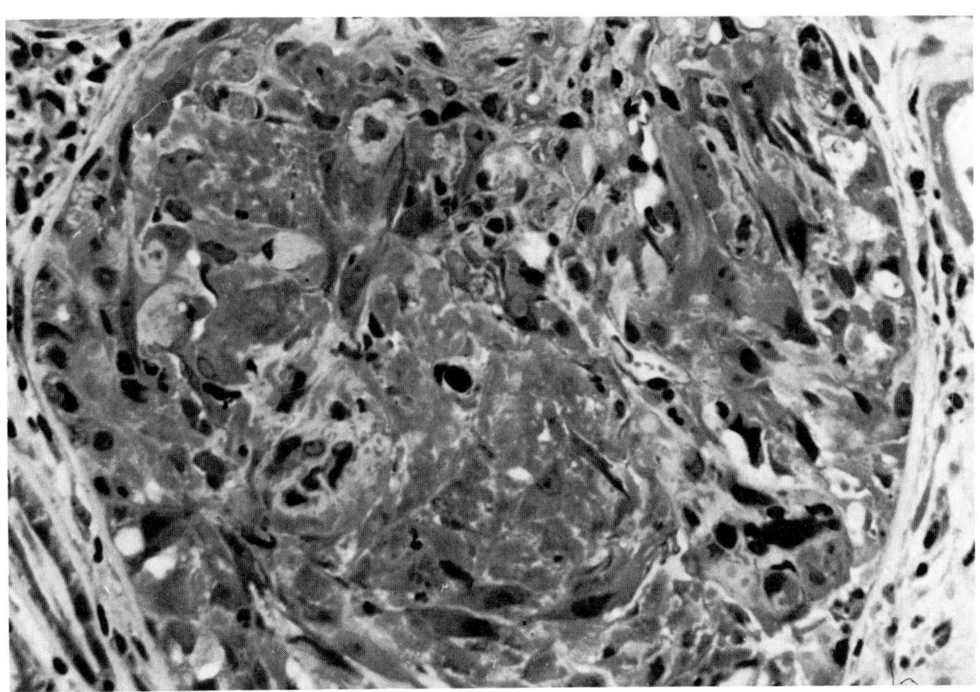

Figure 4–45. The glomerulus is not visible in this mass of proliferating and infiltrating cells and deposits of fibrin. There is extensive necrosis of the glomerulus. (H&E, ×500.)

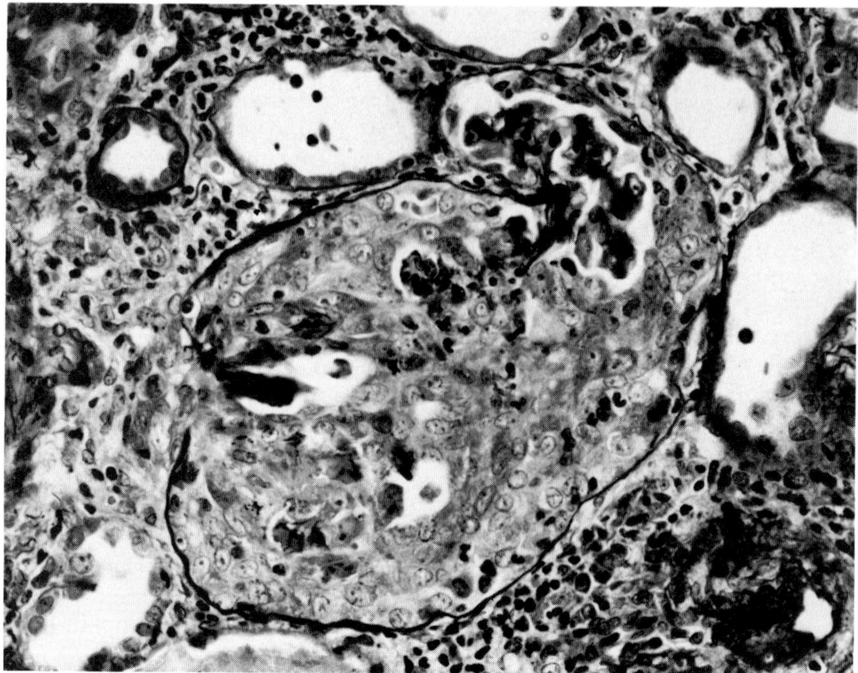

Figure 4–46. The basement membrane of Bowman's capsule is multilaminated in some areas (upper right) and interrupted in others (lower left). (PASM, ×250.)

and collapsed. In this case, the glomerular changes may be difficult to identify. An increased number of intraglomerular cells may result from the accumulation of circulating inflammatory cells or the proliferation of endothelial and mesangial cells. As in the examination of the crescent, the use of monoclonal antibodies to inflammatory cell surface antigens has shown that many of the intraglomerular cells are macrophages. Neutrophils and lymphocytes may also be present.

Immunofluorescence Microscopy

The three distinctive patterns that may be recognized are discussed in the following paragraphs.

Anti-Glomerular Basement Membrane: Linear Pattern

Deposition of IgG along the glomerular basement membranes in a linear, continuous, smooth pattern characterizes the anti-glomerular basement membrane type of crescentic glomerulonephritis. The linear deposition is diffuse, affecting every loop of each glomerulus (Figs. 4–47 and 4–48). Linear IgG deposition may also occur, to a lesser degree, along Bowman's capsule and along occasional tubular basement membranes. In a few cases in the literature, the antibodies to the glomerular basement membrane are of the IgA class, but IgA and IgM are rarely found in this linear fashion.

In association with IgG, C3 has been detected in a linear but interrupted pattern

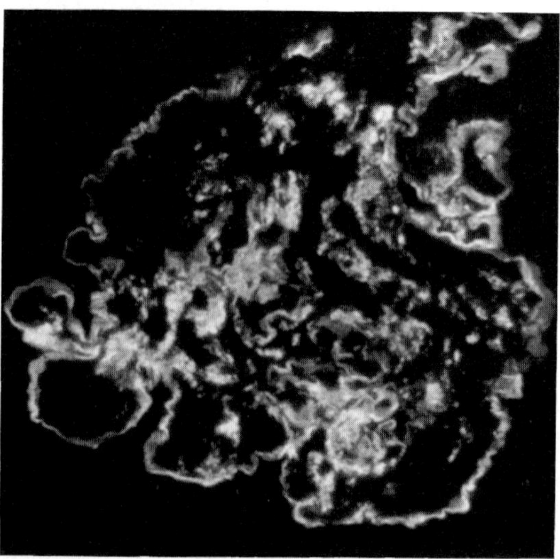

Figure 4–47. Immunofluorescence micrograph, anti-IgG. There are linear deposits along the glomerular basement membranes. The glomerulus is not collapsed in this specimen. (×250.)

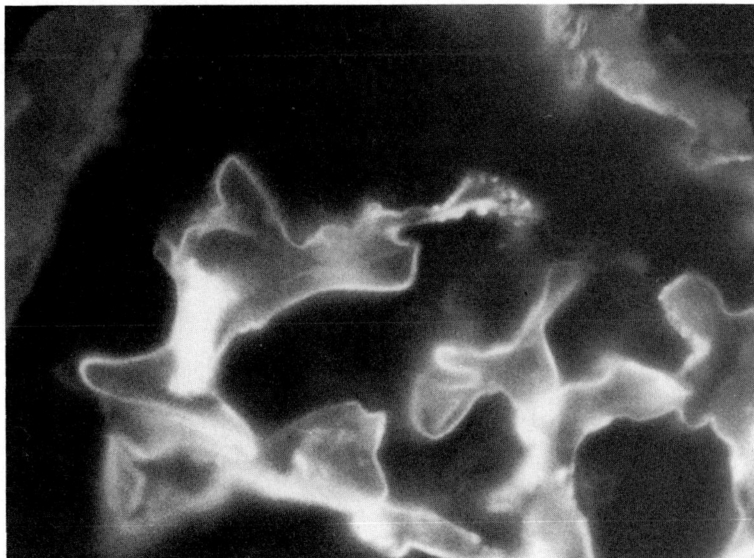

Figure 4–48. Immunofluorescence micrograph, anti-IgG. A high-power photomicrograph showing linear glomerular basement membrane deposits (× 500.)

along the glomerular basement membrane, Bowman's capsule, and tubular basement membranes.

C1q and C4 are not usually present, although there may be some accumulations of these components in areas of sclerosis.

There are only a few circumstances in which the presence of linear deposits of IgG may lead to confusion. First, linear IgG deposits have been found to occur in patients with glomerulosclerosis. This pattern is most commonly seen in patients with diabetes mellitus, but it also occurs in patients with cirrhosis of the liver. However, in both of these circumstances IgG is not the sole immunoglobulin present, and IgA, IgM, and albumin are also present in a similar distribution. Of even more importance is the absence of crescents. Detailed studies of these cases have demonstrated that the immunoglobulins are not autoantibodies directed against the glomerular basement membrane.

Finally, linear deposits of immunoglobulins are occasionally present in light-chain systemic deposition disease, but again the pattern of deposition and the composition of the deposits are different (see Chapter 9). In light-chain systemic deposition disease, the deposits clearly predominate around the tubules and glomerular deposits are found in the enlarged mesangial areas. Finally, the deposits are composed of only one type of light chain, mostly kappa, whereas the deposits in anti-glomerular basement membrane disease are polyclonal.

Fibrin/fibrinogen deposition is a prominent feature of all types of crescentic glomerulonephritis and parallels the extent of necrotizing areas in the glomeruli (Fig. 4–49). Fibrinogen may also be present within the crescents and in the interstitial tissue. In general, masses of fibrin are more conspicuous in fresh "active" lesions and tend to disappear with progression to chronic lesions.

Granular Deposits: Immune Complexes

Granular deposits of immunoglobulins and complement are found in approximately 40% of patients with crescentic glomerulonephritis. The deposits may be present in the mesangial areas as well as along the endothelial or epithelial aspects of the glomerular basement membrane, in a diffuse or focal pattern. Various combinations of immunoglobulins have been reported, including IgG, IgA, and IgM. They are usually found in association with complement components. Fibrin/fibrinogen deposits invariably are found within foci of necrosis or in fresh crescents.

The appearance and distribution of immune reactants vary with the underlying disease. In biopsies of patients with post-streptococcal glomerulonephritis, only IgG and C3 are found in the small granules scattered over the glomerular tufts. In patients with subacute bacterial endocarditis, the deposits contain IgG and IgM in larger amounts and are largely found within the mesangial and subendothelial areas. The deposits in patients

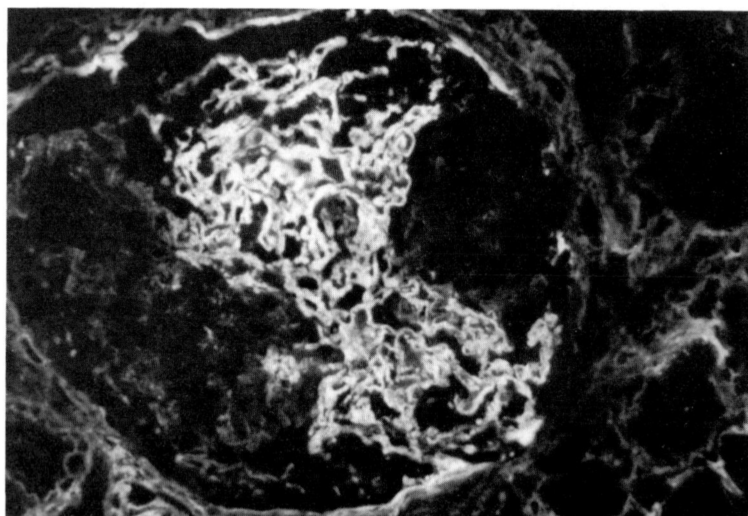

Figure 4–49. Immunofluorescence micrograph, anti-fibrinogen/fibrin. The material that had a pink appearance in H&E sections is stained. (×250.)

with subacute bacterial endocarditis also contain C3, C4, C1q. In patients with visceral abscesses, the deposits may contain IgA, associated with IgG and IgM, in both mesangial and subendothelial areas. When IgA is the predominant immunoglobulin and when the deposits predominate in the mesangial areas, in a patient with crescents, the underlying disease may be either IgA disease (see Chapter 4) or Henoch-Schönlein purpura (see Chapter 6). The latter will be associated with its characteristic clinical syndrome.

Finally, there remains a group of patients who have granular immune deposits but in whom no underlying disease can be ascertained.

Non-Immune Crescentic Glomerulonephritis

In approximately 40% of patients with crescentic glomerulonephritis, no immune reactants can be detected by immunofluorescence microscopic examination. Fibrin/fibrinogen antigens may be present in areas of necrosis or crescents. This group of patients is often considered to represent a variety of vasculitis involving the glomerular vascular bed as its principal target.

Electron Microscopy

Biopsy specimens characteristically show collapse of glomerular capillary loops and an increase in the number of cells in Bowman's space, including epithelial cells and cells resembling macrophages. There is widening of the lamina rara interna and swelling of the endothelial cell cytoplasm. Loose masses of proteinaceous material, including recognizable fibrin, are present between the cells composing the crescent (Fig. 4–50).

There may be interruptions of the peripheral glomerular basement membranes through which the cytoplasm of the adjacent endothelial or epithelial cells may protrude. These have been called gaps and are most frequent in areas of necrosis, in marked hypercellularity, and in early crescents. When such gaps are present in the basement membrane of Bowman's capsule, interstitial inflammatory cells or fibroblasts may be seen either traversing these breaks or may be present in large numbers as a component of the cellular crescent lying within the urinary space. If the biopsy is performed later in the course of the disease, the cells may be separated from one another by extracellular matrix. This matrix is of two varieties. If Bowman's capsule is intact, the intercellular matrix within Bowman's space is composed of homogeneous electron-dense material resembling basement membrane (Fig. 4–51). If the capsular basement membrane has been breached, the matrix contains banded collagen, similar to that found in the interstitium. In both cases, the end result is obsolescence.

Prognosis

Most patients with this group of diseases have severe renal damage at the time of

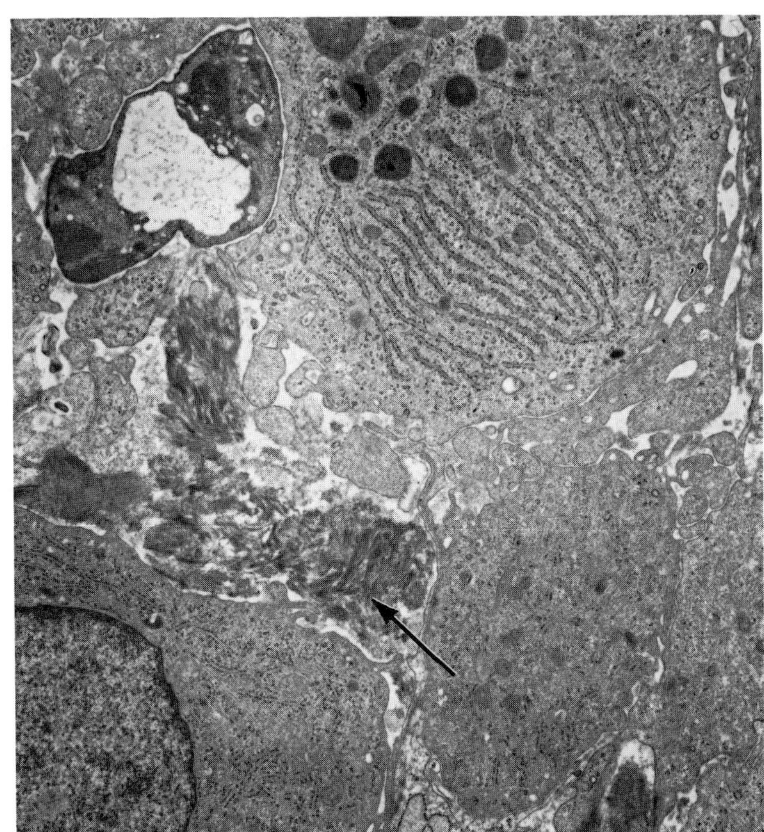

Figure 4–50. The cells of the crescent are of various types. There are strands of fibrin (arrow) between cells. (×5000.)

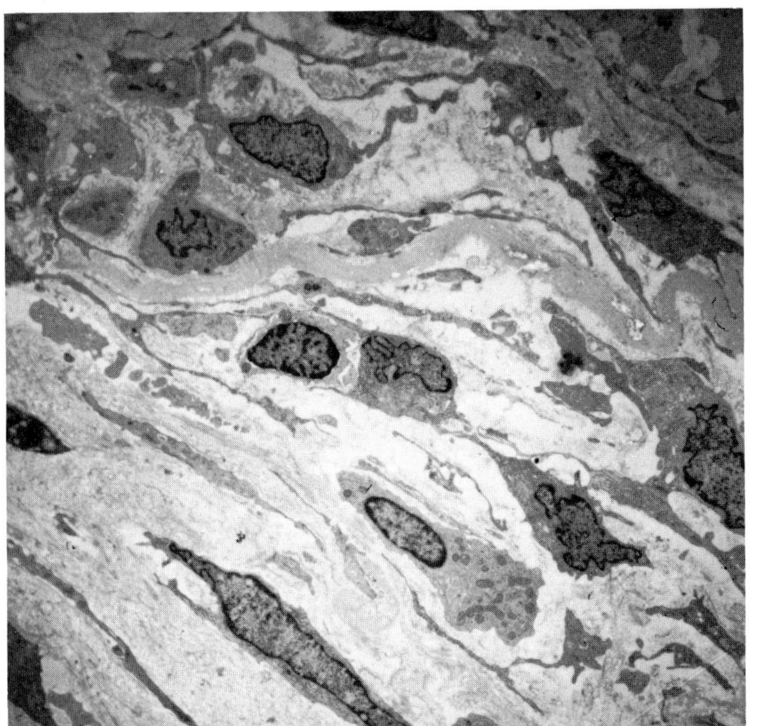

Figure 4–51. There are dense bands of organizing matrix lying between the cells in this organizing crescent. (×1500.)

presentation, and the prognosis largely depends on the degree of irreversible glomerular damage.

The development of crescents in any glomerular disease reflects a severe event and bodes a poor prognosis. It is generally accepted that most patients who have circumferential crescents in 100% of their glomeruli uniformly progress to end-stage renal failure without regaining renal function. If the crescents are not diffuse, there is a greater chance of recovery of some renal function with aggressive therapeutic intervention. Patients who have an underlying endocapillary glomerular hypercellularity seem to also have a better chance of recovering renal function.

As in other glomerular disorders, the extent of interstitial fibrosis correlates with the ultimate outcome. Among the other histologic features that may be prognostic indicators is the presence of extensive fibrinoid necrosis. When this is present, rapid and irreversible deterioration of renal function is likely.

Various therapeutic regimens have been applied, but the small number of cases has prevented the establishment of reliable clinical trials. The worst prognosis is generally associated with antibodies against the glomerular basement membranes. Patients with granular immune deposits seem to have a better response to treatment because they often have a treatable form of infectious disease. Recognition of this form of the disease is essential to avoid inappropriate and undesirably aggressive therapeutic approaches.

Treatment protocols are varied and comprise pulse steroids, high-dose methylprednisolone, and/or immunosuppressive drugs. Finally, plasma exchange has been widely used in an attempt to remove the anti-glomerular basement membrane antibodies in the plasma.

Repeat renal biopsies have been used after the therapeutic trial to determine if the acute lesions have been ameliorated and whether sclerosis has supervened. This is the only reliable means to determine the amount of fixed renal damage and may provide an estimate of the need and potential for response in any remaining active disease process.

SELECTED READINGS

1. Bacani R, Velasquez F, Kanter A, et al: Rapidly progressive (non-streptococcal) glomerulonephritis. Ann Intern Med 69:463, 1968.
2. Couser WG: Idiopathic rapidly progressive glomerulonephritis. Am J Kidney Dis 2:57, 1982.
3. Lerner R, Glassock R, Dixon F: The role of antiglomerular basement membrane antibody in the pathogenesis of human glomerulonephritis. J Exp Med 126:989, 1967.
4. Magil AB: Histogenesis of glomerular crescents. Am J Pathol 120:222, 1985.
5. Stejskal J, Pirani CL, Okada M, et al: Discontinuities (gaps) of the glomerular capillary wall and basement membrane in renal diseases. Lab Invest 28:149, 1973.
6. Striker L, Killen PD, Chi E, et al: The composition of glomerulosclerosis. I. Studies in focal sclerosis, crescentic glomerulonephritis, and membranoproliferative glomerulonephritis. Lab Invest 51:181, 1984.
7. Whitworth J, Morel-Maroger LJ, Mignon F, et al: The significance of extracapillary proliferation: Clinicopathological review of 60 patients. Nephron 16:1, 1976.

Chapter

5

PRIMARY GLOMERULAR DISEASE OF KNOWN ETIOLOGY

BACTERIAL INFECTIONS

GLOMERULONEPHRITIS FOLLOWING STREPTOCOCCAL INFECTIONS

Acute glomerulonephritis is the term used to designate glomerulonephritis associated with bacterial infections in sites distant from the kidney. The best example is post-streptococcal glomerulonephritis, which has been considered to be the prototype of an immune complex disease. It is characterized by the development of a diffuse, proliferative glomerulonephritis after a latent period of 8 to 14 days in patients with a streptococcal infection of the upper respiratory tract or skin.

Pathogenesis

Post-streptococcal glomerulonephritis was the first type of nephritis considered to be an immunologic disease. This conclusion was based on the association of circulating immune complexes, a low serum complement level at initiation of the renal lesion, and the finding of immune reactants in the glomeruli. This postulate was further supported by the presence of similar clinical and laboratory observations in patients with serum sickness. Finally, a similar set of findings could be reproduced in experimental animals by eliciting a humoral immune response.

The largest number of cases of acute post-streptococcal glomerulonephritis is now reported from developing countries. This lesion has been almost eradicated from many other regions by the widespread use of antibiotics in the treatment of respiratory tract infections and the institution of proper sanitary conditions.

Patient Presentation

The most common presenting signs and symptoms are hematuria, edema, hypertension, and azotemia. There is a history of a recent infection, often culture positive for streptococci, in the patient or a family member. An elevated and rising titer to streptococcal antigens establishes the streptococcal infection as the most likely cause of the renal lesion, especially in children. The serum complement levels are low, and circulating antigen-antibody complexes may be detectable during the early phases of the process. The exact pathogenesis of the disease is poorly understood, but factors relating to both the host and the pathogen are important. For instance, several family members may have protein and red blood cells in the urine during an episode of upper respiratory tract infections, but most often only one member develops the rest of the symptoms and signs of renal disease. In addition, there are "nephritogenic" strains of streptococci. Finally, few of the patients who develop acute post-streptococcal glomerulonephritis develop long-term renal sequelae. Beta-hemolytic streptococci are not the only bacteria to be associated with post-infectious glomerulonephritis, but they are the most frequent pathogen.

The renal signs are not always typical. Some patients have only hematuria, and others may have anuria at the clinical onset. Very few patients have the nephrotic syndrome at the outset, but when it is present, it appears to portend a poor prognosis. Finally, some patients have acute oliguric renal failure at the onset.

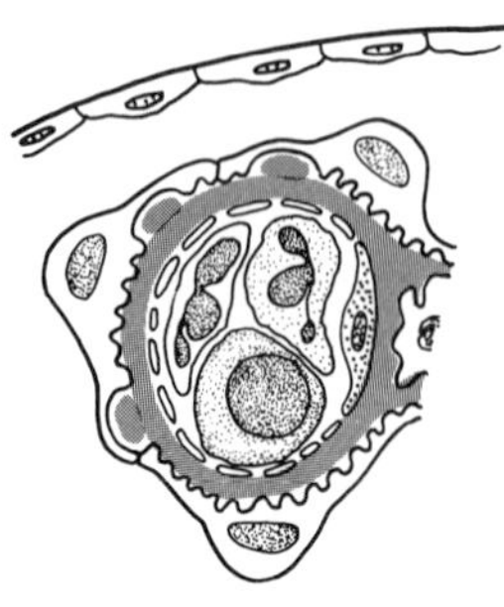

Figure 5–1. Diagram of an acute proliferative glomerulonephritis with subepithelial deposits, proliferation, and exudation.

Histology

Light Microscopy

The glomeruli are the principal site of the lesion and are characteristically large, diffusely hypercellular, and infiltrated with neutrophils (Fig. 5–1). The hypercellularity consists of both resident glomerular cells and infiltrating mononuclear and polymorphonuclear inflammatory cells. Mesangial and endothelial cells are thought to be the principal glomerular cell types involved in the proliferation. The term *exudative glomerulonephritis* has been used to designate this early lesion.

The infiltrating inflammatory cells and the increased number of glomerular cells lead to almost complete obliteration of the glomerular vascular spaces (Fig. 5–2).

The glomerular basement membranes are not altered, for the most part, although occasional areas of "splitting" may be observed. In some patients who are examined during the exudative phases of the disease, subepithelial deposits may be visualized (Fig. 5–3). These large subepithelial deposits are seen by light, immunofluorescence, and electron microscopy and have been called humps because of their shape. They are best seen on trichrome-stained sections in paraffin-embedded specimens or on silver stains on plastic embedded sections (Fig. 5–4).

Visceral epithelial cells are not frequently

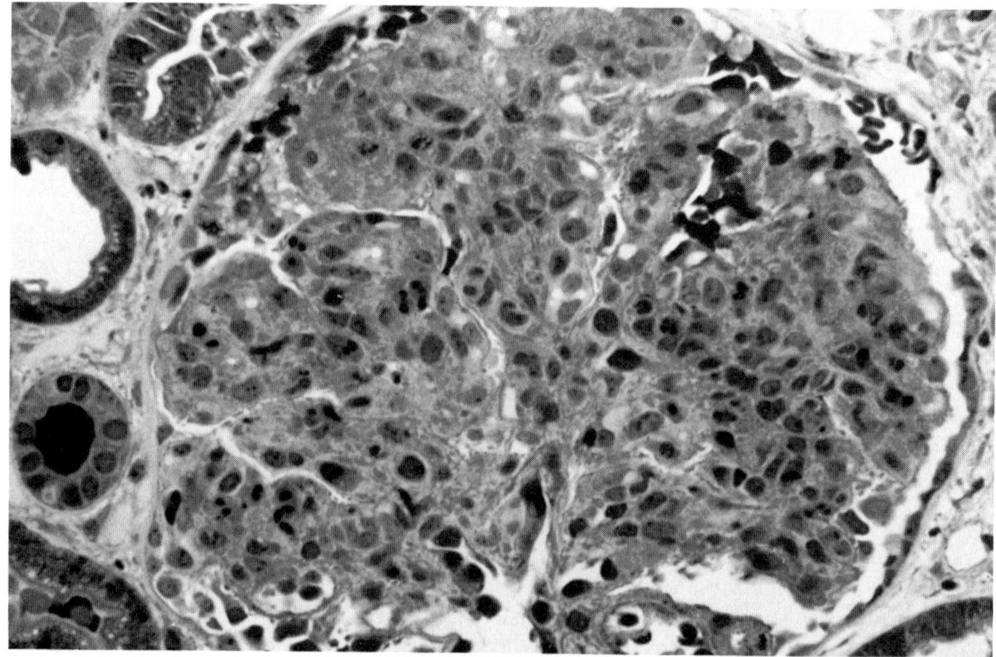

Figure 5–2. The glomerulus is hypercellular and contains many inflammatory cells. (H&E, ×300.)

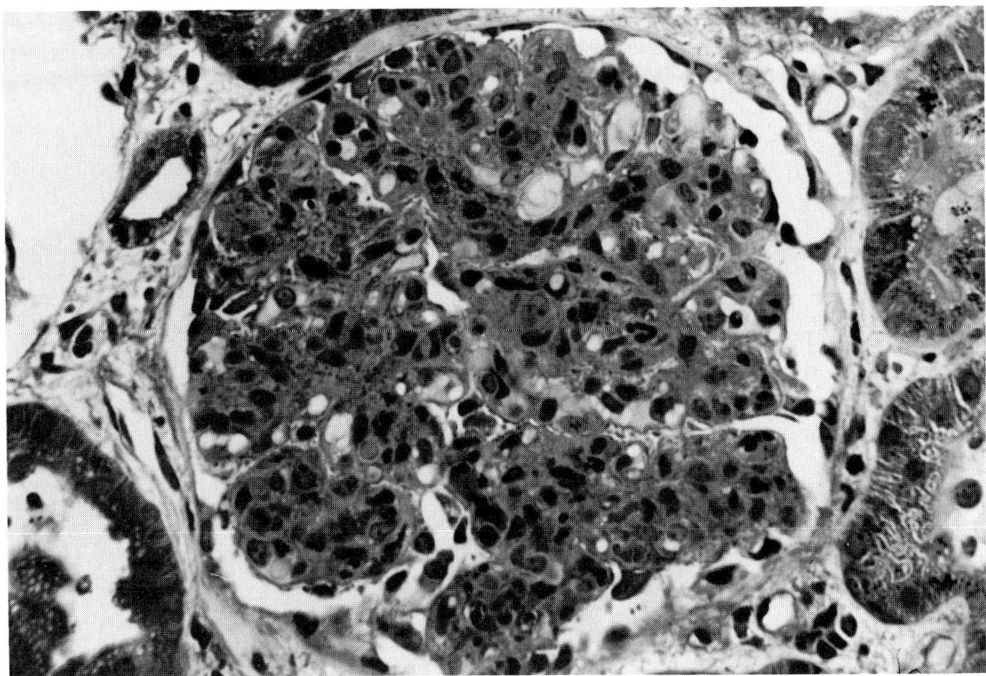

Figure 5–3. The parietal and visceral epithelial cells are also prominent in this acute glomerulonephritis. (H&E, ×300.)

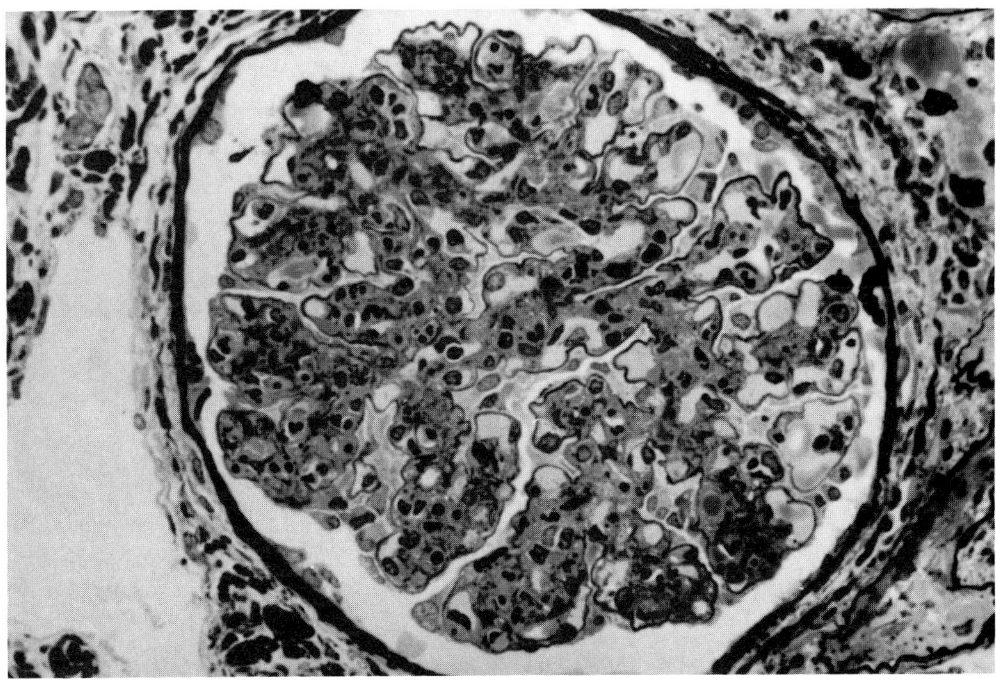

Figure 5–4. The glomerular basement membranes are clearly outlined, and most of the increased number of cells lie within their confines. (PASM, ×300.)

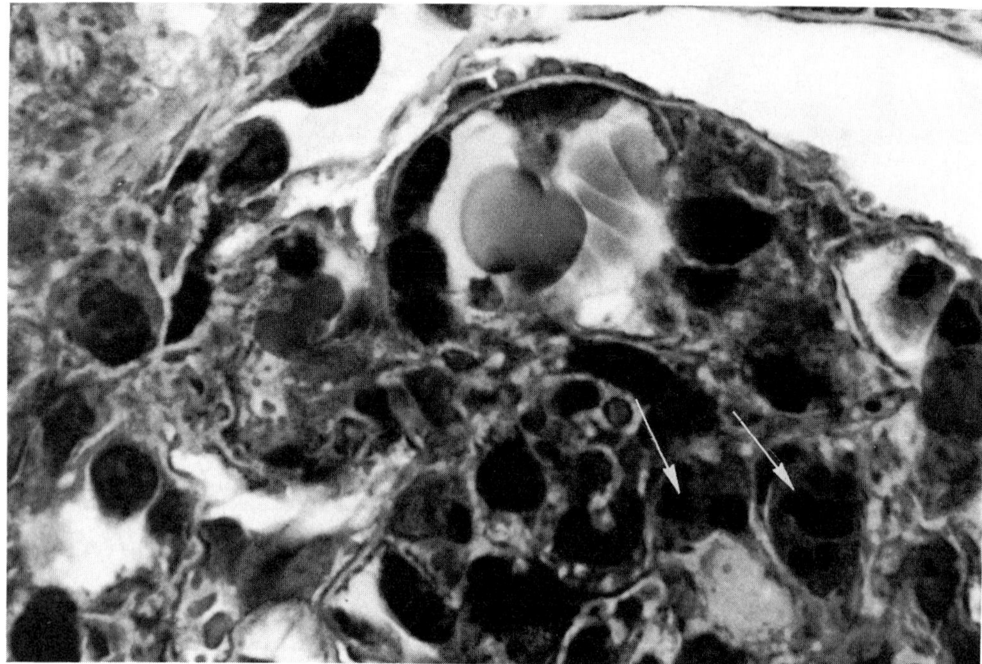

Figure 5–5. Multiple deposits are present on the subepithelial aspects of the glomerular basement membranes. Neutrophils are present within the glomerular tufts (arrow). (H&E, ×1200.)

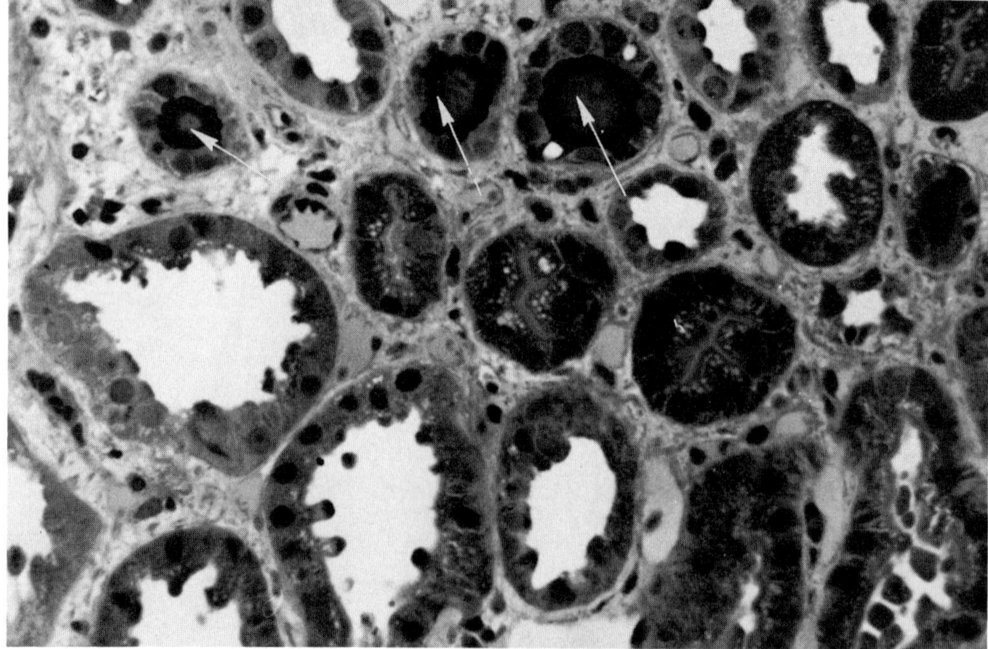

Figure 5–6. The interstitium is widened and contains edema and an increased number of interstitial cells. Red blood cells embedded in a protein matrix are noted in distal tubules and collecting ducts. (H&E, ×300.)

increased in number, although their cytoplasm may be prominent. In patients with marked epithelial proliferation (i.e., those with diffuse crescents) the lesion has a different prognosis and should not be considered different from other types of immune-mediated crescentic glomerulonephritis (see Chapter 4).

Within a few weeks after onset of the illness, the glomerular lesions change significantly. The inflammatory cell infiltrate disappears, and the number of deposits is sharply limited. At this stage, the cellular proliferation involves only the mesangial regions (Fig. 5–5). The mesangial matrix may be moderately increased in amount. The glomerular vascular loops are patent, and the glomerular basement membranes are normal. At this stage, the lesion is a diffuse mesangial proliferative glomerulonephritis.

The tubules contain many hyalin and cellular casts composed of mixtures of red and white blood cells (Fig. 5–6). Proximal tubular cells may contain protein-laden lysosomes, but necrosis is uncommon.

The interstitium is often widened by edema, but inflammatory cell infiltrates are more prominent in cases in which there is crescentic glomerulonephritis.

Immunofluorescence Microscopy

The glomerular basement membranes are outlined by small, granular aggregates of IgG and C3 (Fig. 5–7). These deposits are more widely spaced and more irregular in shape than those present in membranous glomerulonephritis. The mesangial regions may also contain granular deposits of immunoglobulins and complement components. IgM may be present, but it is seldom prominent.

Electron Microscopy

The centrilobular regions are filled with cells, and many of the usual anatomic landmarks are not recognizable. There is an increase in the number of endothelial cells, and their cytoplasm is prominent and filled with organelles. Their usual fenestrated, thin cytoplasm is so altered that it is often difficult to separate the endothelial cells from infiltrating mononuclear cells or proliferating mesangial cells (Fig. 5–8).

The mesangial regions are expanded, and their boundaries may be difficult to discern. Adjacent mesangial zones often appear to be joined, leaving the impression of the presence of mesangiolysis. Dead cells and cellular debris may be seen, admixed with the increased number of mesangial cells.

The electron-dense deposits on the subepithelial aspects of the glomerular basement membrane are separated from the lamina densa and from the podocytes by a clear zone (Fig. 5–9). The peripheral glomerular basement membrane is otherwise unremarkable.

There are also many deposits within the substance of the mesangial matrix. In the paramesangial area, deposits may be found

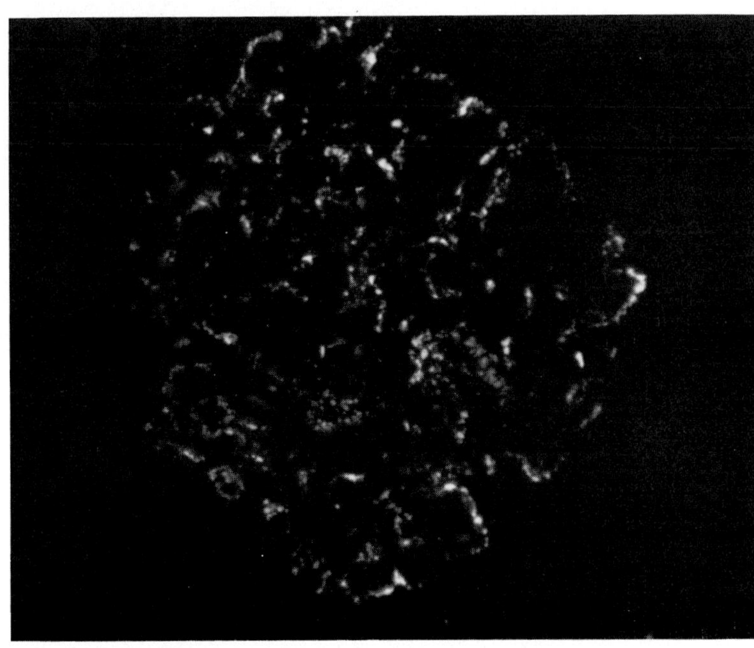

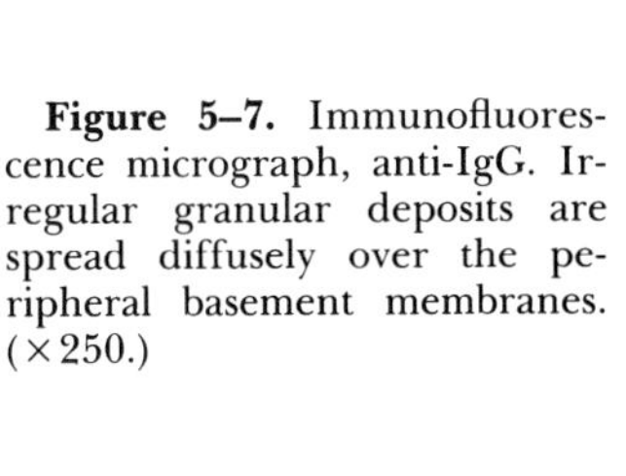

Figure 5–7. Immunofluorescence micrograph, anti-IgG. Irregular granular deposits are spread diffusely over the peripheral basement membranes. (×250.)

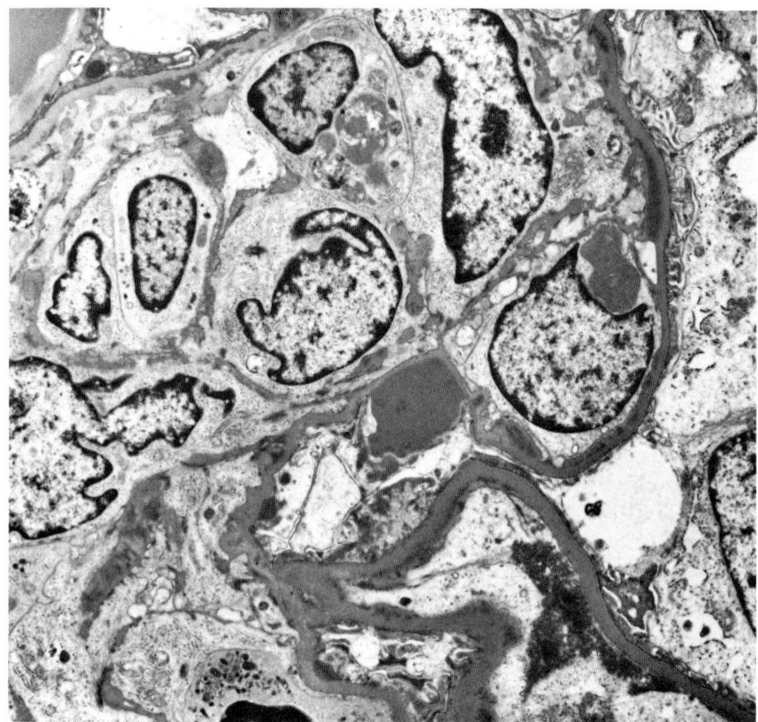

Figure 5–8. The usual anatomic landmarks may be effaced by the presence of infiltrating inflammatory cells as well as an increased number of glomerular cells. There are also subepithelial and mesangial deposits. (×2200.)

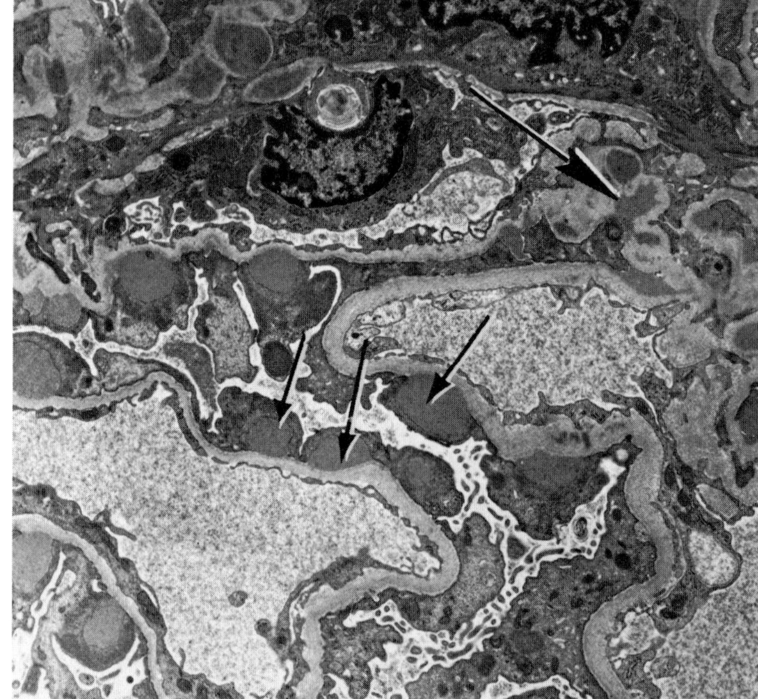

Figure 5–9. The subepithelial spaces are studded by irregularly spaced deposits (arrows). Deposits are also present in the mesangium (arrowhead). (×2200.)

within the glomerular basement membranes. As noted earlier, the mesangial matrix may be unrecognizable in some areas, and adjacent mesangial areas may coalesce.

The podocytes are prominent, and their cytoplasmic outlines are considerably altered. There is irregular effacement of the pedicels, and many villi are seen on the urinary surface (see Fig. 5–9). The number of cytoplasmic organelles is considerably increased, especially in the regions of the pedicels, and the normal dense layer of microfibrils near the glomerular basement membrane is no longer evident.

Prognosis

The immediate prognosis is usually excellent, even when anuria is present at the onset. The exudative response disappears quickly, and the proliferative lesions defervesce thereafter. All signs of renal disease disappear in most patients within a few weeks. However, in children, proteinuria and hematuria may reappear for several months after upper respiratory tract infections. The prognosis in adults is not as well established, but few cases are reported to progress to end stage, except for those with persistent hypertension.

GLOMERULONEPHRITIS DUE TO OTHER BACTERIAL INFECTIONS

Many bacterial infections have been associated with the development of glomerulonephritis. Although the exact cause of the glomerulonephritis remains unproven, it has been assumed that the renal lesions are due to the deposition (or local formation) of immune complexes derived from circulatory components. This supposition is supported by animal studies using protein antigens, but there have been few reports of an identified bacterial antigen in glomerular deposits in humans. The epidemiologic evidence for such a link is clear, however, and most accept the notion that glomerular deposits are related to the infectious agent and the antibody response to it. It is less well documented that the type, titer, or even presence of circulating antigen-antibody complexes is directly related to the renal disease.

The type of glomerular lesions that may be found as a consequence of these bacterial infections covers the spectrum of inflammatory renal diseases. There is some consistency within general categories of infection, allowing positive correlations to be made. These are considered in the following sections.

Acute Endocarditis

Introduction and Presentation

Acute endocarditis is now most frequently seen in drug abusers or patients who have undergone invasive vascular surgery. The patient's condition deteriorates rapidly unless the infection is recognized early and treated effectively. The renal lesions are often not detected or are recognized only by finding a few casts and a small amount of protein in the urine of an otherwise hectically ill patient. Very few patients develop evidence of renal failure.

Pathogenesis

The renal lesions are due to the formation and/or deposition of immune complexes in the glomeruli.

Histology

Light Microscopy

The glomeruli are diffusely hypercellular, containing a number of intrinsic glomerular cells and leucocytes (Fig. 5–10). The number of neutrophils, interestingly, is often quite small. This stands in sharp contrast to poststreptococcal glomerulonephritis, in which neutrophils are a major component of the hypercellularity at this stage. Localized crescents and synechiae may be present. The intraglomerular lesion is infrequently focal and segmental, thus it seldom mimics that seen in subacute bacterial endocarditis. The glomerular basement membranes are not thickened, but subepithelial deposits may be recognizable in thin sections stained with periodic acid-Schiff (PAS).

Scattered foci of interstitial infiltrates and tiny foci of tubular necrosis are often seen.

Immunofluorescence Microscopy

IgG and IgM are found in scattered granular deposits along the peripheral glomerular basement membranes and in the mesangium. The most prominent deposits consist of large granules of C3 in the same distribution as

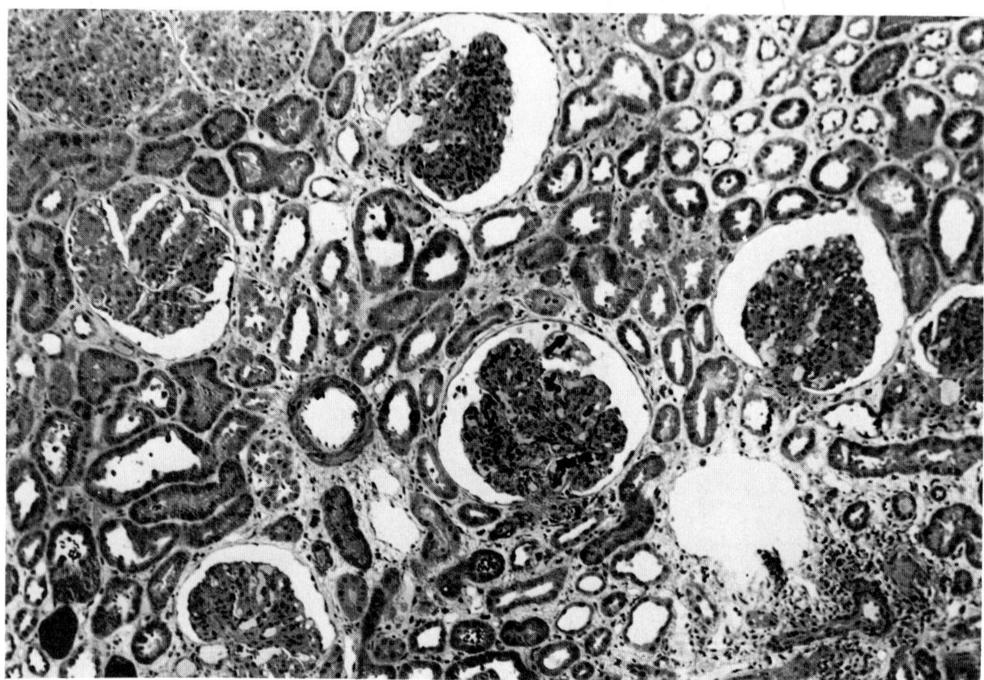

Figure 5–10. The glomeruli are diffusely hypercellular. The interstitium is diffusely edematous and contains many inflammatory cells. (H&E, ×75.)

the immunoglobulins. When the glomerular lesions are modest by light microscopy, the deposits may be limited to the mesangial regions.

Electron Microscopy

The irregularity of the immune deposits is confirmed by electron microscopy. Quite large but localized electron-dense deposits are seen in the subepithelial and mesangial regions.

Prognosis

The prognosis is excellent if appropriate therapy is instituted early in the course.

Subacute Bacterial Endocarditis

Introduction and Patient Presentation

As with acute bacterial endocarditis, this lesion is now most commonly encountered in intravenous drug abusers and patients who have had intravascular operative procedures. The organisms most frequently implicated are streptococci *(Streptococcus viridans),* but valvular infections with staphylococci have also been reported. Patients with acute valvular infections present with a vivid, rapidly progressive illness, whereas those with subacute endocarditis often have a more indolent disease. Renal lesions are much more frequent in the subacute disease, and they become evident within a few weeks after the onset of the intravascular infection. The urine sediment contains red blood cells, white blood cells, and casts containing one or both cell types. Proteinuria is also present. These urine findings suggest an active underlying glomerulonephritis. Renal failure or the nephrotic syndrome is uncommon but may appear if the lesion is not recognized and treated promptly.

The extrarenal signs consisting of fever, rash, splenomegaly, and weakness may lead to the erroneous diagnosis of an autoimmune disease.

Pathogenesis

The renal lesions are due to the formation and/or deposition of immune complexes in the glomeruli. The difficulty in separating an infectious from an immune cause may be a particular problem in patients with repeatedly negative blood cultures, because they may also have plasma findings that contribute to further obfuscation of the true diagnosis.

These include hypocomplementemia, low titers of antinuclear factors, mixed polyclonal cryoglobulins, and rheumatoid factor. The diagnosis depends on the finding of a positive blood culture and a high level of suspicion.

Histology

Light Microscopy

The glomerular lesions are initially focal and segmental in most patients. This observation led to the initial, erroneous notion that they were due to emboli derived from the heart valve vegetations. The lesions consist of segmental and focal proliferation coexisting with focal sclerotic (healed) lesions (Fig. 5–11). Diffuse glomerular lesions are present in a smaller number of patients. Both focal and diffuse glomerular lesions may be associated with localized crescents. The crescents and the areas of increased cellularity within the tufts characteristically contain large numbers of macrophages. This unique finding helps to differentiate this lesion from other clinical and histologic types of renal disease.

The interstitium contains multifocal areas of interstitial infiltrate, composed of mononuclear cells.

The blood vessels are usually not involved. Patients with vasculitic lesions have been reported, but this is an exceptional finding.

Immunofluorescence Macroscopy

Deposits of IgG, IgM, C3, C1q, and C4 are invariably diffuse, even when the light microscopic lesions appear focal. Those that had focal lesions by light microscopy most frequently have deposits restricted to the mesangium, whereas both mesangial and subendothelial deposits are found in the diffuse lesions (Fig. 5–12).

Electron Microscopy

Electron-dense deposits are present within the mesangial regions. In the diffuse form, deposits are also found in the subendothelial zones, less commonly in the subepithelial areas, and rarely within the substance of the peripheral basement membranes.

Prognosis

If the lesions are promptly diagnosed and treated, the proteinuria and hematuria disappear. It is assumed that the inflammatory glomerular lesions also diminish and ultimately resolve, leaving sclerotic zones. The most severe sequelae are related either to perforation or deformity of a cardiac valve.

Infected Shunts (Infected Intravascular Catheters and Prostheses)

Introduction and Patient Presentation

Infected shunts were first described in children who had hydrocephalus and had atrioventricular shunts. Similar lesions have subsequently been reported in patients who have other types of chronic, indwelling intravascular prostheses. The most common bacterium cultured from the prosthesis or blood is *Staphylococcus albus*. These infections often do not come to the attention of the clinical team until some time after the prosthesis has been placed, and often long after the disease has started, because the infection pursues such an indolent course. The renal lesion is recognizable by the presence of significant proteinuria and hematuria. Impairment of renal function is not present early in the course but may appear in the absence of appropriate therapy.

Pathogenesis

The renal lesion is thought to be a consequence of the formation of immune complexes. Thus, plasma levels of complement components are decreased and circulating immune complexes are present.

Histology

Light Microscopy

The glomerular lesions are reminiscent of those in type I membranoproliferative glomerulonephritis. There is an increased number of cells within the tuft, composed of macrophages and mesangial cells. Crescents, either local or diffuse, are commonly seen. The peripheral glomerular basement membranes are frequently thickened and duplicated in a diffuse manner.

The interstitium, tubules, and blood vessels do not differ from those in subacute bacterial endocarditis.

Immunofluorescence Microscopy

The glomeruli have diffuse mesangial and peripheral glomerular basement membrane

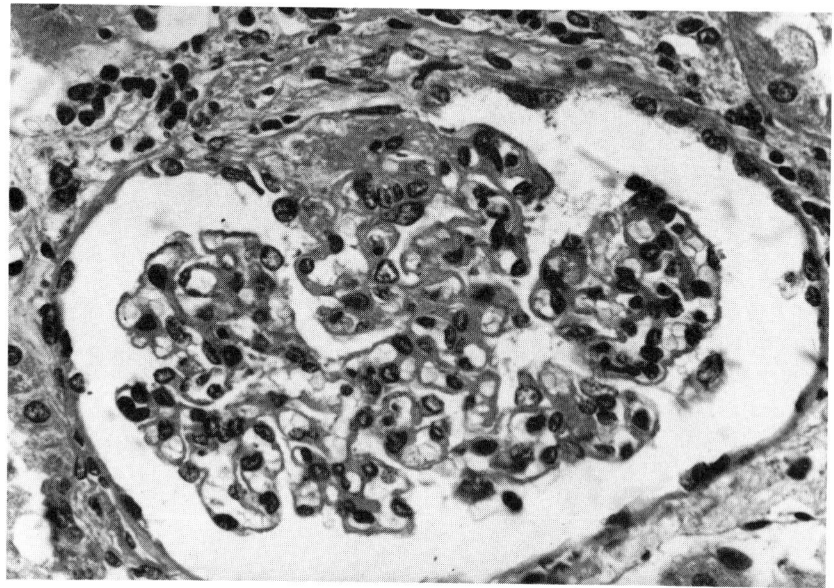

Figure 5–11. There is an area of segmental proliferation and sclerosis, with a partially organized synechia. (Masson's trichrome, ×250.)

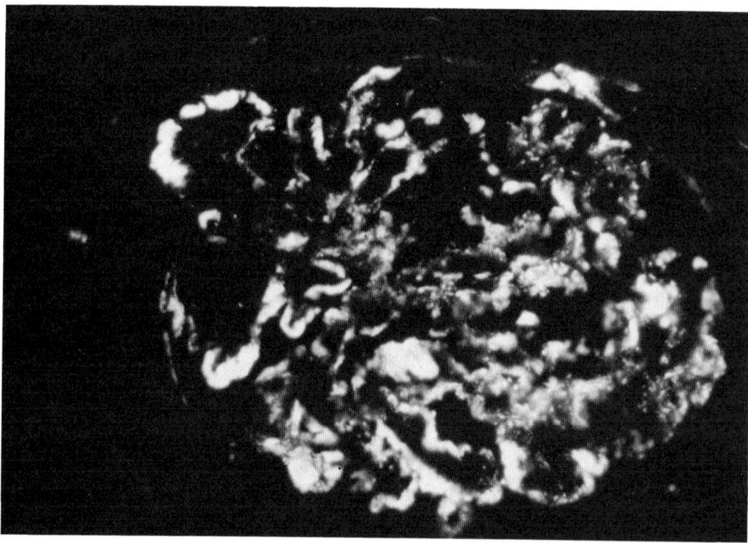

Figure 5–12. Immunofluorescence micrograph, anti-C1q. There are diffuse subepithelial and subendothelial deposits. (×259.)

(intramembranous, subendothelial, and less commonly subepithelial) deposits of IgM, C3, C1q, and C4, with a smaller amount of IgG.

There are no deposits associated with the tubules or interstitium.

Electron Microscopy

The location of the deposits is confirmed. The architecture of the glomerular basement membrane is even more altered than appreciated by light microscopy.

Prognosis

As with subacute endocarditis, the signs of renal damage recede and then disappear with appropriate therapy. Patients with severe sclerosing lesions may, however, continue to have proteinuria. Long-term studies on which to gauge the ultimate prognosis are not available, but renal failure is not a common outcome.

SELECTED READINGS

1. Arze RS, Hashid H, Morley R, et al: Shunt nephritis: Report of two cases and review of the literature. Clin Nephrol 19:48, 1983.
2. Beaufils M, Gibert C, Morel-Maroger L, et al: Glomerulonephritis in severe bacterial infections with and without endocarditis. Adv Nephrol 7:217, 1978.
3. Beaufils M, Morel-Maroger L, Sraer JD, et al: Acute renal failure of glomerular origin during visceral abscesses. N Engl J Med 295:185, 1976.
4. Black JA, Challacombe DN, Ockenden BG: Nephrotic syndrome associated with bacteraemia after shunt operations for hydrocephalus. Lancet 2:921, 1965.
5. Boulton-Jones JM, Sissons JGP, Evans DS, et al: Renal lesions of subacute infective endocarditis. Br Med J 2:11, 1974.
6. Gutman RA, Striker GE, Gilliland BC, et al: The immune-complex glomerulonephritis of bacterial endocarditis. Medicine (Baltimore) 51:1, 1972.
7. Kaufmann DB, McIntosh R: The pathogenesis of the renal lesion in a patient with streptococcal disease, infected ventriculoatrial shunt, cryoglobulinemia and nephritis. Am J Med 50:262, 1971.
8. Kim Y, Michael AF: Chronic bacteremia and nephritis. Ann Rev Med 29:319, 1978.
9. Leonard CD, Nagle R, Striker GE, et al: Acute glomerulonephritis with prolonged oliguria. Ann Intern Med 73:703, 1970.
10. Morel-Maroger L, Sraer JD, Herreman G, et al: Kidney in subacute endocarditis: Pathological and immunofluorescent findings. Arch Pathol 94:205, 1972.
11. Neugarten J, Gallo GR, Baldwin DS: Glomerulonephritis in bacterial endocarditis. Am J Kidney Dis 3:371, 1984.

VIRAL INFECTIONS

HEPATITIS B

Among the numerous viral diseases thought to be associated with specific renal lesions, hepatitis B is the most extensively documented. Nonetheless, the mechanisms and even the type of renal damage induced by the hepatitis B virus have not been elucidated, and it is not clear whether the association currently described will remain as an established entity.

Pathogenesis

Hepatitis B antigenemia has been considered to be a pathogenic factor in diseases as diverse as polyarteritis nodosa, membranous glomerulonephritis, membranoproliferative glomerulonephritis, and mixed cryoglobulinemia. There appear to be marked geographic variations between the incidence of hepatitis B virus infections and the proportion of patients who develop an associated renal disease. Furthermore, the type and course of renal diseases associated with infections with hepatitis B virus have been so diverse that the relationship has been questioned, as has the validity of the association.

It has been generally accepted that the individuals infected with the virus develop circulating immune complexes. The role of circulating immune complexes in the pathogenesis of the many renal lesions associated with hepatitis B virus infection is not well established, and most of the evidence is indirect.

Patient Presentation

The findings vary with the type of renal diseases. Those associated with polyarteritis nodosa and mixed cryglobulinemia will be described respectively in Chapters 6 and 9.

Hepatitis B surface antigen has most frequently been reported in the serum of children with the nephrotic syndrome and more rarely in nephrotic adults. In these patients, liver symptoms are either absent or not prominent. The renal symptoms in patients who have developed renal disease usually appear after a long delay. Proteinuria is almost always present, and some patients have the nephrotic syndrome.

Histology

Light Microscopy

Membranous glomerulonephritis and membranoproliferative glomerulonephritis are the varieties of glomerulonephritis most commonly associated with infection with hepatitis B virus (see Chapter 4). The lesions do not show any specific features that could differentiate them from their idiopathic counterparts. In addition to membranous and type I membranoproliferative glomerulonephritis, which are by far the most common patterns, patients have been reported to have endocapillary proliferation and crescentic glomerulonephritis.

Immunofluorescence Microscopy

In patients with membranous glomerulonephritis, deposits of IgG are invariably found in a regular granular pattern along the glomerular basement membranes. This pattern of deposition characterizes the disease. C3 usually codistributes with the IgG. It is interesting that a few patients have been reported to have had mesangial deposits of IgA and IgG in the typical membranous pattern.

In membranoproliferative glomerulonephritis, IgG and complement components have always been detected with the coarse granular pattern that characterizes this disease. In addition, most are associated with small deposits of IgM and IgA.

Many researchers have examined biopsy specimens for the presence of hepatitis B related antigens. These antigens have been demonstrated in membranous glomerulonephritis by some investigators. Hepatitis B surface antigens have not been found consistently, although some early reports claimed the contrary. It seems that the diagnosis of the condition relies more on the association between serologic markers and the clinical association than on the local detection of hepatitis B viral antigens in the glomeruli.

Electron Microscopy

In most cases, the ultrastructural features are not different from those in idiopathic glomerular diseases. Some investigators have described spherical particles of 400 to 600 Å in the basement membranes.

Prognosis

In children, the disappearance of the carrier state of the virus has been associated with disappearance of proteinuria.

SELECTED READINGS

1. Brzosko WJ, Krawzynski K, Nazarewicz T, et al: Glomerulonephritis associated with hepatitis-B surface antigen immune complexes in children. Lancet 2:477, 1974.
2. Collins SB, Bhan AK, Dienstag JL, et al: Hepatitis B immune complex glomerulonephritis: Simultaneous glomerular deposition of hepatitis B surface and e antigens. Clin Immunol Immunopathol 26:137, 1983.
3. Hirschel BJ, Benusiglio LN, Favre H, et al: Glomerulonephritis associated with hepatitis B. Report of a case and review of the literature. Clin Nephrol 8:404, 1977.
4. Southwest Pediatric Nephrology Study Group—Dallas, Texas: Hepatitis B surface antigenemia in North American children with idiopathic membranous glomerulonephritis. J Pediatr 106:571, 1975.
5. Yoshikawa N, Ito H, Yamada Y, et al: Membranous glomerulonephritis associated with hepatitis B antigen in children: A comparison with idiopathic membranous glomerulonephritis. Clin Nephrol 23:28, 1985.

AIDS NEPHROPATHY

Acquired immunodeficiency syndrome (AIDS) was first described in 1978. The role of human immunodeficiency virus (HIV) as the causal agent was recognized in 1984. The manifestations of AIDS are protean, and the presence of an AIDS-related nephropathy was demonstrated in 1984. During the ensuing 5 years, several issues concerning the association of AIDS and renal disease have been clarified. However, the cause and, in particular, the potential role for the virus in these syndromes remain unknown.

Several autopsy studies have shown that approximately 10% of patients with AIDS have some type of renal abnormality. The presence of significant renal lesions in some patients with AIDS is underscored by the

Table 5–1. Risk Factors for AIDS

Risk Factors	San Francisco *% with AIDS*	Miami *% with AIDS*	Miami *% with AIDS Nephropathy*
Homosexual/bisexual	85%	53%	3%
Intravenous drug users	1%	17%	45%
Race			
Black	6%	48%	87%
White (including Hispanic)	94%	52%	13%

observation that almost 45% of the patients at a New York nephrology service consisted of AIDS patients. However, the experience on the West Coast was very different, in that the incidence of renal disease was quite low and the principal renal syndrome was acute renal failure. Analysis of the risk factors leading to AIDS in the patient populations on the two coasts may help to explain the differences (Table 5–1).

Examination of Table 5–1 may provide clues to the differences between the incidence of renal disease in AIDS patients on the two coasts. First, the risk factors in the two groups of AIDS patients are quite different. On the West Coast, most of the AIDS patients are homosexuals or bisexuals, whereas there is a higher proportion of intravenous drug abusers among the AIDS patients on the East Coast, a trend that continues. Another major difference between the two coasts is the proportion of black patients. Examination of the risk factors in the Miami patients with renal disease as compared with the Miami AIDS population further accentuates the disparate risk for renal involvement among the patient groups. A disproportionate number of blacks are affected with AIDS as compared with whites, suggesting that blacks may be particularly susceptible to the development of renal lesions. The prevalence of renal disease in patients who are intravenous drug abusers is greater, as might be expected, because focal glomerulosclerosis has been reported in this population. Some investigators have suggested that AIDS nephropathy is identical to heroin-associated nephropathy because it is only encountered in intravenous drug abusers with AIDS. Although this view has merit and may account for some of the renal disease in this group, cases of focal glomerular sclerosis have appeared in some patients who have AIDS but who deny intravenous drug abuse. Further evidence in support of this postulate is the fact that it may be seen in young children with AIDS who are not intravenous drug abusers. Furthermore, the Miami figures also show increased risk of renal disease in heterosexual partners of patients who have AIDS and who are not intravenous drug abusers. One other factor that supports a separate AIDS-associated nephropathy is the accelerated course to renal failure and death in these patients as compared with those with heroin-associated nephropathy without AIDS.

Pathogenesis

The pathogenesis of AIDS-associated nephropathy is an area of current active research and remains largely undefined. In part, this is because of a lack of knowledge about the etiology of focal and segmental glomerulosclerosis in general (see Chapter 4). It seems likely that race is an important factor. Intravenous drug abuse clearly increases the risk for development of this lesion in patients with AIDS. Moreover, it should be noted that the incidence of focal and segmental glomerulosclerosis in intravenous drug abusers with AIDS is higher than in such patients without AIDS. It is possible, but unlikely, that viral infection of renal cells is responsible for the glomerular lesion. Electron microscopic studies have been said to show evidence of viral infection in endothelial cells (see below) in patients with glomerular lesions. The inclusions have been shown to be related to the action of interferon. Thus, these changes may represent the renal response to a systemic infection, rather than to specific viral products. It is likely that there are many causative factors in the genesis of the renal disease.

Patient Presentation

Four renal syndromes have been recognized, including acute renal failure, nephrotic syndrome, glomerular lesions without clinical renal disease, and post-dialysis acquisition of AIDS accompanied by failure to thrive in intravenous drug abusers. Because many patients with AIDS are septic or are treated with potentially nephrotoxic drugs, they may develop acute renal failure on the basis of ischemic or drug-induced acute tubular necrosis. The ischemia may be related to the high frequency of diarrheal syndromes in these patients. It has not been determined whether AIDS patients are more likely to develop acute tubular necrosis in the setting of sepsis or drug toxicity than other patients.

The renal lesion in patients who have the nephrotic syndrome with or without renal insufficiency is most often focal and segmental glomerulosclerosis. This may be the initial manifestation of an HIV infection.

Ten per cent of AIDS patients without clinical evidence of renal disease have mesangial proliferative lesions. Finally, a small group of hemodialysis patients who were intravenous drug abusers and became infected with HIV have developed a syndrome characterized by failure to thrive and rapid progression to death.

Histology

Light Microscopy

Two types of glomerular changes have been described. Most patients with the nephrotic syndrome have focal and segmental glomerulosclerosis. The lesions may be identical to those in idiopathic focal and segmental glomerulosclerosis (Chapter 4). The differences relate principally to the degree of severity and the fact that the sclerosis may not have a prominent component of hyalinotic lesions. The second pattern is moderate mesangial cell proliferation and prominent epithelial cell hypertrophy (Fig. 5–13). When this pattern is a conspicuous feature, it is associated with collapse of the glomerular tuft (Fig. 5–14). As the sclerotic lesions ad-

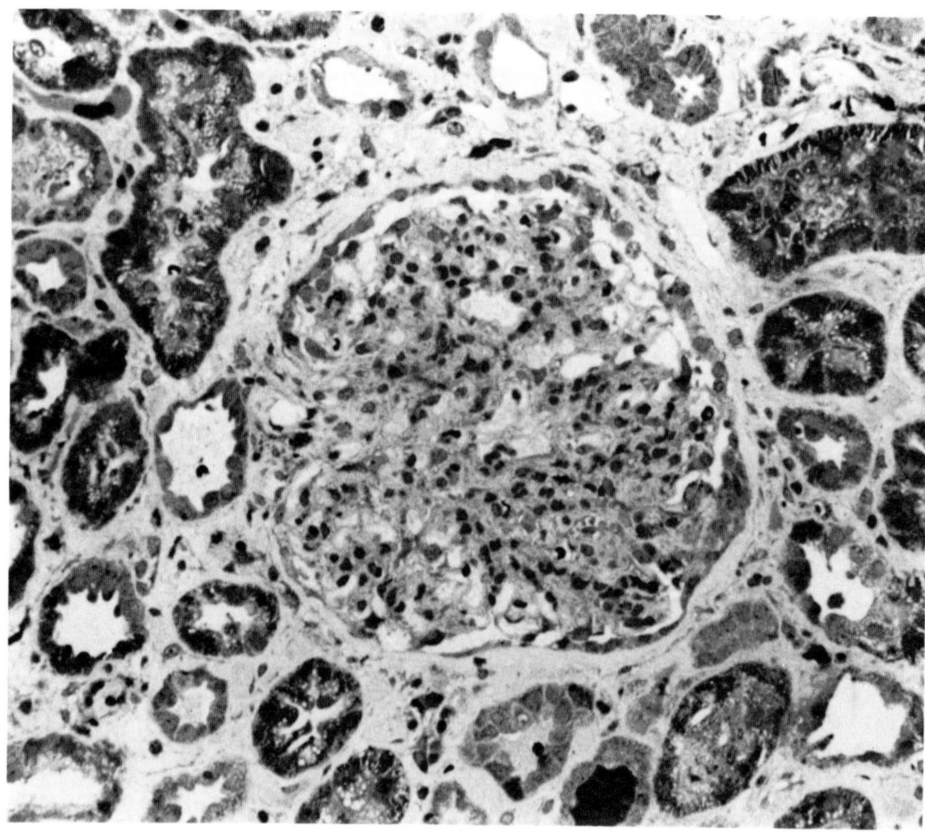

Figure 5–13. Note the diffuse intraglomerular proliferation and infiltration with inflammatory cells. The epithelial cells are also prominent. (H&E, ×250).

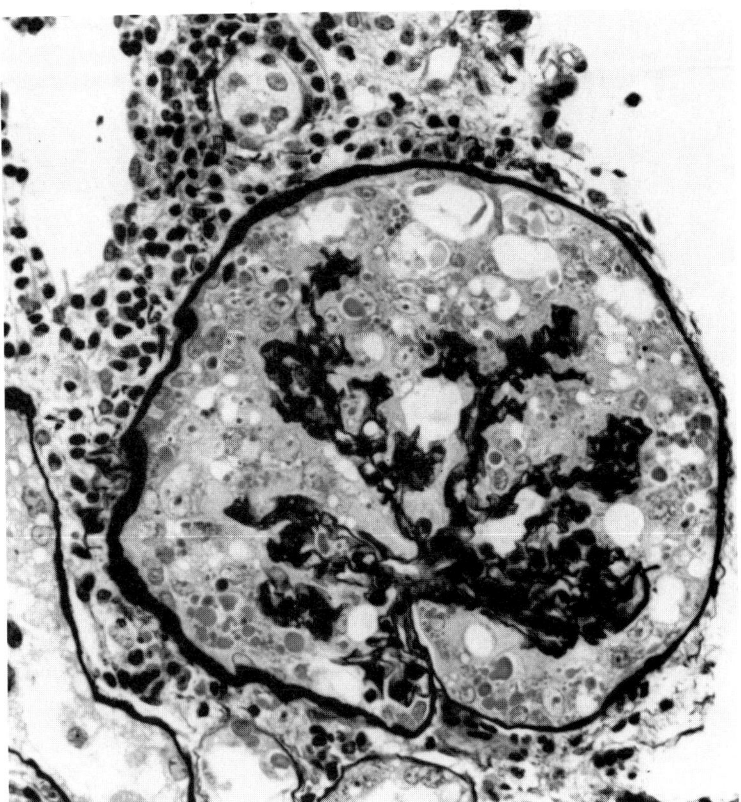

Figure 5–14. Bowman's space is filled with cells. The glomerular basement membranes are collapsed. (PASM, ×250.)

vance, it may be difficult to determine that the original lesion was focal and segmental.

A peculiarity of the focal and segmental glomerulosclerotic lesion in patients with AIDS is the presence of widespread marked tubular dilation and formation of hyalin casts (Fig. 5–15). As the glomerulosclerosis advances, there is accompanying tubular atrophy with interstitial fibrosis.

A patchy interstitial infiltrate composed chiefly of lymphocytes and plasma cells is occasionally found. The infiltrate may be marked in some biopsy specimens (Fig. 5–15).

There are no vascular lesions of note.

At Johns Hopkins University, kidney sections taken at autopsy in patients who had AIDS but had no clinical evidence of renal disease were found to have diffuse mesangial proliferative glomerular lesions in 10% of the cases. This lesion was thought to represent an early stage of focal and segmental glomerulosclerosis.

Patients with AIDS may develop glomerular lesions that are independent of the HIV infection, because they have many comcomitant medical problems.

Immunofluorescence Microscopy

IgM and C3 may be found in areas of sclerosis; otherwise, no deposits are present.

Electron Microscopy

The alterations are almost identical to those described for focal and segmental glomerulosclerosis (see Chapter 4). There are several reports on the presence of various tubulo-reticular inclusions and cylindric confronting cisternae, chiefly within endothelial cells (Fig. 5–16). Tubulo-reticular inclusions are thought to represent cytoplasmic alterations due to the presence of interferon. They have been found in patients with systemic lupus erythematosus, associated with several viral infections, and in patients with a variety of neoplasms. Cylindric confronting cisternae have also been described in non-A non-B hepatitis infections and multiple sclerosis. Therefore, neither structure is specific for HIV infection. Verifiable HIV particles have not been unequivocally demonstrated. Furthermore, because patients without renal disease have not been studied, the causal asso-

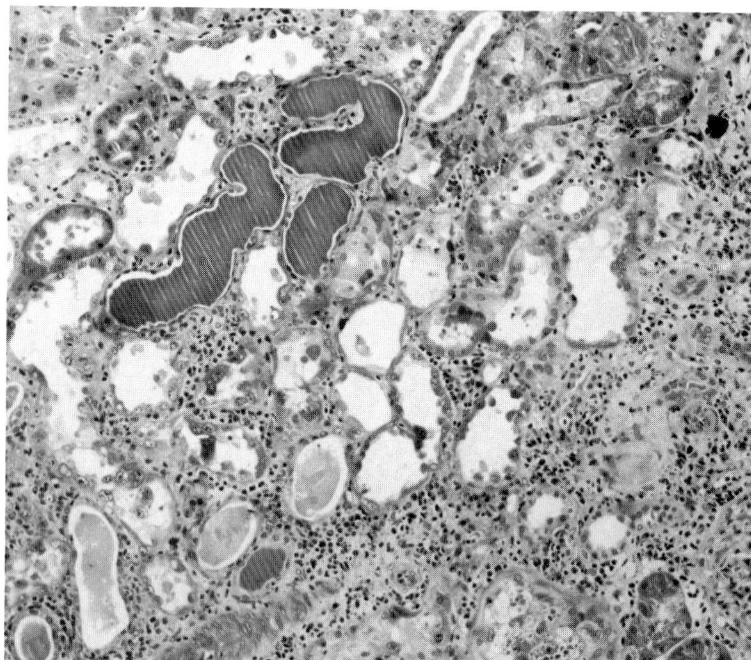

Figure 5–15. The interstitium contains a diffuse inflammatory cell infiltrate composed of lymphocytes and plasma cells. There is also marked tubular atrophy and dilation. (H&E, ×100.)

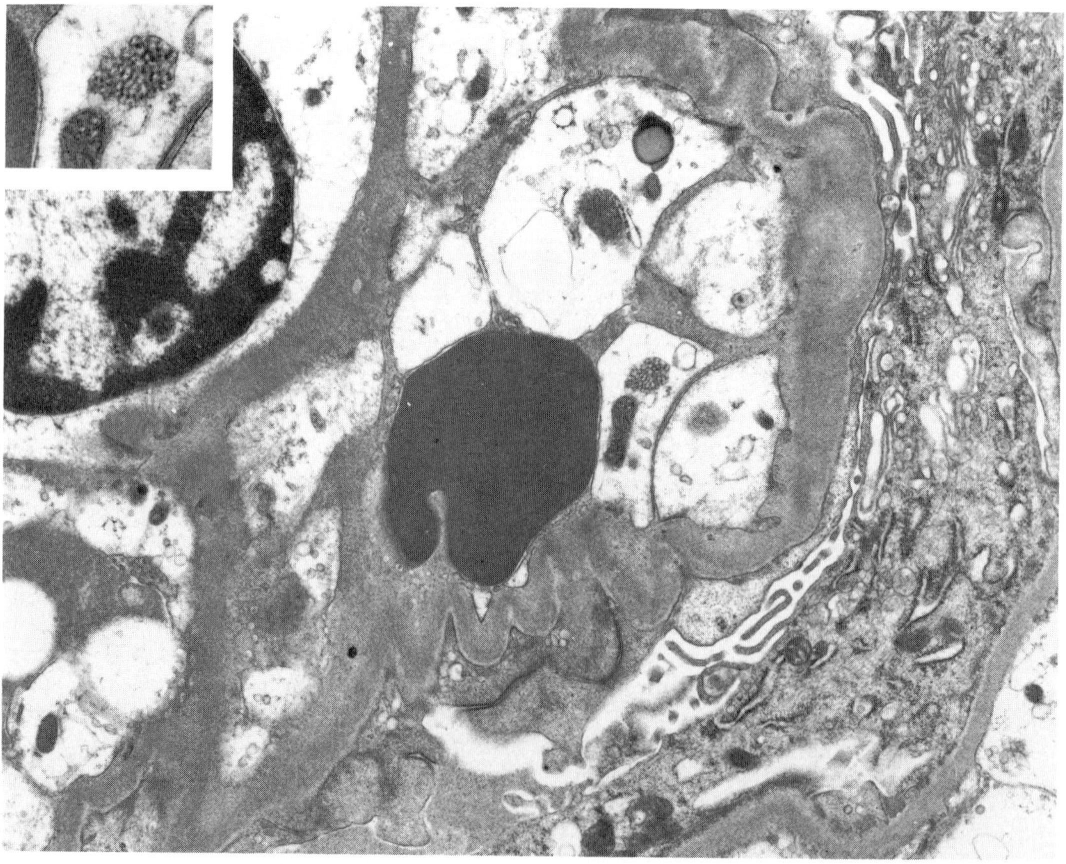

Figure 5–16. Glomerular sclerosis with wrinkling and thickening of the basement membranes, particularly near the mesangium. Tubulo-reticular inclusions are found within endothelial cells (insert, top left). (×13,000, insert ×28,000.)

ciation between these structures and the renal disease has not been established.

Although deposits are not usually present in patients with focal and segmental glomerulosclerosis, mesangial deposits are frequently observed in AIDS patients with either focal and segmental glomerulosclerosis or mesangial proliferative disease.

Prognosis

The overall prognosis in patients with AIDS is improving, but it remains poor. Patients who develop acute renal failure may recover normal renal function. However, the appearance of the nephrotic syndrome in patients with AIDS is associated with a shortened life expectancy. Most die within 6 months of the onset of the nephrotic syndrome, even if chronic hemodialysis therapy is instituted. Patients who are on dialysis and who develop AIDS die within weeks, with a syndrome of failure to thrive.

The natural history of the mesangial proliferative disorder is not delineated.

SELECTED READINGS

1. D'Agati V, Suh J-I, Carbone L, et al: Pathology of HIV-associated nephropathy: A detailed morphologic and comparative study. Kidney Int 35:1358, 1989.
2. Soni A, Agarwal A, Chander P, et al: Evidence for an HIV-related nephropathy: A clinico-pathological study. Clin Nephrol 31:12, 1989.
3. Humphreys MH, Schoenfeld PY: Renal complications in patients with the acquired immune deficiency syndrome (AIDS). Am J Nephrol 7:1, 1987.
4. Pardo V, Meneses R, Ossa L, et al: AIDS-related glomerulopathy: Occurrence in specific risk groups. Kidney Int 31:1167, 1987.
5. Rao TKS, Friedman EA, Nicastri AD: The types of renal disease in the acquired immunodeficiency syndrome. N Engl J Med 316:1062, 1987.

PARASITIC DISEASES

Although glomerular lesions due to parasitic infestation are unusual in the United States and Western Europe, they represent a major cause of renal disease in developing countries. It is generally considered that parasitic infestation may induce an immune complex glomerulonephritis. Three groups of parasites have been implicated in the development of glomerulonephritis: those that cause malaria, schistosomiasis, and leishmaniasis.

MALARIA

Patient Presentation and Pathogenesis

Quartan malaria has been reported to be a cause of an immune complex glomerulonephritis. Patients with quartan malaria have a high incidence of the nephrotic syndrome. They may present with massive edema, pleural effusions, and anasarca. Hypertension and hematuria are uncommon in the early stages of the disease; however, within the first 5 years of the disease, most patients develop decreased renal function that is followed by hypertension. Quartan malaria nephropathy is mainly a disease of childhood.

Although the lesions described later are known as quartan malaria nephropathy and were initially described in areas where quartan malaria was endemic, comparable lesions have been reported in areas where quartan malaria is essentially unknown. Thus, the specificity of the lesion is unknown, and we prefer to use the term *tropical nephropathy.*

Histology

Light Microscopy

The glomerular lesions are characteristic but can be easily overlooked if the pathologist is not familiar with the condition. There is a diffuse alteration of the glomerular basement membranes consisting of a plexiform alteration of the lamina densa. This results in a double layering of the peripheral glomerular basement membranes by silver stain. The lesions may superficially resemble membranoproliferative glomerulonephritis, but the glomerular lesions in quartan malaria do not have a proliferative component. In addition to the glomerular basement membrane lesions, segmental areas of glomerulosclerosis are irregularly dispersed within and between glomeruli. The glomerulosclerotic lesions gradually increase in amount and frequency, eventuating in end-stage glomerulosclerosis. The peripheral glomerular basement membrane thickening also slowly advances, resulting in obliteration of the vascular spaces.

Immunofluorescence Microscopy

The findings are quite variable. Diffuse deposits of immunoglobulins, including IgG and IgM, may be seen in a mixed pattern of both linear and granular distribution. There are a few reports of malarial antigens in the glomeruli. Complement components are almost always present with immunoglobulin deposits. On the other hand, in patients who have tropical nephropathy and in whom there are no deposits of immune reactants, the etiologic and the pathogenetic linkage of the disease to quartan malaria has been called into question.

Electron Microscopy

The glomerular basement membranes are of irregular thickness and contain lacunae, often filled with electron-dense material. The amount of extracellular matrix in the mesangium is increased, and there is often a subendothelial layer of similar material.

SCHISTOSOMIASIS

Patient Presentation and Pathogenesis

Schistosoma mansoni has frequently been reported as a cause of renal disease, but infestation with the other schistosomes does not appear to result in renal parenchymal lesions. Renal disease has only been well documented in the hepatosplenic form of *S. mansoni* disease. This is a common parasite in certain regions of South America, and the renal lesions in Brazil have been well studied. In regions of endemic schistosomal disease, the frequency of glomerular lesions in infected patients has been estimated to be approximately 15%. The cause of the renal lesion has been thought to be the deposition of circulating immune reactants in the glomeruli. In support of this concept are the observations that the patients have circulating immune complexes and the glomeruli contain large deposits of immune reactants.

Histology

Light and Electron Microscopy

The glomerular lesions may be identical to those in type I membranoproliferative glomerulonephritis, but focal glomerulonephritis and membranous glomerulonephritis have also been identified.

Immunofluorescence Microscopy

The lesions are similar to that of type I membranoproliferative glomerulonephritis, but the deposits of IgG, IgM, and C3 may be larger. The deposits are mixed—that is, they are both coarse and finely granular.

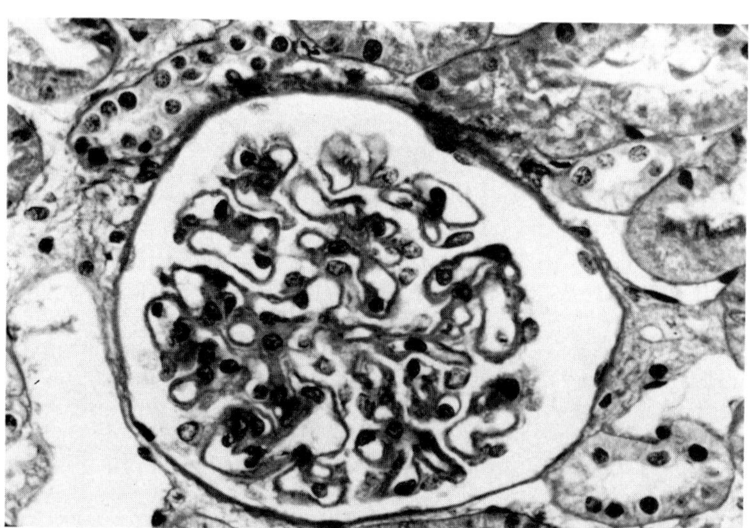

Figure 5–17. Biopsy from a patient with filariasis showing diffuse glomerular basement membrane thickening (membranous glomerulonephritis). (Masson's trichrome, ×250.)

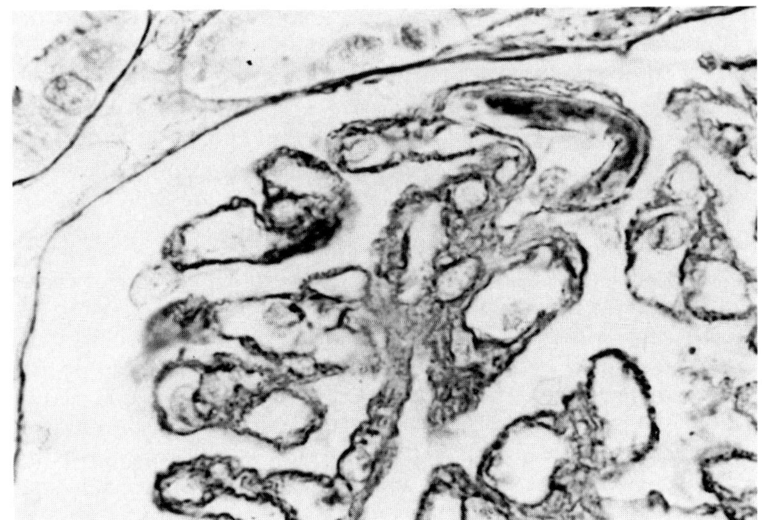

Figure 5–18. In the same patient as in Figure 5–17, a microfilaria is visible within the vascular space at 1 o'clock. The glomerular basement membrane lesions consist of subepithelial spikes, thickening, and focal duplication. (PASM, ×1000.)

FILARIASIS

The filariasis that has most often been reported to be associated with renal disease is loiasis, and the lesion reported is membranous glomerulonephritis (Figs. 5–17, 5–18).

SELECTED READINGS

1. Andrade ZA, Rocha H: Schistosomal glomerulopathy. Kidney Int 16:23, 1979.
2. Andrade AZ, Andrade SG, Sadifursky M: Renal changes in patients with hepatosplenic schistosomiasis. Am J Trop Med Hyg 20:77, 1971.
3. Hendrickse RG, Adeniyi A: Quartan malarial nephrotic syndrome in children. Kidney Int 16:64, 1979.
4. Kibukamusoke JW, Hutt MSR, Wikls NE: The nephrotic syndrome in Uganda and its association with quartan malaria. Q J Med 36:393, 1967.
5. Martinelli R, Carlos A, Noblat B, et al: *Schistosoma mansoni*-induced mesangiocapillary glomerulonephritis: Influence of therapy. Kidney Int 35:1227, 1989.
6. Morel-Maroger L, Saimot AG, Sloper JC, et al: Tropical nephropathy and tropical extramembranous glomerulonephritis of unknown etiology in Senegal. Br Med J 1:541, 1975.
7. Ngu JL, Chatelanat F, Leke R, et al: Nephropathy in Cameroon: Evidence for filarial derived immune-complex pathogenesis in some cases. Clin Nephrol 24:128, 1985.

DRUG-INDUCED

HEROIN-ASSOCIATED NEPHROPATHY

Glomerular lesions of many types have been reported in drug abusers. The frequency with which one encounters patients with glomerular disease related to drug abuse appears to vary widely between different populations and regions within a country. At present, most studies in the literature are of patients in the United States. This uneven distribution is far from completely understood. There are many causes of glomerular diseases, other than the drug itself. For instance, intravenous drug abusers are exposed to drugs of widely varying composition and purity, and the means by which they are administered lead to a serious hazard of acquiring infectious diseases. The complications from these causes include infections from unsterile needles and syringes and impurities in the injected materials. For instance, there is a high frequency of subacute bacterial endocarditis in these patients. (For a description of the renal lesions in subacute bacterial nephritis see the earlier section in this chapter.) In addition, AA amyloid is also one of the potential complications of long-term substance abuse. Finally, AIDS occurs with a high frequency in the population who abuse intravenous drugs. Thus, it may be difficult to determine whether the renal disease is due to the effects of the drugs, a viral (HIV) infection, malnutrition, bacterial infection, or some combination of these processes.

Pathogenesis

The term that is used to describe the renal lesion thought to be directly related to heroin abuse is *heroin-associated nephropathy.* This renal lesion occurs exclusively in addicts who inject drugs, either subcutaneously or intravenously. There is no direct evidence that heroin, by itself, causes the renal lesion.

Thus, although heroin is the drug most frequently associated with nephropathy, it is not clear whether the renal manifestations are restricted to this drug or are part of a general, nonspecific response to drug abuse. There is agreement that the most common renal lesion associated with heroin abuse is focal glomerulosclerosis, which often progresses to diffuse glomerulosclerosis. It has become prevalent in areas where drug abuse is endemic and in some metropolitan areas is a major cause of the nephrotic syndrome and end-stage renal failure. The disease seems to predominantly affect black males. It has therefore been speculated that this population may have a susceptibility for the development of sclerosing glomerular diseases that is uncovered by the substance abuse. However, the exact pathogenesis of the lesions remains unknown.

The second major cause of glomerular disease in heroin addicts is systemic amyloidosis of the AA type. Amyloidosis is a complication in persons who inject the drug subcutaneously, leading to the suspicion that the amyloid disease is secondary to long-lasting infections in multiple cutaneous sites.

Patient Presentation

Proteinuria is almost always present, and the nephrotic syndrome is very common. Patients who have glomerulosclerosis also have microscopic hematuria. Those with amyloidosis may also present with hypertension. Many patients already have evidence of significant renal failure at the time of presentation, and almost all show rapid and progressive loss of renal function.

FOCAL GLOMERULOSCLEROSIS

Histology

Light Microscopy

The glomerulosclerosis initially consists of segmental obliteration of glomerular vascular loops by focal sclerosis (Fig. 5–19). The sclerosis is often accompanied by synechiae. There is seldom evidence of proliferation; rather there tends to be a paucity of nuclei

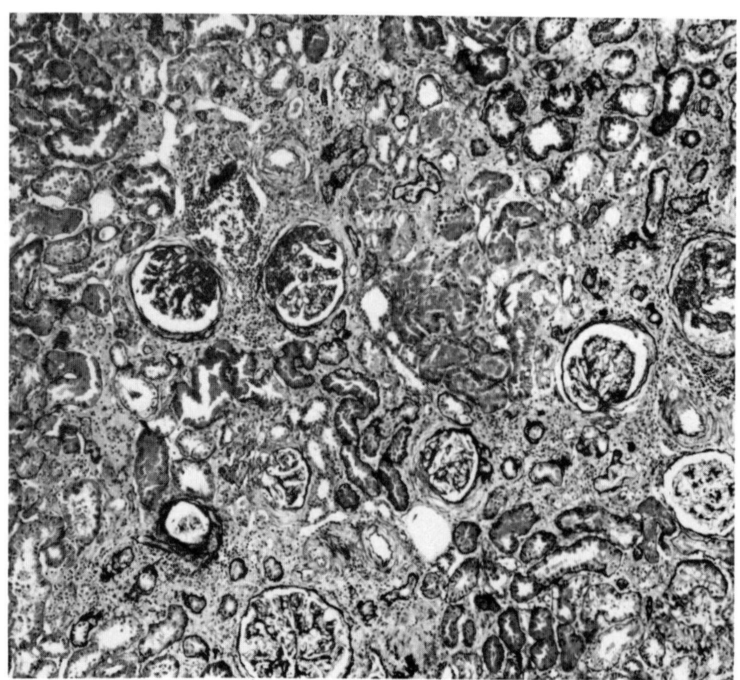

Figure 5–19. There are focal and segmental sclerosing lesions with synechiae. The interstitium contains an increased amount of connective tissue, especially in areas of tubular atrophy. (PASM, ×40.)

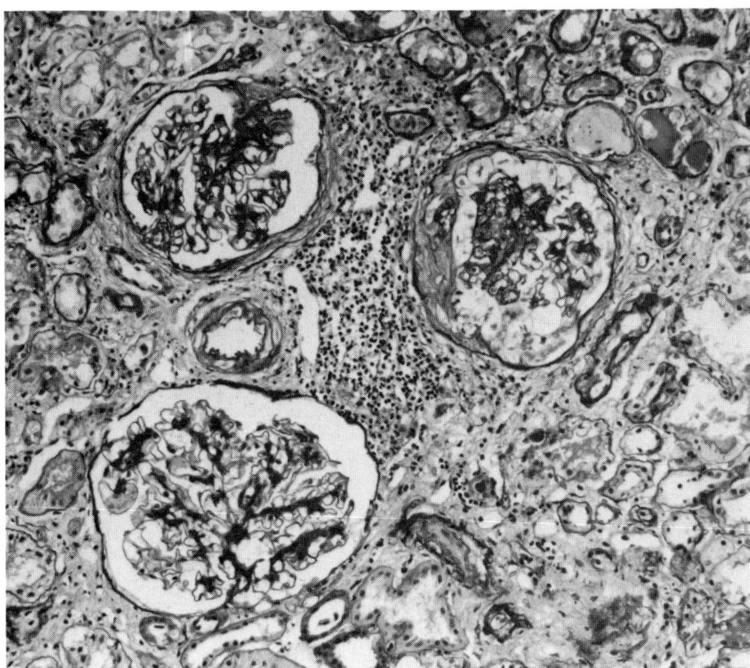

Figure 5–20. The focal and segmental nature of the glomerular lesions is evident. There are few nuclei in the sclerotic areas. (PASM, ×100.)

in and near the areas of sclerosis. The basement membranes near the sclerotic areas are thickened and wrinkled, and the vascular spaces are diminished in size, a picture reminiscent of chronic ischemia. As the lesions progress, larger areas of the glomeruli are affected, and the lesions that initially appeared to be focal and segmental are now replaced by diffuse sclerosis (Fig. 5–20). Foam cells and large hyalin deposits may be found in the areas of sclerosis. The end result is complete replacement of normal glomerular structures by sclerosis—that is, glomerular obsolescence. The mesangial matrix is seldom increased in amount, but when present, the sclerosis is usually mild and local. Bowman's capsule is multilaminated adjacent to the synechiae. The visceral epithelial cells often appear swollen, in early stages, and they may appear to be increased in number.

Tubular atrophy associated with interstitial fibrosis accompanies and is in rough proportion to the glomerular lesions. Similarly, arteriolar and small artery lesions are found in these biopsy samples, appearing to be a part of the overall glomerulosclerotic process.

These lesions are very similar to those seen in idiopathic focal glomerulosclerosis. There is one important distinguishing feature in addicts—namely, in these patients there is considerable wrinkling and thickening of the glomerular basement membranes near the sclerotic zones. This is far more pronounced than in the idiopathic form and is useful in the differentiation of the two lesions. Another differential feature is the more frequent presence of interstitial infiltrates in heroin-associated nephropathy.

Immunofluorescence Microscopy

Large, coarsely granular aggregates of IgM and C3 are found in a segmental distribution corresponding to the areas of glomerular sclerosis. Other immunoglobulins are usually absent. However, there are reports of weak linear deposits of IgG along the glomerular basement membranes, similar to the distribution and intensity reported in some patients with other chronic sclerosing lesions, such as diabetes mellitus.

Electron Microscopy

The glomerular basement membranes are wrinkled and thickened near the sclerotic zones. The pedicels of the podocytes in these areas are partially effaced or detached, similar to the findings in the idiopathic variety of focal and segmental glomerulosclerosis. Electron-dense material resembling immune deposits is not seen, although there often is material resembling hyalin on the endothelial aspect of the glomerular basement membrane and in the vascular spaces as well as in and abutting the mesangium.

Prognosis

The renal lesions most often relentlessly and rapidly progress to complete obliteration of the glomeruli. Renal failure, requiring renal replacement therapy, is therefore the usual outcome.

AMYLOIDOSIS

Amyloidosis of the AA type is the second most common renal pathologic entity encountered in heroin addicts.

Histology

The renal lesions do not differ histologically from those with other underlying diseases leading to the deposition of AA amyloid. The type of amyloid in the deposits was determined to be AA in these patients by both immunofluorescence microscopic techniques and biochemical analysis.

Prognosis

The development of amyloid deposits in the kidneys is associated with a rapid and progressive loss in renal function. Although the deposition does not appear to be altered or reversed by the interruption of drug abuse, proteinuria markedly abated in one recently reported patient after drug abuse was stopped. The renal amyloid deposits did not visibly decrease in this patient.

OTHER LESIONS

Several other types of glomerular disease have been described in heroin addicts. Some appear to be the consequence of the infectious diseases that are common in addicts, such as subacute bacterial endocarditis. There have also been reports of focal and segmental glomerulonephritis, membranoproliferative glomerulonephritis, and membranous glomerulonephritis. In addition, several reports state that minimal change nephrotic syndrome is common in these patients. The latter reports appeared at a time when the diagnosis of the minimal change nephrotic syndrome included mild, focal sclerotic changes and thus could have represented addicts in the early stages of the glomerulosclerotic process.

Thus, if there are renal lesions specific to heroin addiction, other than focal glomerulosclerosis, their nature and pathogenesis have not been fully elucidated.

SELECTED READINGS

1. Arruda J, Kurtzmann N: Heroin addiction and renal disease. Contrib Nephrol 7:69, 1977.
2. Cunningham EE, Brentjens JR, Zielezny MA, et al: Heroin nephropathy. A clinicopathologic and epidemiologic study. Am J Med 68:47, 1980.
3. Fillastre JP, Mery JP, Druet P: Nephropathies glomerulaires medicamenteuses. Nephrologie 4:1, 1983.
4. Liach F, Descoeudres CM, Massry SG: Heroin-associated nephropathy: Clinical and histological studies in 19 patients. Clin Nephrol 11:7, 1979.
5. Menchel S, Cohen D, Gross E, et al: AA protein-related renal amyloidosis in drug addicts. Am J Pathol 112:195, 1983.
6. Neild GH, Gartner HV, Bohle A: Penicillamine-induced membranous glomerulonephritis. Scand J Rheumatol 79:90, 1979.

TOXIN EXPOSURE

Glomerular diseases are a much less frequent complication of toxin exposure than are tubular or interstitial lesions. Unlike many tubulo-interstitial diseases, however, the glomerular lesions tend to either remit or stabilize when the offending agent is removed from the patient's environment. Thus, recognition of this entity may be of considerable clinical importance.

Heavy Metals

Membranous glomerulonephritis is the lesion most frequently described to be associated with prolonged exposure to heavy metals. The following list is in approximate order of reported frequency:

Gold salts
Mercury salts
Silver salts
Bismuth salts

A small number of patients have also developed a histologic pattern consistent with minimal lesion after exposure to gold salts.

Drugs with a Free Sulfhydryl Group

Penicillamine

Penicillamine is the major drug in this category that is associated with glomerular disease. Other drugs with a similar structure have been reported, but they are quite rare. Penicillamine has been implicated in the development of several different types of glomerular lesions, but the most common is membranous glomerulonephritis. The following is a brief description of the renal lesions.

Membranous Glomerulonephritis

Most patients with proteinuria have a pattern consistent with membranous glomerulonephritis. The lesions are often difficult to detect without careful assessment of the specimen by immunofluorescence microscopy, because there are often few or no basement spikes and the lesions may be quite irregular in distribution.

Membranoproliferative Glomerulonephritis

Membranoproliferative glomerulonephritis is an uncommon occurrence, and some researchers believe that the presence of epimembranous deposits in these patients, in addition to those in the basement membranes and the mesangial regions, casts the diagnosis of membranoproliferative glomerulonephritis in doubt.

Minimal Lesions and Focal Necrotizing Glomerulonephritis

Very few patients have been reported in either of these histologic categories.

Crescentic Glomerulonephritis

Several patients have been reported to have developed a clinical course resembling that of Goodpasture's syndrome with pulmonary hemorrhage and rapidly progressive renal failure. One patient had linear glomerular basement membrane deposits of IgG, whereas the rest had granular deposits. Thus, although they all appeared to have an immune-mediated crescentic glomerulonephritis, it was of two different varieties.

Captopril

Very few patients have been reported, but the renal lesion appears to be membranous glomerulonephritis.

Other Drugs

Two other drugs, pyrithioxine and thiopronine, have been reported to be associated with the development of membranous glomerulonephritis. Again, the total number of reported cases is small.

Antineoplastic Drugs

Glomerular lesions resembling those present in the hemolytic-uremic syndrome have been reported in patients receiving mitomycin-C (see Chapter 6). One patient treated with alpha-interferon has been reported to have developed minimal lesion nephrotic syndrome.

NON-STEROIDAL ANTI-INFLAMMATORY DRUGS

Several patients who have developed the nephrotic syndrome following therapy with non-steroidal anti-inflammatory agents have been reported. The histologic pattern of renal involvement is principally that of interstitial involvement, but it has been reported that in some patients there appears to be effacement of the pedicels. The spreading of the pedicels is not as uniform and diffuse as in minimal lesion nephrotic syndrome, although the patients may have proteinuria. In these cases, the most common agent has been fenoprofen.

Other Drugs

Other drugs have been implicated in the development of proteinuria or a lupuslike syndrome. The following is a list of the most common associations and the general type of histologic lesion reported:

Drug	Lesion
Lithium	Minimal change
Procainamide	Lupuslike
Hydralazine	Lupuslike
Phenindione	Minimal change
Levamisole	Minimal change

HEPATIC CIRRHOSIS

The occurrence of glomerular lesions in patients with cirrhosis has been recognized for decades. However, this association has received little attention because the renal lesions seldom require intervention and do not lead to significant sequelae. The most frequent urinary finding is the presence of modest proteinuria and hematuria. The nephrotic syndrome is extremely uncommon.

Pathogenesis and Patient Presentation

Renal lesions have most often been described in patients with alcoholic liver disease. The presence of IgA deposits in glomeruli has suggested that the lesions have an immune complex pathogenesis. In autopsy studies of patients with cirrhosis, it is common to find a wide variety of asymptomatic renal lesions. However, few of these lesions were of significance during life.

Histology

Two histologic patterns have been described, mesangial sclerosis and membranoproliferative glomerulonephritis.

Mesangial Sclerosis

Light Microscopy

Many histologic patterns have been described. The mesangial sclerosis is so characteristic that it has been called hepatic glomerulosclerosis (Fig. 5–21). It may superficially resemble the early changes present in patients with diabetes mellitus, but the peripheral glomerular basement membranes are usually of normal thickness in cirrhotic patients whereas they are nearly always thickened in diabetic patients. Foci of hyalin deposits have been described but are uncommon. Bowman's capsular basement membrane may be thickened, and obsolescent glomeruli are sometimes present. These changes are most likely not directly related to the hepatic lesion, rather being reflective of a general underlying atherosclerotic process.

The interstitium contains patchy areas of fibrosis and tubular atrophy with basement membrane thickening.

Hyalin deposits in small arterioles are a frequent finding.

In summary, the light microscopic changes all are relatively mild and nonspecific. The kidney is not normal, however, and the find-

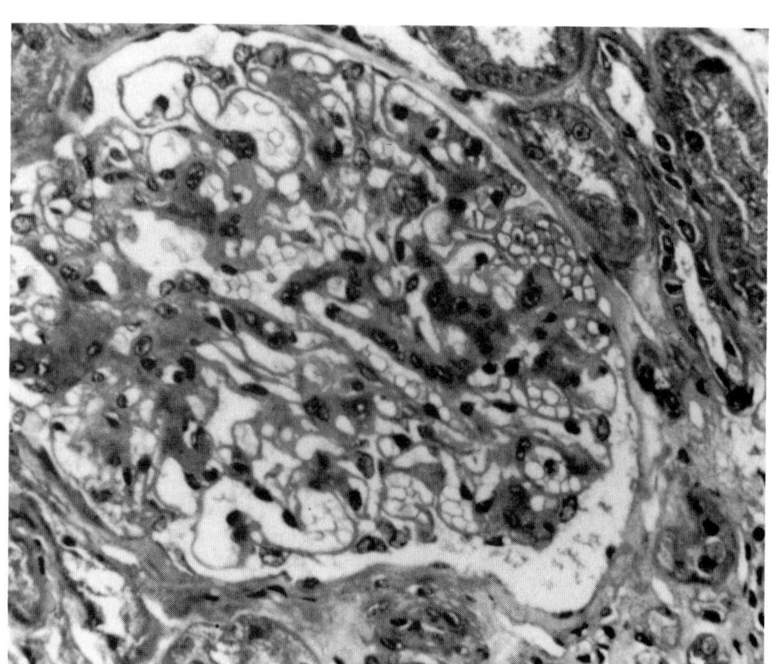

Figure 5–21. Diffuse mesangial sclerosis. (Masson's trichrome, ×400.)

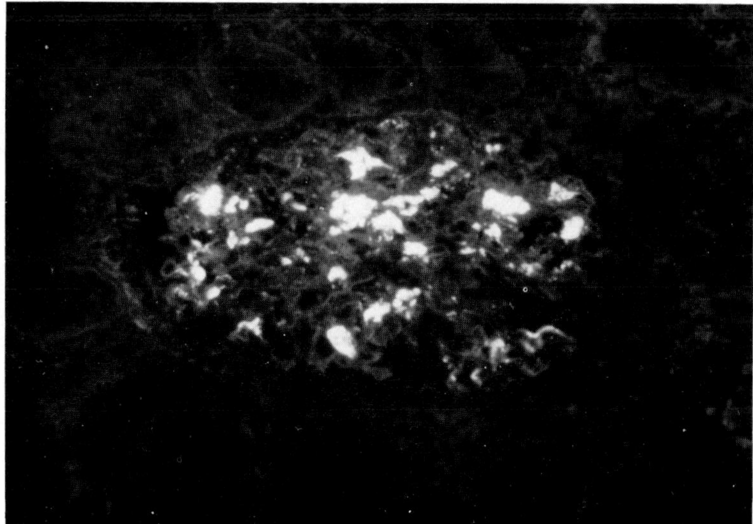

Figure 5–22. Immunofluorescence micrograph: IgA deposits in the mesangial area. (×250.)

ings suggest that there is some mild, chronic renal damage.

Immunofluorescence Microscopy

Most patients with mesangial changes by light microscopy have mesangial deposits of IgA (Fig. 5–22). The deposits are diffuse, often quite small, and frequently codistribute with C3. Less commonly, IgG is present in the same distribution as IgA. However, IgG is commonly found in a faint linear pattern, outlining the peripheral glomerular basement membranes. In such cases, IgA and albumin may be found in the same linear pattern. This distribution seems characteristic of sclerotic lesions rather than being specific for cirrhosis, because a similar pattern is sometimes seen in patients with diabetes mellitus.

Electron Microscopy

The mesangial regions are sclerotic, but there are no definable electron-dense deposits. The peripheral glomerular basement membranes are normal, as are the epithelial and endothelial cells.

Membranoproliferative Glomerulonephritis

A small number of patients have been described to have developed a renal lesion resembling membranoproliferative glomerulonephritis after the placement of a portacaval shunt.

Light Microscopy

The light microscopic features are identical to those in patients without cirrhosis and are described in Chapter 4.

IMMUNOFLUORESCENCE MICROSCOPY

The pattern of deposits in membranoproliferative glomerulonephritis associated with cirrhosis is unique. The predominant immunoglobulin found in the mesangial and subendothelial deposits is IgA. The IgA deposits are abundant, diffuse, and codistribute with C3. IgG and IgM are present in the same distribution, but in much lesser quantity. Fibrin/fibrinogen deposition is inconspicuous.

The only other clinical syndrome associated with the light microscopic features of membranoproliferative glomerulonephritis and IgA deposits by immunochemical analysis is the Schönlein-Henoch syndrome. The major difference between these two entities is the abundance of fibrin/fibrinogen deposits in the Schönlein-Henoch syndrome and their paucity in patients with cirrhosis.

Electron Microscopy

On light microscopy, the lesions at the ultrastructural level do not differ from those in other patients with membranoproliferative glomerulonephritis (see Chapter 4).

Prognosis

Although the renal lesions are overshadowed by those in the liver, at the present time, they may assume more importance as the number of liver transplants increases and patients survive for longer periods. In addition, it will be important to recognize the possibility of preexisting renal lesions in patients who are recipients of liver transplants and who are being considered for drug therapy that has the potential for renal toxicity.

SELECTED READINGS

1. Berger J, Yaneva H, Nabarra B: Lesions glomerulaires des cirrhotiques. *In* Grunfeld JP, Corvol P (eds): Actualites Nephrologiques de l'Hopital Necker Flammarion, Paris, 1977, pp 165–176.
2. Bloodworth JMB, Sommers SC: Cirrhotic glomerulosclerosis, a renal lesion associated with hepatic cirrhosis. Lab Invest 8:962, 1959.
3. Callard P, Feldman G, Prandi D, et al: Immune-complex type glomerulonephritis in cirrhosis of the liver. Am J Pathol 80:329, 1975.
4. Manigand G, Morel-Maroger L, Simon J, et al: Lesions glomerulaires et cirrhoses du foie. Note preliminaire sur les lesions histologiques du rein au cours des cirrhoses hepatique, d'apres 20 prelevements biopsies. Rev Eur Etud Clin Biol 15:989, 1970.

Chapter

6 GLOMERULAR DISEASES ASSOCIATED WITH SYSTEMIC DISEASES

SYSTEMIC LUPUS ERYTHEMATOSUS (AND MIXED CONNECTIVE TISSUE DISEASE, POLYMYOSITIS, AND RHEUMATOID ARTHRITIS)

Systemic lupus erythematosus is a renal disease in which immune complexes are assumed to have a major role. It is by no means an exceptional disease, and several thousand cases are newly recognized in the United States each year. The symptoms, renal histopathology, and outcome are quite diverse, but uremia has been the leading cause of death. The development of working classifications of the renal disease in systemic lupus erythematosus has allowed the comparison between different patients as well as between different centers. Refinements in the treatment regimens and steady improvement in the renal prognosis have resulted.

Pathogenesis

Systemic lupus erythematosus is considered to be the prototype of immune complex diseases and in fact represents one of the best examples of human diseases in which animal studies have led both to further understanding of the basic processes and to many advances in clinical therapeutic approaches.

The composition of the immune complexes has proved to be more complicated than originally envisioned. The antigens thus far identified include double-stranded DNA, single-stranded DNA, and ribonucleoproteins. There usually is evidence of the systemic activation of complement, and the glomerular deposits contain large amounts of complement components. The type and nature of the antibodies appear to be important in determining the course of the renal disease. It has been been proposed that antibodies to DNA are more likely to be nephrotoxic if they are of high avidity. High concentrations of precipitating antibodies to DNA are thought to be more likely to be associated with mesangial and subendothelial deposits. On the contrary low-avidity antibodies are more commonly associated with subepithelial deposits, and the associated renal lesions are much less likely to progress rapidly.

Recent studies have investigated the possibility that the first phase of the formation of glomerular immune deposits is the formation or deposition of antigens in the glomerulus, at a time before antibodies are involved. It was found that DNA binds to glomerular basement membranes. Thus DNA might localize to the glomerular basement membrane and lead to the fixation of anti-DNA antibodies in the glomerulus. Immune complexes would therefore result from in situ formation.

A similar mechanism has been proposed for the formation of some types of subepithelial deposits.

Another recent observation is that some monoclonal antibodies to DNA react with glomerular antigens, suggesting that humoral autoimmunity may also have a role in the glomerulonephritis. The development of cellular autoimmunity has been extensively studied in animal models of systemic lupus erythematosus. In these models, it has been strongly suggested that hyperreactivity of T- and B-lymphocytes and defective T-cell suppression contribute to the disease.

Defects in the clearance of immune complexes from the circulation also contribute to the disease. There may be both impaired clearance of complexes by the mononuclear system and impaired opsonization of immune complexes by complement.

Finally, both genetic and hormonal factors play a part in the pathogenesis of systemic lupus erythematosus. A substantial female: male preponderance (9:1) exists, and blacks are much more susceptible. The age range is quite broad in women, usually commencing between the ages of 16 and 50.

Patient Presentation

Although multiple systems are always involved, the range of severity between individual sites may vary significantly. The diagnosis of systemic lupus erythematosus requires a combination of clinical and laboratory findings that have been defined by the American Rheumatism Association. These criteria do not rely on the presence of renal disease.

The clinical and laboratory findings vary widely among patients, and there is not a close correlation between involvement of other organs and the kidney. Unfortunately, the laboratory findings do not accurately reflect the underlying renal disease. In fact, this is one of the most important examples of glomerular diseases in which the urinary sediment is an unreliable indicator of the underlying nephritis. Urinary findings generally tend to underestimate the glomerular diseases, but in the case of focal active lesions, the sediment may overestimate both the distribution and severity of the glomerulonephritis. For this reason, renal biopsy is an important part of both the diagnosis and the therapeutic management in these patients. Even though the urine sediment is not an accurate guide, asymptomatic proteinuria and microscopic hematuria characterize the mildest forms of nephritis, and the nephrotic syndrome signals a more severe renal lesion.

Hypertension is found in 25 to 45% of the patients, a significant number considering the relatively young age of the affected population.

The onset of the renal disease is often difficult to pinpoint, but it is often stated to be within 4 years of recognition of the syndrome. However, the renal lesion may be the first disease manifestation in young women. The renal disease rarely presents as rapidly progressive glomerulonephritis.

Classification of Glomerular Lesions

The extreme variability and irregularity of the distribution of the lesions have led investigators to attempt some form of classification and quantification. The classification most widely accepted and endorsed by the World Health Organization groups patients into five different categories (see below) and assumes that the biopsy is evaluated by light, immunofluorescence, and electron microscopy. It has proved to be a useful classification scheme because each of the five categories has a different prognosis. The classification provides a framework of reference, but its utility is most clear in newly diagnosed, untreated patients. It is much less applicable to the histologic findings in patients who have been treated, because the categories become much less distinct and separable. Currently available potent and effective therapeutic agents lead to rapid and often dramatic changes in the renal histopathology, and many researchers have sought to develop more accurate means to evaluate renal biopsy samples by including quantitative measurements for the purpose of comparing repeat biopsies in the same patient.

We have proposed a simple method based on systematically separating the renal changes into those that appear reversible (active) and those that appear to be fixed (sclerotic). The schema is shown in Table 6–1.

The lesions are scored (0 to 3+) for severity and distribution. The sum of the active lesions is obtained and is a measure of the disease activity. The sum of the sclerotic lesions is also obtained and is an indication of the amount of fixed damage. This sum has been called the index of chronicity. The method allows for a rough comparison to be made between different stages of the disease in one patient and between different patients.

The classification that is currently used combines that proposed by the World Health Organization and some form of quantitation

Table 6–1. Scoring System for Renal Lesions in Systemic Lupus Erythematous

Active Lesions	*Sclerotic Lesions*
Endocapillary proliferation	Tubular atrophy/ interstitial fibrosis
Nuclear debris	Glomerular obsolescence
Hematoxylin bodies	Fibrous crescents
Hyalin thrombi	***Lesions of Unknown Significance***
Necrosis	Membranous glomerulonephritis
Cellular crescents	
Inflammatory cells (interstitial)	
Acute tubular necrosis	
Necrotizing angiitis	

using light, immunofluorescence, and electron microscopy. The description that follows is the one we currently use (Table 6–2).

Minimal Lesions or No Changes: Class I

Histology

Light, Immunofluorescence, and Electron Microscopy

There are no deposits or lesions. This category can only be used when the patient's biopsy sample has been studied with light, immunofluorescence, and electron microscopy. Most renal specimens in this category are obtained from patients who underwent biopsy during the course of a prospective study in which all patients with systemic lupus erythematosus are subjected to renal biopsy, since these patients have no urinary sediment changes.

Mesangial Change: Class IIA or IIB

Introduction and Patient Presentation

Patients with mesangial change have urine sediment abnormalities, but their renal function is otherwise normal. They may occasionally develop more severe lesions. The first evidence of such a transition may be the involvement of the peripheral vascular loops by immune deposits.

Histology

Light Microscopy

There is a slight increase in mesangial cellularity or sclerosis. The difference between class IIA and IIB is that no mesangial lesions are identified by light microscopy in the former, whereas either a moderate increase in the number of mesangial cells or in the amount of the mesangial matrix is observed in class IIB (Fig. 6–1).

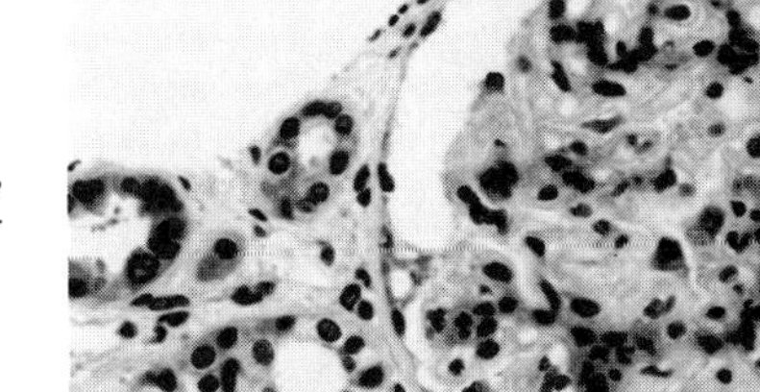

Figure 6–1. There is diffuse, moderate mesangial cell proliferation. (H&E, ×250.)

Table 6–2. Glomerular Lesions in Systemic Lupus Erythematosus

World Health Organization Class	Light Microscopy	Immunofluorescence Microscopy	Electron Microscopy
I	No lesions		
IIA	No lesions	Mesangial, diffuse	Few mesangial deposits
IIB	Mesangial cell and matrix increase, mild	See IIA	See IIA
III	Focal proliferative	Mesangial, diffuse, subepithelial, focal	Mesangial deposits, few subepithelial deposits, mesangial thickening
IV	Diffuse proliferative	Mesangial, subendothelial, and subepithelial deposits	Diffuse deposits, mesangial and glomerular basement membrane thickening
V	Membranous	Epimembranous and a few mesangial deposits	Subepithelial deposits, diffuse; mesangial deposits, few, and glomerular basement membrane thickening

Immunofluorescence Microscopy

There are deposits exclusively localized to the mesangial areas, detectable by immunofluorescence and electron microscopy in both class IIA and IIB. The glomerular mesangial deposits contain IgG, C1q, and C3 (Fig. 6–2). IgA, IgM, and C4 may also be found in the same distribution, but they are most often of lesser amount. IgG and Clq may be found in the interstitium.

Electron Microscopy

The deposits are localized to the paraendothelial mesangial regions and are quite small.

Focal Proliferative: Class III

Introduction and Patient Presentation

In contrast to class II lesions, this group is at great risk for developing more extensive lesions, and they often have proteinuria and hematuria at the onset.

Histology

Light Microscopy

The lesions are focal and segmental, and at least 50% of the glomerular tufts appear normal (Fig. 6–3). The mixture of active and chronic lesions may vary considerably be-

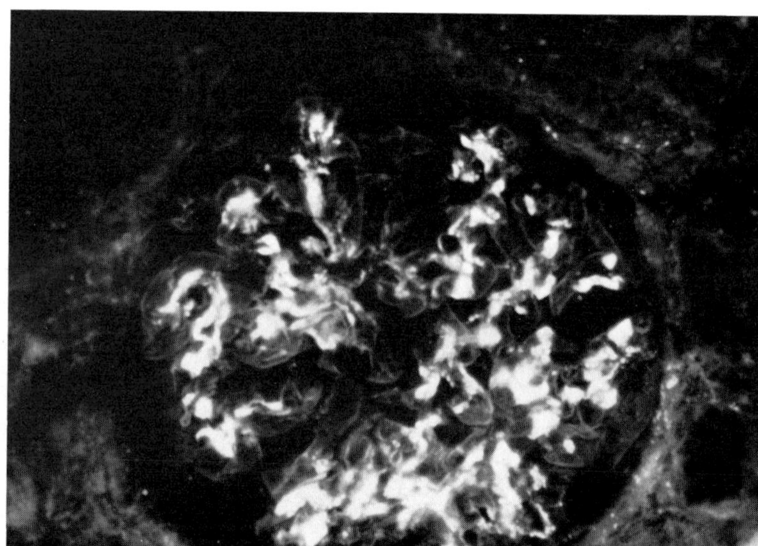

Figure 6–2. Immunofluorescence micrograph, anti-IgG. The mesangial regions all contain deposits. (×250.)

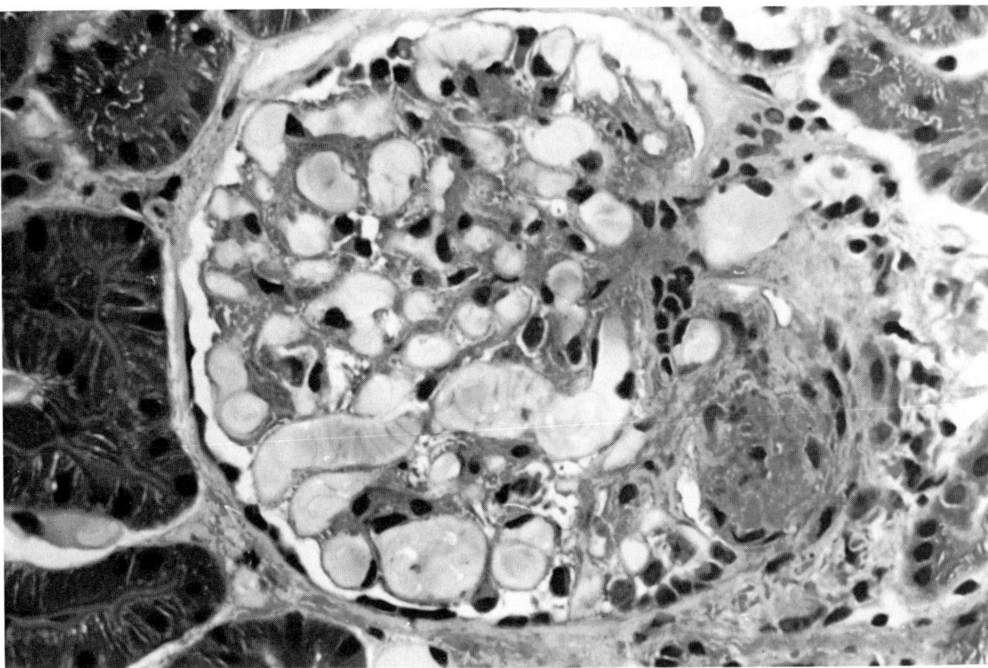

Figure 6–3. This focal and segmental lesion (right lower quadrant) consists of an increased number of cells, infiltration with inflammatory cells, and deposition of matrix and serum proteins. (H&E, ×300.)

tween different areas of the same biopsy sample; thus multiple sections must be examined and scored semi-quantitatively to provide an accurate estimate of the renal lesion.

The glomeruli may show various degrees of intracapillary proliferation. The presence of nuclear debris in the areas of proliferation, an indication of active disease, appears as an ill-defined area of dark material, of smaller size than the surrounding nuclei. Nuclear debris may also be associated with necrotic foci. The foci of necrosis are often poorly delimited, but they are usually restricted in size, rarely involving more than one lobule.

Limited crescents and cellular synechiae are frequently encountered. They are often associated with areas of necrosis and are rapidly replaced by sclerosis (Fig. 6–4).

Hematoxylin bodies are small, regular, oval or round, DNA-containing structures that are stained lilac by hematoxylin and eosin (H&E). They are quite rarely found but are pathognomonic of systemic lupus erythematosus.

The mesangial and subendothelial regions contain deposits that often appear brightly eosinophilic by H&E, red by trichrome stains, and purple with periodic acid-Schiff (PAS) stains. When subendothelial deposits are large and occupy the entire circumference of the vascular loop, they are called wire-loops.

The peripheral basement membranes are not thickened, but occasional small, scattered subepithelial spikes and deposits may be seen by silver staining.

Hyalin thrombi may be seen in areas of segmental lesions. They are recognizable as intraluminal masses of amorphous material that fill the lumen. They can be shown to contain aggregates of immune complexes. Fibrin is occasionally present, justifying the retention of the term *thrombi* for this histologic finding. Some groups have reported conspicuous intravascular coagulation and consider this to be a major cause of progression. This has not been a prominent finding in our experience.

The mesangial spaces are diffusely affected, whereas the vascular loops are normal in many areas.

The irregularly distributed tubulo-interstitial lesions appear to correlate directly with the extent and stage of the glomerular changes. Inflammatory cells in the interstitium may be prominent, in which case a careful search by immunofluorescence microscopy may reveal granular deposits scattered along the tubular basement membranes.

The arterioles and arteries often shown intimal proliferation and medial lesions consisting of hyalinosis and smooth muscle cell hypertrophy. These are far in excess of what

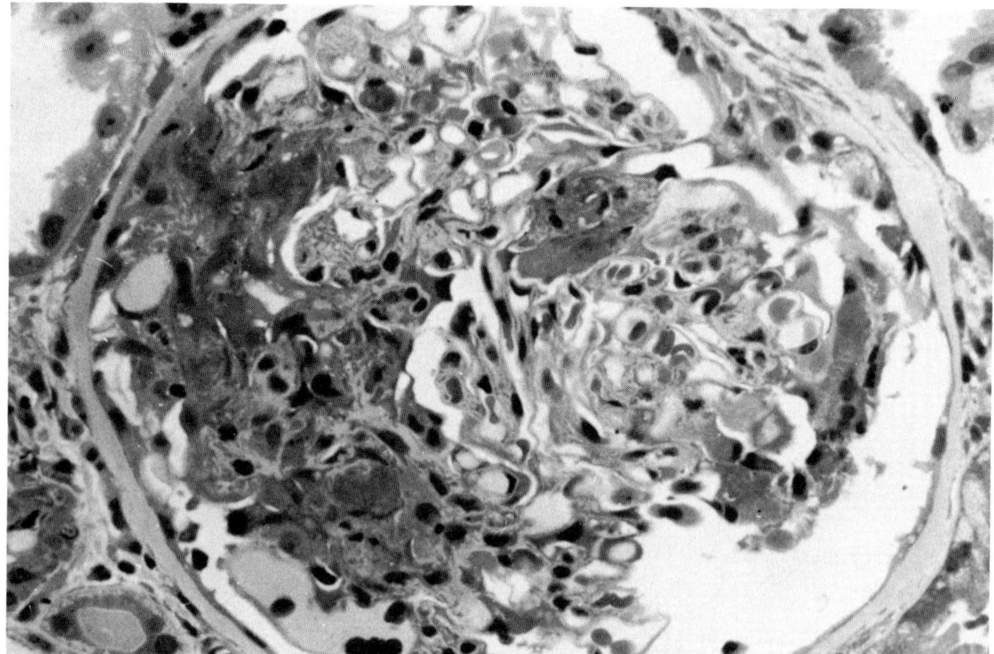

Figure 6–4. The cellular proliferation is more marked in Bowman's space than within the tuft. The partial crescent contains fibrin, which is homogenously pink. (H&E, ×300.)

might be expected on the basis of either the patient's age or blood pressure.

Immunofluorescence Microscopy

Immunoglobulins and complement components are always found in biopsy samples with active lesions. They may largely disappear as the active lesions resolve and sclerosis develops. The deposits invariably include IgG and C1q and often IgM. IgA is found in smaller amounts. Fibrin/fibrinogen is often abundant in the areas of necrosis.

A characteristic of these biopsy specimens is the uniform and diffuse presence of mesangial deposits. The peripheral vascular walls may also contain focal and segmental deposits, either in the form of large granular subendothelial deposits or with a regular granular pattern suggesting subepithelial deposits. The deposits along the peripheral glomerular basement membrane are not often extensive, distinguishing this category from class IV or VI (Fig. 6–5).

The frequency of extraglomerular deposits, although not specific for systemic lupus erythematosus, is a much more frequent associated finding in this disease than in other glomerular diseases. The tubular basement membrane deposits consist of small, scattered granules. The interstitial capillary basement membranes and those of the arterioles may also contain deposits. The deposits are usually accompanied by interstitial infiltrates. The nuclei of tubules and arteries may have a finely speckled distribution of IgG.

Electron Microscopy

The finding of deposits in multiple glomerular regions is typical of systemic lupus erythematosus, although it is not diagnostic. The deposits are mainly localized to the mesangial regions and are scattered throughout the extracellular matrix. Nuclear debris may be found in the deposits (Fig. 6–6). A number of different organizational patterns have been described in the deposits of patients with systemic lupus erythematosus, including "fingerprints" and microtubules (Fig. 6–7). These microtubules have also been described in the cytoplasm of endothelial cells. Neither of these findings is specific for systemic lupus erythematosus but should suggest the diagnosis. Deposits are found in the subendothelial and subepithelial spaces but usually in much smaller amounts. The presence of large subendothelial deposits suggests that the true category is class IV rather than III.

Deposits are often found along Bowman's capsular basement membranes and those of the tubules and interstitial capillaries.

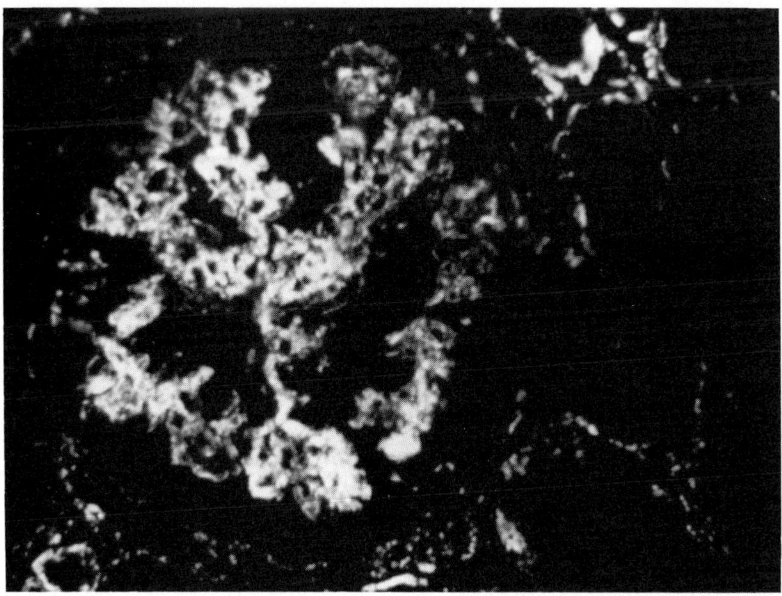

Figure 6–5. Immunofluorescence micrograph, anti-IgG. The mesangial regions contain large deposits. Note the granular deposits outlining the basement membranes of tubules and Bowman's capsules. (×250.)

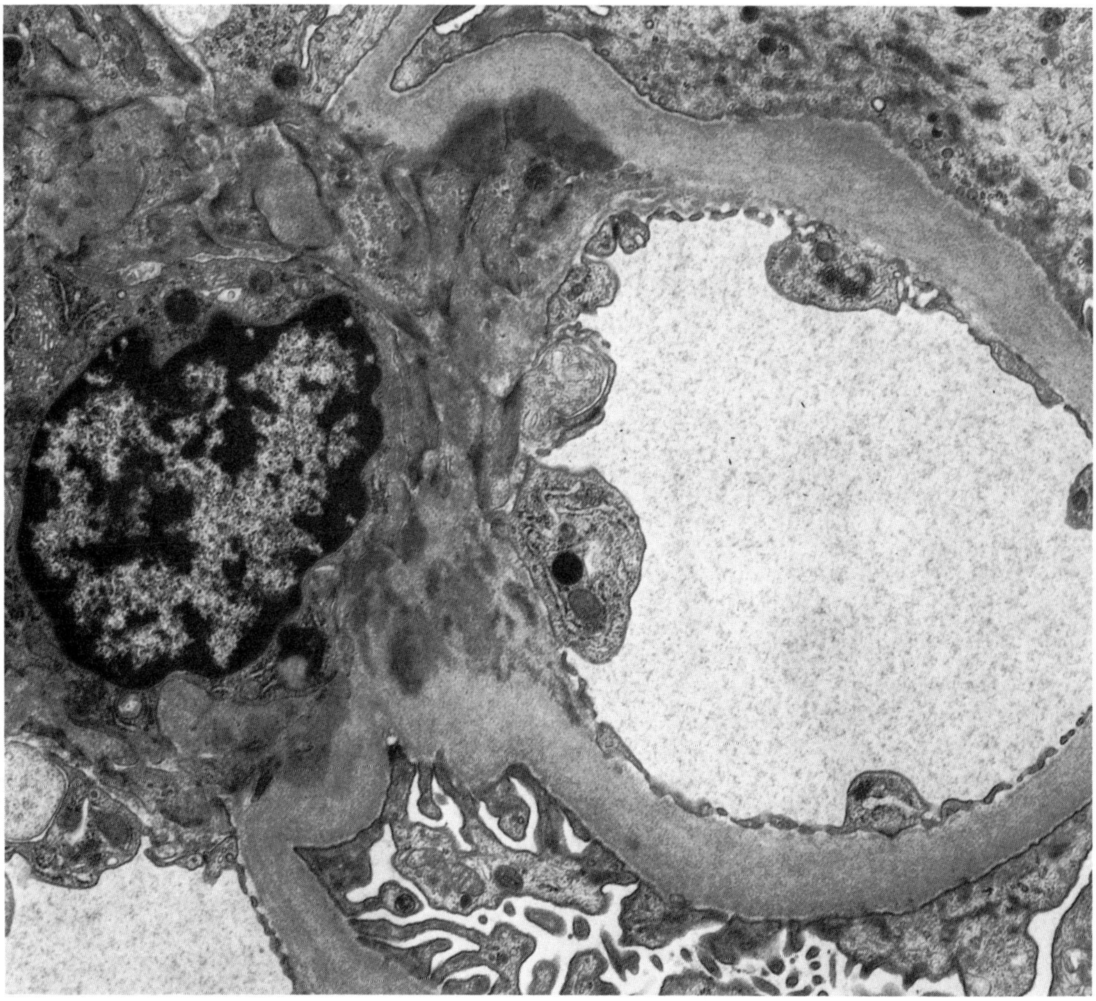

Figure 6–6. There are a large number of deposits in the mesangial matrix. (×3000.)

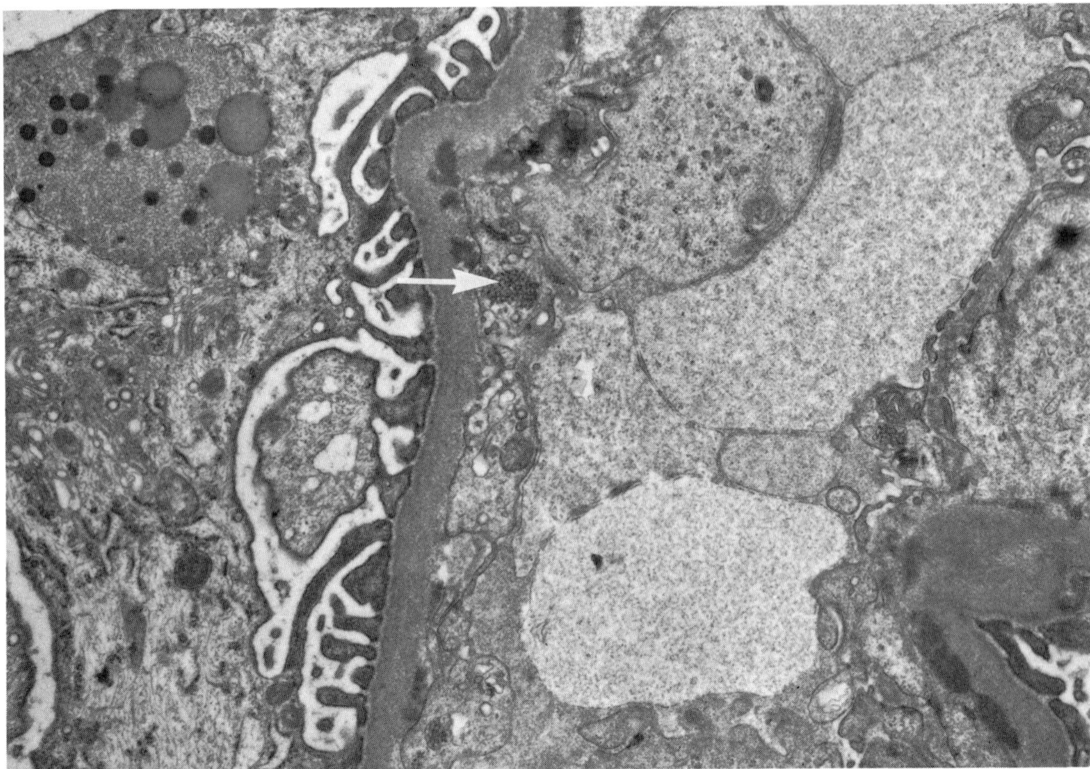

Figure 6–7. The endothelial cells contain tubulo-reticular inclusions (arrow). (×3200.)

Diffuse: Class IV

Introduction and Patient Presentation

When the focal and segmental lesions (class III) are severe and widespread, it may be difficult to decide whether or not they should be placed into the category of diffuse glomerulonephritis (class IV). In fact, the division is artificial and arbitrary, because it has now been documented by repeat renal biopsies that there is a continuum between the two groups. In fact, transition can occur in both directions, either with focal becoming diffuse as a result of progression or with diffuse becoming focal in response to therapeutic intervention. In the latter case, the lesions may appear as irregular sclerotic foci alternating with focal, active lesions. As has been noted with the earlier categories, the renal lesions vary in their distribution and severity.

Histology

Light Microscopy

The diffuse lesion is the most common histologic pattern encountered in renal biopsies performed before treatment, reflecting in part a selection bias based on the fact that patients with relatively severe renal disease are the ones most frequently subjected to renal biopsies. It is therefore also the variety of renal lesion that has been most extensively studied and has the clearest and most successful response to therapy.

The histologic pattern typical of untreated patients with the diffuse form of systemic lupus erythematosus consists of mesangial hypercellularity, neutrophil infiltration, focal areas of necrosis, nuclear debris, and markedly thickened peripheral vascular loops (Fig. 6–8), resulting in a sharply reduced vascular lumen.

Hematoxylin bodies are present in 1 to 2% of the biopsies.

The thickening of the peripheral vascular loops is due to either duplication of the basement membranes or large subendothelial deposits (Fig. 6–9). In addition, scattered subepithelial deposits are common. Hyalin thrombi are frequently found in the zones of the most active lesions (Fig. 6–10).

The most common visceral epithelial cell lesion is cytoplasmic hyalin droplets. Localized crescents or synechiae may be present,

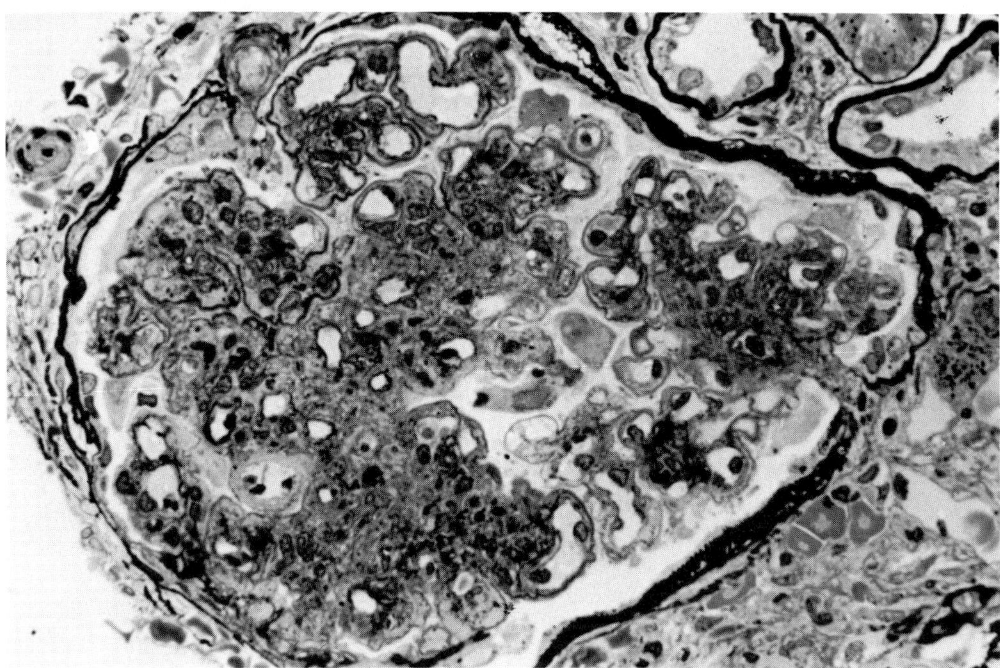

Figure 6–8. There is diffuse thickening of the glomerular basement membranes, cellular proliferation, many profiles of nuclear debris, and segmental necrosis. An organized synechia is present in the right quadrant. (PASM, ×500.)

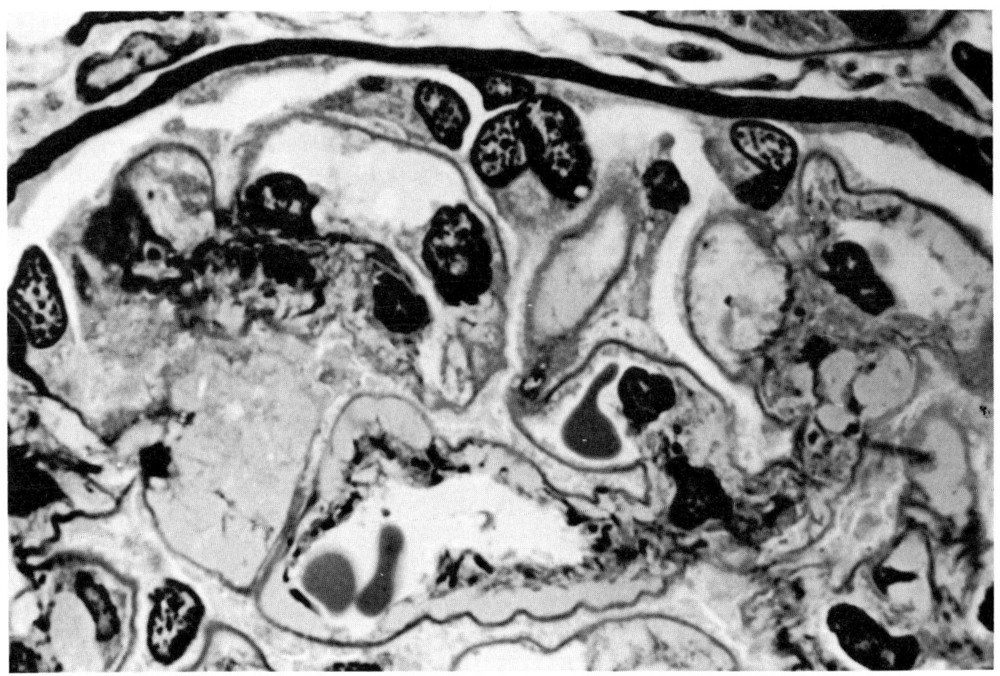

Figure 6–9. Large subendothelial deposits are present in most vascular loops. (PASM, ×1000.)

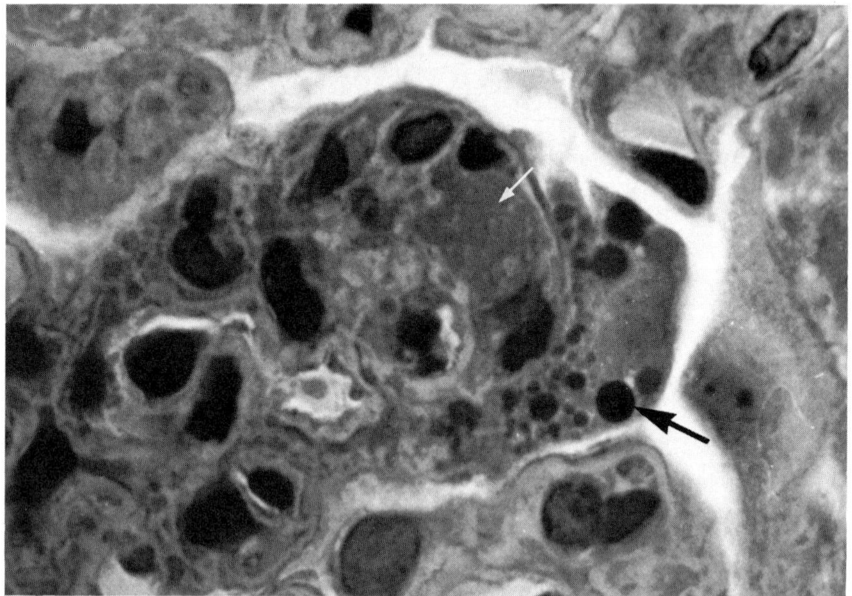

Figure 6–10. A large subendothelial deposit occupies almost the entire vascular space (light arrow). The podocyte cytoplasm contains many dark lysosomal protein droplets (dark arrow). (H&E, ×1200.)

but they are usually limited to areas adjacent to necrotic foci. Necrotic foci are frequent and are irregularly distributed between and within glomeruli. A diffuse crescentic lesion is uncommon and is generally only found at the initial presentation in patients with rapidly progressive glomerulonephritis.

The lesions often appear to be of different ages, with obsolescent glomeruli and focal sclerosing lesions admixed with active lesions. For this reason, patients with diffuse sclerotic glomerular lesions are often classified as having diffuse glomerulonephritis (class IV), even in the absence of active lesions.

Also included in this category are the biopsy samples that have the histologic features of type I membranoproliferative or lobular glomerulonephritis. Some investigators have proposed that a separate subcategory be developed for these biopsies, but this suggestion has not been widely adopted.

Interstitial lesions are usually prominent. The interstitium contains significant infiltrates of inflammatory cells. The tubular lesions consist of epithelial cell swelling, cytoplasmic hyalin droplets, and casts. Acute tubular necrosis has been reported, but it is rare.

The small arteries and arterioles often show intimal proliferation and medial thickening. When severe, these lesions may resemble those of scleroderma. An acute necrotizing angiitis is uncommon and is limited to those biopsy specimens with severe, active lesions in the other compartments. In these cases, occasional areas of necrosis and hemorrhage may be associated with thrombi in the lumen.

Immunofluorescence Microscopy

These biopsy specimens present a nearly unique appearance because of the markedly abundant and diffusely spread deposits in almost all anatomic compartments. Large immunoglobulin deposits (principally IgG and IgM) are always present along the glomerular basement membranes, often in a coarsely granular pattern. Many vascular loops appear occluded by the deposits (Fig. 6–11). The mesangial spaces may also contain large amounts of immune reactants. IgG is always present associated with IgM, C1q, and C3 (Fig. 6–12). IgA and C4, although present, are usually much less abundant. Fibrin/fibrinogen deposits are found in association with the areas of necrosis and/or crescents.

Extraglomerular granular deposits are often found along the basement membranes of Bowman's capsule, interstitial capillaries, and the tubules.

The arteriolar walls may contain IgG and IgA. As noted previously, there may be speckled nuclear deposits of IgG.

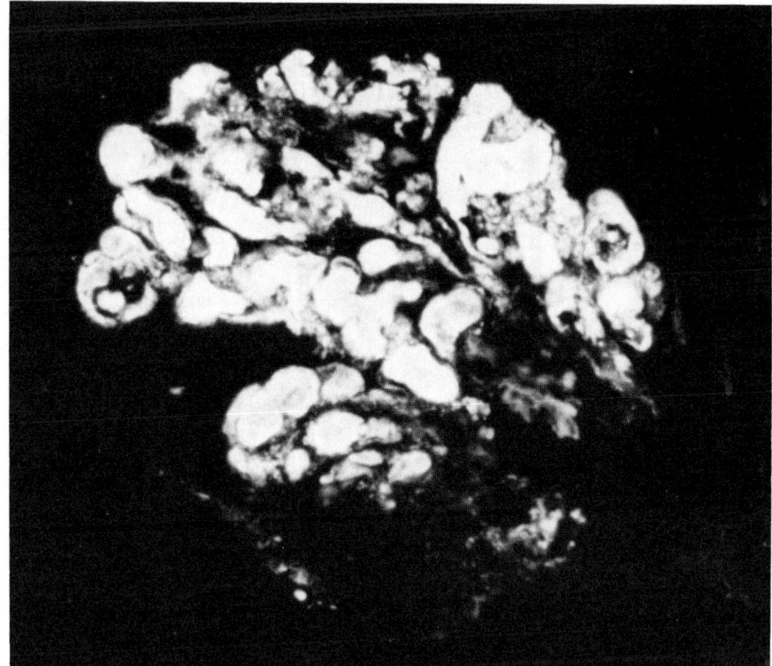

Figure 6–11. Immunofluorescence micrograph, anti-IgG. Large deposits occlude the vascular spaces and fill the mesangium. (×250.)

Electron Microscopy

The electron microscopic findings confirm those obtained by light and immunofluorescence methods. Massive deposits are present in all glomerular areas; subendothelial, subepithelial, and mesangial (Figs. 6–13 and 6–14). Cellular changes are marked, and both nuclear debris and neutrophils are prominent in the mesangium. The whole architecture of the glomerulus may be so distorted that it becomes difficult to be sure of the anatomic segment under investigation. As noted for the focal lesions, the deposits may contain structures resembling fingerprints or pseudotubules. Such structures are more frequently observed in this histologic class than in the milder lesions.

The size and extent of subendothelial deposits are directly correlated with a poor prognosis. Those in the subepithelial and mesangial regions do not have this close association.

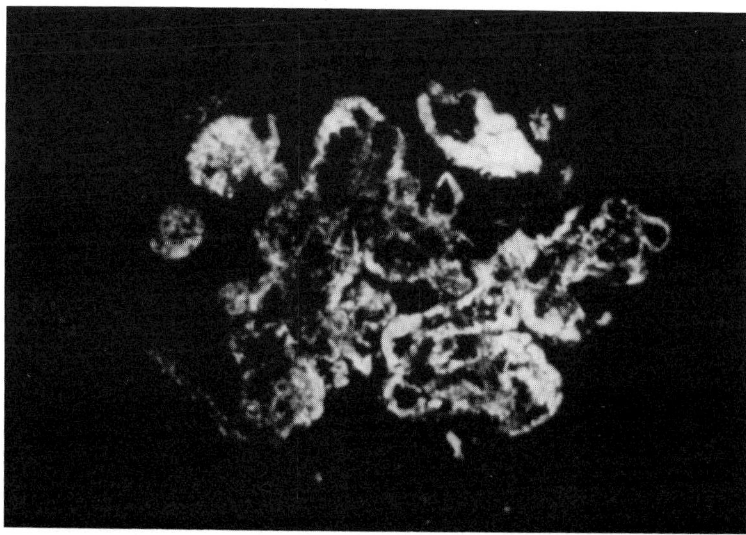

Figure 6–12. Immunofluorescence micrograph, anti-IgA. The deposits are quite large, but have a granular appearance. Bowman's capsule is weakly stained. (×250.)

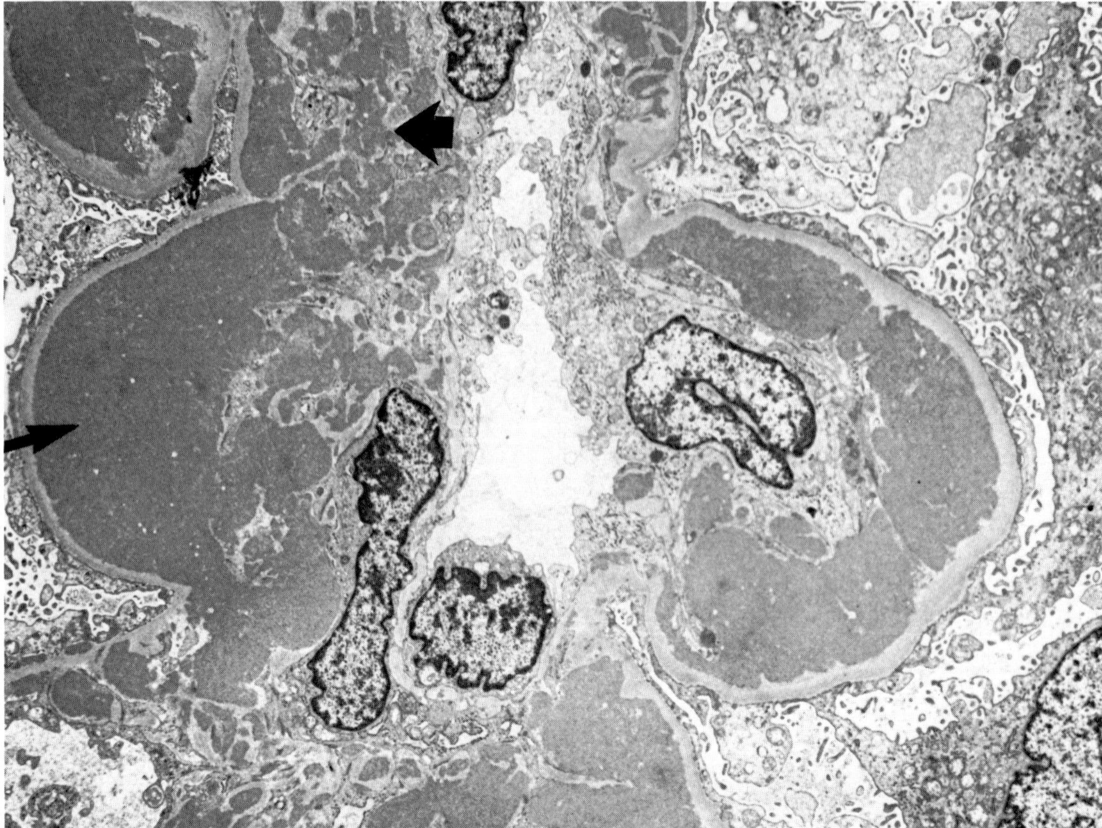

Figure 6–13. The extensive subendothelial (light arrow) and mesangial (heavy arrow) deposits are easily visualized. (×5000.)

Membranous: Class V

Introduction and Patient Presentation

This category represents no more than 10% of the patients in most series, and even this number may be an overestimate because it depends on how strictly the pathologist has adhered to the morphologic criteria. The exactness of the categorization is important because patients with a pure membranous lesion steadily progress, although rather more slowly than those in the focal or diffuse categories. On the other hand, the membranous lesions do not respond to the drugs that are used for the other histologic types of nephritis in lupus erythematosus. The most confusing factor in the definition of this category is the fact that significant numbers of subepithelial deposits are found in most biopsy samples with diffuse lesions. However, we believe that the category of membranous glomerulonephritis should be reserved for those specimens that have diffuse subepithelial deposits as their *main* morphologic feature and in which deposits in the mesangial and subendothelial regions are relatively inconspicuous and mesangial proliferation is lacking or modest.

Histology

Light Microscopy

The H&E appearance is that of membranous glomerulonephritis—that is, bright, thick peripheral basement membranes. Silver stains reveal diffuse, regular subepithelial spikes of basement membranelike material. In some cases, the amount of mesangial matrix or cells is slightly increased.

Some authors have insisted that a large number of leukocytes in the vascular loops and stasis in patients with membranous glomerulonephritis indicate the coexistence of renal vein thrombosis. This association has not been clear-cut in our experience.

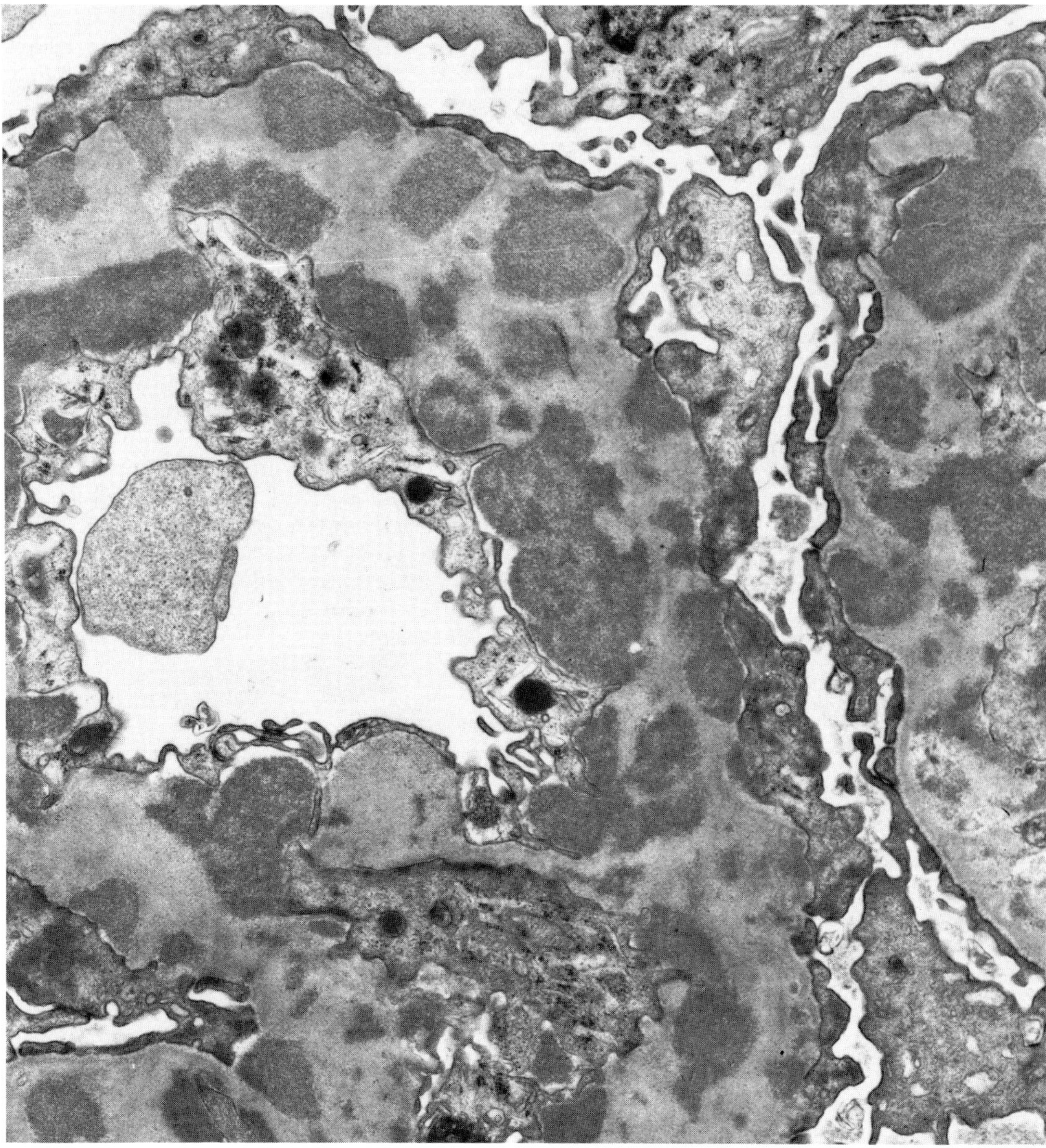

Figure 6–14. The glomerular basement membranes contain large, irregular deposits that occupy all areas from the urinary to the vascular aspects. The mesangial matrix also contains many deposits. The endothelial cell cytoplasm is prominent and contains tubulo-reticular inclusions. (×4800.)

Immunofluorescence Microscopy

The composition and sometimes the distribution of immune reactants should lead the pathologist to suspect systemic lupus erythematosus in what might otherwise appear to be membranous glomerulonephritis. In addition to IgG these include the almost universal presence of C1q, and often C4, IgM, and IgA. In addition, there are often small mesangial deposits (Fig. 6–15). Finally, there frequently are deposits of immunoglobulins in the peritubular basement membranes. None of these findings are present in the usual case of idiopathic membranous glomerulonephritis.

Electron Microscopy

Diffuse subepithelial deposits are the hallmark of this category. They are often associated with smaller deposits in either the subendothelial or mesangial regions (Fig. 6–16). The pedicels are irregularly but diffusely spread. The substructure of the electron-dense deposits shares the features of the other categories.

Transformation from One Category to Another

The use of repeat biopsies in large series of patients has made it clear that multiple types of transformation may occur. For instance, mesangial lesions may develop into diffuse lesions, membranous into proliferative, and mesangial or diffuse into membranous. The exact time frame required for these transformations to occur is unknown, but it has been dramatically modified by the availability of effective therapy. For this reason, renal biopsy has frequently been used not only to guide therapy, but also as a part of the investigation of the pathogenesis of this renal disease.

Prognosis

Patients who have lesions restricted to the mesangium may occasionally suffer more severe renal disease, but this outcome is much less common than in those who have focal proliferative lesions at the onset. It also seems likely that therapy has improved the course of illness in patients with focal proliferative lesions. In this case, treatment appears to prevent the transformation of focal lesions into diffuse disease.

The prognosis for patients with diffuse, active lesions has been transformed by treatment with high-dose steroids and/or cytotoxic drugs. Although these patients frequently progressed to renal failure in the past, repeat biopsy studies have shown that therapy results in a decrease in active lesions and a decrease in the deposits of immune reactants in almost 80% of the patients. These changes are accompanied by an improvement in the patient's overall clinical well-being.

Diffuse crescentic lesions in this disease portend a poor prognosis, in common with the outcome for this histologic category of renal disease when it is associated with other etiologies.

In a large prospective study, some refinements were recently introduced into the classification of the renal lesions of systemic lupus erythematosus. Investigators confirmed the bleak prognosis in the most severe lesions. They showed that patients with focal and segmental lesions with active lesions affecting more than 50% of the glomeruli have a prognosis comparable to those with diffuse lesions. Finally, they showed that patients with membranous lesions in association with proliferation respond in a manner identical to those who have diffuse glomerulonephritis.

MIXED CONNECTIVE TISSUE DISEASE

A group of patients present with manifestations that seem to overlap those of systemic lupus erythematosus, scleroderma, and polymyositis. These patients have circulating antibodies to extractable nuclear antigen (ribonuclear trypsin-sensitive antigen) in the absence of the SM antigen. They rarely have a renal lesion. In the few reported cases in which a renal lesion is present, the glomerular lesions have been of a wide variety of histologic types including focal and diffuse glomerulonephritis as well as membranous glomerulonephritis. The renal lesions are indistinguishable from those in systemic lupus erythematosus. The vascular lesions resemble those in scleroderma (see later in this chapter).

POLYMYOSITIS

Renal lesions are very uncommon in patients with polymyositis. In those few cases in

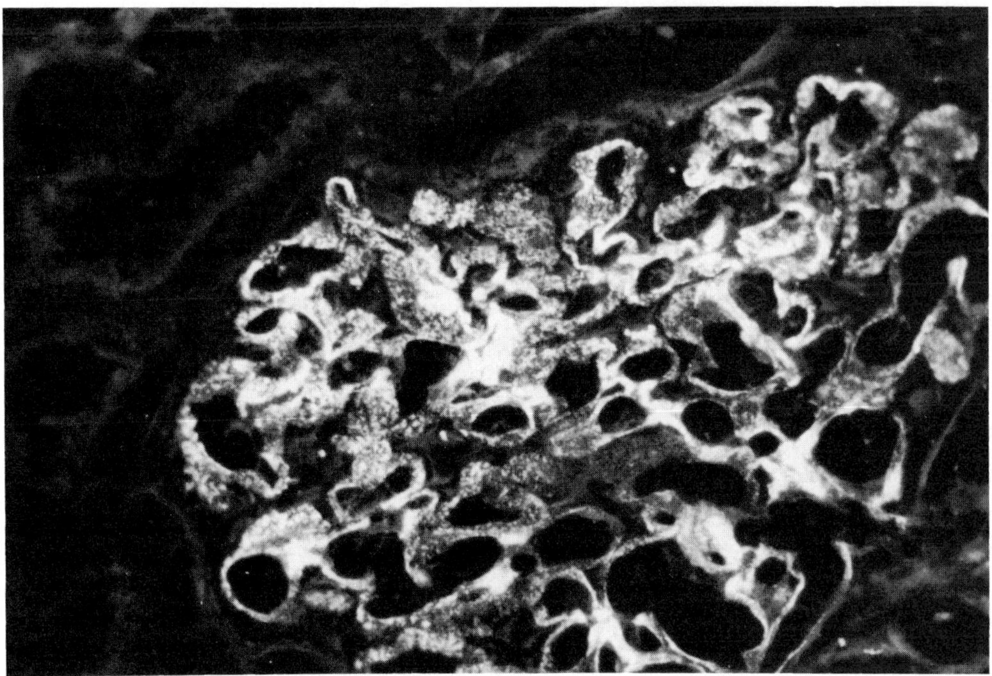

Figure 6–15. Immunofluorescence micrograph, anti-IgG. There are large numbers of subepithelial deposits. There are also deposits in the mesangial and subendothelial regions. (×400.)

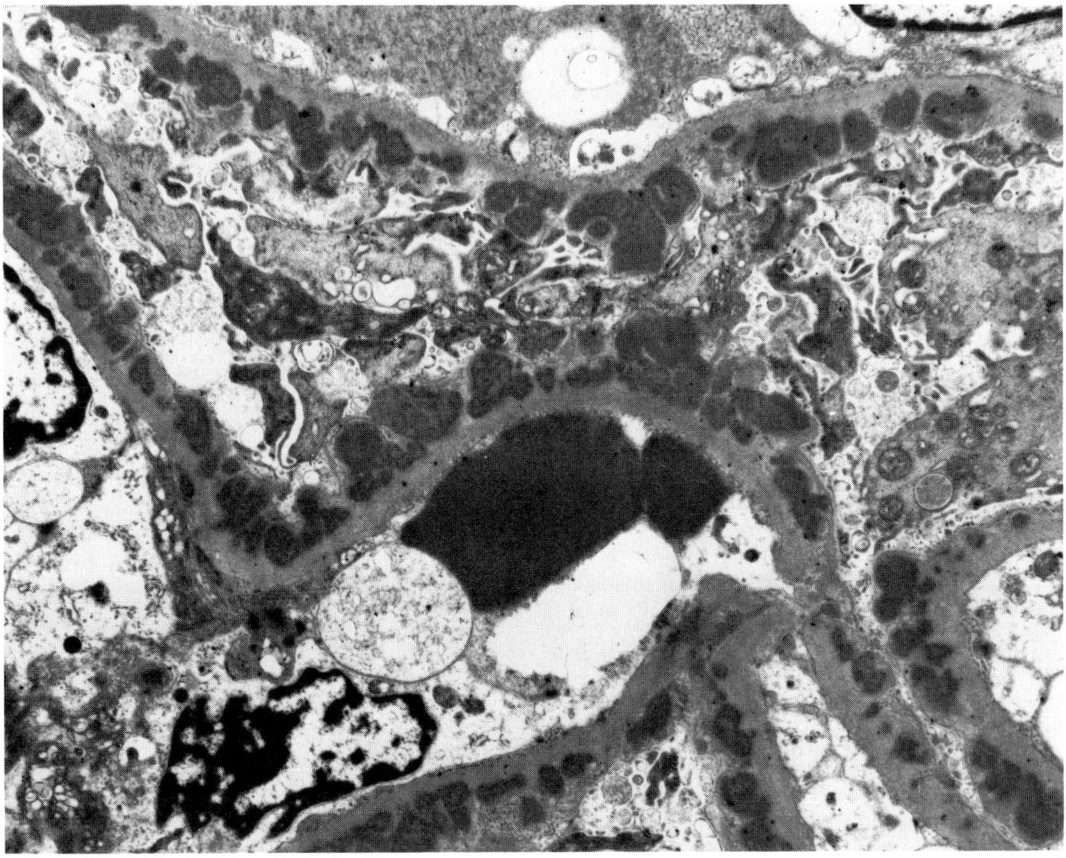

Figure 6–16. The diffusely distributed subepithelial deposits vary widely in their size and shape. (×7500.)

which urinary sediment abnormalities have occasioned a renal biopsy, the glomeruli have shown a mild, focal mesangial proliferative and sclerotic lesion. Immunofluorescence microscopic examination of these biopsies revealed granular deposits of IgG, IgM, IgA, and complement. Electron microscopic examination confirmed the presence of deposits in the mesangium and their absence in other sites.

RHEUMATOID ARTHRITIS

Patients with rheumatoid arthritis seldom have renal lesions related to the primary disease. Almost all of the renal lesions reported in these patients are due to a complication of therapy. However, AA amyloidosis may complicate long-standing disease. The following list includes the common causes:

1. Renal lesions directly related to rheumatoid arthritis
   a. Amyloidosis
   b. Glomerulosclerosis (rare and mild)
   c. Vasculitis (rare)
2. Renal lesions associated with therapeutic agents
   a. Gold salts: membranous glomerulonephritis
   b. Penicillamine: membranous glomerulonephritis
   c. Non-steroidal anti-inflammatory drugs: minimal lesion and acute interstitial nephritis
   d. Analgesics: chronic interstitial nephritis (See Chapter 5 for a description of the lesions associated with these.)

SELECTED READINGS

1. Appel G, Cohen D, Pirani C, et al: Long-term follow-up of patients with lupus nephritis. Am J Med 83:877, 1987.
2. Appel GB, Silva FG, Pirani LL, et al: Renal involvement in systemic lupus erythematosus. Medicine 57:371, 1978.
3. Balow JE, Austin HA, Muenz LR, et al: Effect of treatment on the evaluation of renal abnormalities in lupus nephritis. N Engl J Med 311:491, 1986.
4. Brentgens JR, Sepulveda M, Baliah T, et al: Interstitial immune complex nephritis in patients with systemic lupus erythematosus. Kidney Int 7:342, 1975.
5. D'Agati VD, Appel GB, Estes D, et al: Monoclonal antibody identification of infiltrating mononuclear leucocytes in lupus nephritis. Kidney Int 30:573, 1986.
6. Font J, Torras A, Cervera R, et al: Silent renal disease in systemic lupus erythematosus. Clin Nephrol 27:283, 1987.
7. Hill GS, Hinglais N, Tron F, et al: Systemic lupus erythematosus. Morphologic correlations with immunologic and clinical data at the time of biopsy. Am J Med 64:61, 1978.
8. Magil AB, Ballon HS, Chan V, et al: Diffuse proliferative lupus glomerulonephritis. Determination of prognostic significance of clinical, laboratory, and pathologic factors. Medicine 63:210, 1984.
9. McCluskey RT: Lupus nephritis. *In* Sommers SC (ed): Kidney Pathology Decennial. Appleton-Century-Crofts, New York, 1975, p 456.
10. Morel-Maroger L, Mery J, Droz D, et al: The course of lupus nephritis: Contribution of serial renal biopsies. Adv Nephrol 76:118, 1976.
11. Schwartz MM, Kawaia K, Roberts JL, et al: Clinical and pathological features of membranous glomerulonephritis of systemic lupus erythematosus. Am Nephrol 4:301, 1984.
12. Schwartz MM, Shu-Ping Lan MA, Bonsib SM, et al: Clinical outcome of three discrete histologic patterns of injury in severe lupus glomerulonephritis. Am J Kidney Dis 13:273, 1989.
13. Sellars L, Siamopoulos K, Wilkinson R, et al: Renal biopsy appearances in rheumatoid disease. Clin Nephrol 20:114, 1983.
14. Tan EM, Cohen AS, Fries JF, et al: The 1982 revised criteria for the classification of systemic lupus erythematosus. Arthritis Rheum 25:1271, 1982.

GOODPASTURE'S SYNDROME

Goodpasture's syndrome is characterized by the association of crescentic glomerulonephritis and acute pulmonary disease (often with massive hemorrhage). Long after its first description, it was recognized that this syndrome was often accompanied by circulating antibodies that react with glomerular (and other) basement membranes. At present, the term *Goodpasture's syndrome* is reserved for those patients with all three components—that is, crescentic glomerulonephritis, pulmonary involvement, and circulating anti-glomerular basement membrane antibodies. Because there are other forms of crescentic glomerulonephritis and these may have pulmonary involvement, it is imperative that the renal biopsy specimen be examined by immunofluorescence microscopy, paying special attention to the presence and distribution of glomerular immunoglobulin deposits.

Pathogenesis (see Chapter 4)

Patient Presentation

Goodpasture's syndrome is more common in males and is frequently preceded by a flulike illness. Despite attempts to document viral infection, either by culture or by change in serum antibody titers, the association with a viral agent remains unproven. Similarly, a small number of case reports suggest a relationship between solvent exposure and this syndrome. Again, the evidence in humans does not support such a conclusion, and the disease cannot be reproduced in experimental animals.

The antibodies are directed against the non-helical portion of the type IV collagen molecules in the glomerular basement membrane. This antigen has now been isolated and studied in detail and has been called the Goodpasture's epitope. This antigen is common to all patients with this syndrome and is lacking in patients with Alport's syndrome.

A small amount of epidemiologic data are available on this syndrome. As noted previously, it is most common in males and in Caucasians. Although it is found in all age-groups except young children, it is most common between the second and fourth decades of life. There appears to be a seasonal incidence, peaking in spring or summer, and many pathologists with referral renal biopsy practices have commented on the fact that the outbreaks tend to be geographically localized.

Pulmonary hemorrhage is a serious complication. It is essentially restricted to patients who are smokers or who are exposed to pulmonary injury. The pulmonary lesion begins early in the disease course and may precede the renal symptoms.

Hypertension is not often severe, unless there is marked fluid overload.

Macroscopic hematuria and loin pain may be the first signs of the syndrome and cause the patient to consult a physician. Shortly thereafter, oliguria or anuria becomes evident. The urine sediment is filled with casts of all types, cellular compositions, and sizes (the so-called telescope urine sediment). The amount of protein per unit volume is large, but because patients are often severely oliguric, the 24-hour urine protein excretion may not be greatly elevated.

Histology

Light Microscopy

The classic lesion is a crescentic glomerulonephritis (Figs. 6–17 and 6–18). The glomerular tufts are collapsed, and a large mass of cells occupies Bowman's space. It should be recognized, however, that a spectrum of glomerular lesions may be associated with this syndrome, and the renal lesions may not be as severe as those in the pulmonary tract. Thus, the glomerular crescents may be irregular in distribution and severity, with some glomeruli occupied by crescents and others with focal epithelial cell lesions (Fig. 6–19).

There are rarely intraglomerular changes. In fact, the presence of proliferation or exudation pathologic within glomerular tufts should raise the question of some other process. The only caveat is that we have seen a few patients whose initial biopsy revealed rather modest lesions and who developed a severe glomerular disease shortly thereafter.

Bowman's capsule remains intact in many cases. When it is interrupted, the crescent resolves only by sclerosis. Thus there may be prognostic significance in determining the state of its integrity, because it is thought that some cellular crescents may resolve with appropriate therapy.

Immunofluorescence Microscopy

The diagnosis of Goodpasture's syndrome rests entirely on the presence of linear glomerular basement membrane deposits of IgG. Essentially all patients with circulating anti-glomerular basement membrane anti-

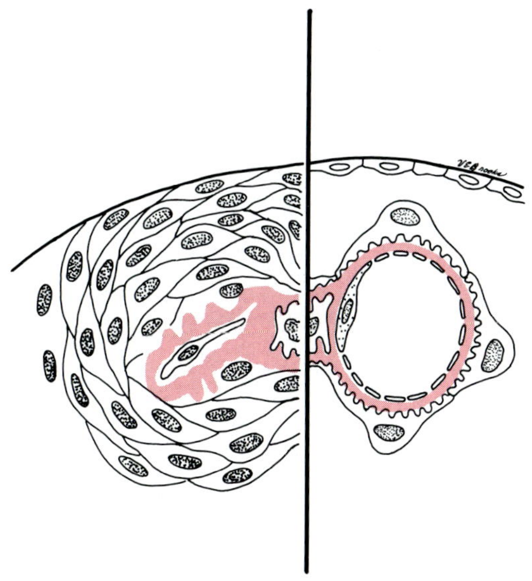

Figure 6–17. Diagram of diffuse epithelial cell proliferation.

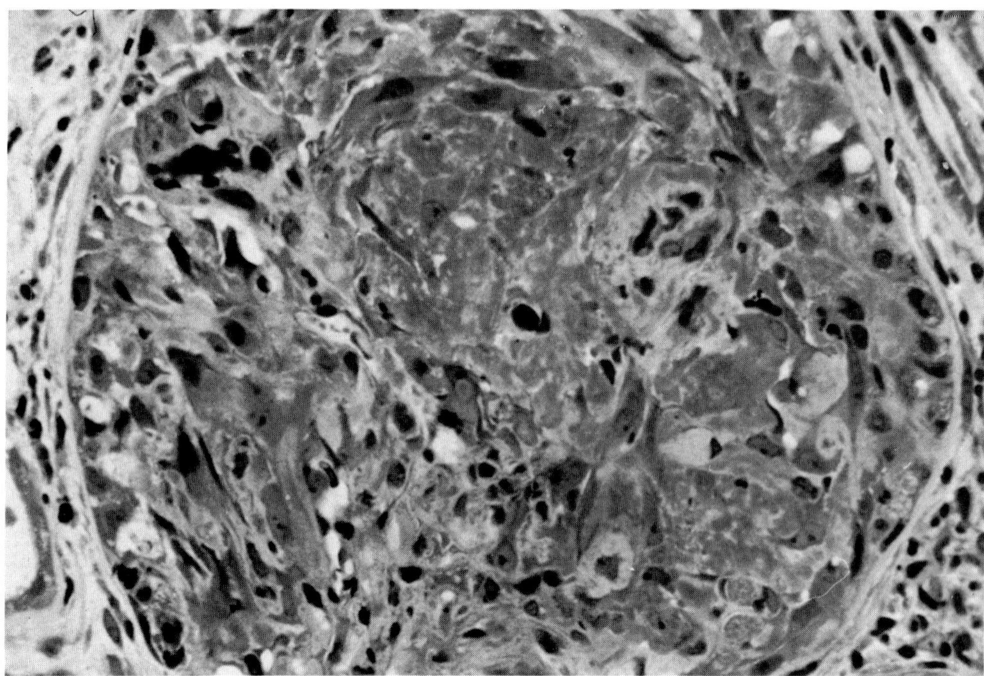

Figure 6–18. Diffuse crescent formation occupying the urinary space. There are large amounts of fibrin lying between the cells. The glomerular tufts are collapsed and barely visible within the crescent. (H&E, ×400.)

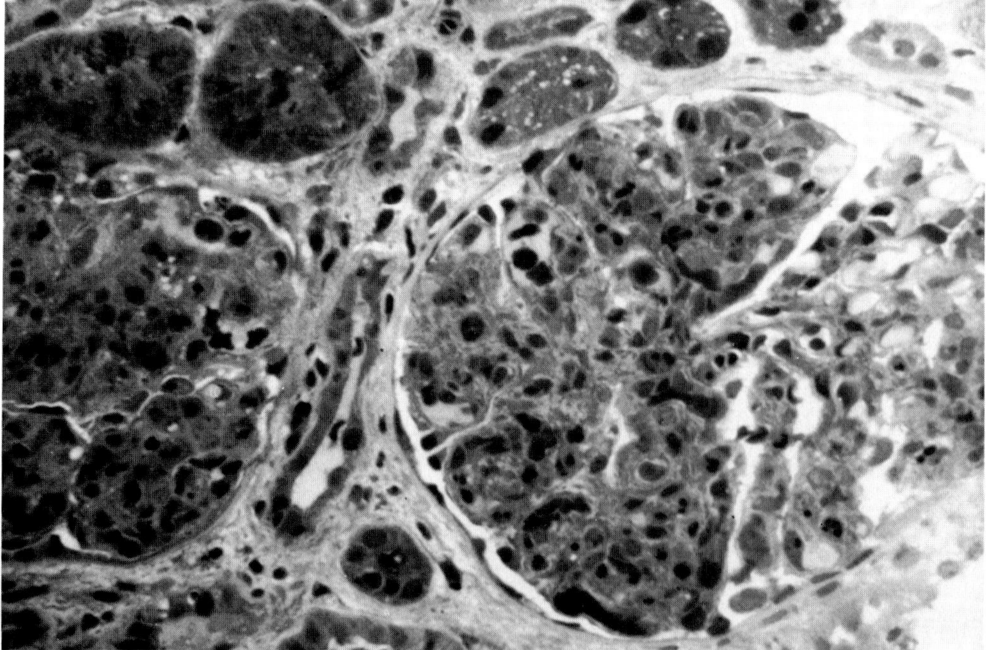

Figure 6–19. Two glomeruli that are irregularly affected by a proliferative and exudative lesion. The epithelial cell proliferation is irregular in distribution and not as prominent as that in Figure 6–18. (H&E, ×300.)

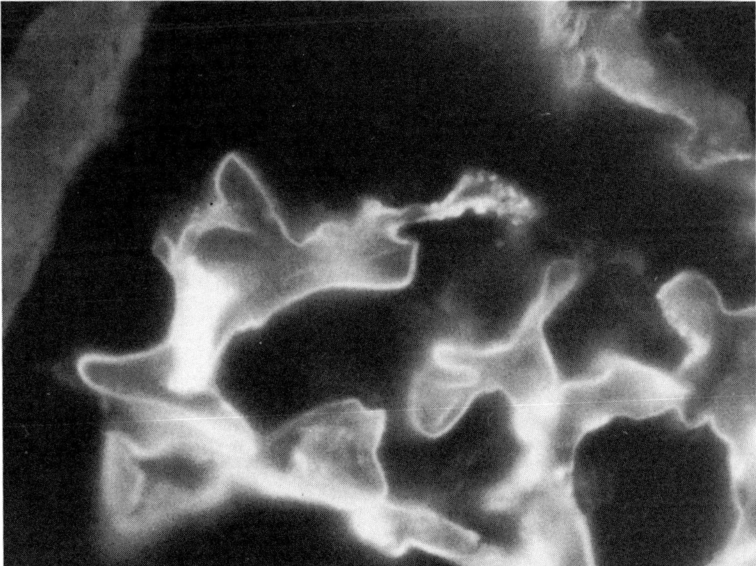

Figure 6–20. Immunofluorescence micrograph, anti-IgG. There is a linear deposit outlining the glomerular basement membranes. (×500.)

body have linear deposits (Fig. 6–20). Note, however, that some patients with linear glomerular basement membrane deposits of IgG have either low or undetectable levels of serum antibodies. The immunofluorescence findings are also important to rule out other causes of crescentic glomerulonephritis, such as antigen-antibody complex diseases, nonimmune glomerulonephritis, and vasculitis (see Chapter 4 and later in this chapter).

The patient's serum can be used to stain frozen sections of normal kidney and lung tissue as a preliminary, crude screening test for anti-glomerular basement membrane antibodies.

Electron Microscopy

The electron microscopic findings are useful to rule out the presence of immune deposits in those biopsies in which there is no tissue available for immunofluorescence analysis.

Prognosis

A number of new therapeutic strategies have been introduced in the past decade, including plasmapheresis, high-dose pulse steroids, and cytotoxic drugs. Each form has its proponents, and good results have been obtained when the underlying renal lesions have either been early in the course or when the underlying extracellular matrix architecture has been preserved. As mentioned earlier, the disruption of basement membranes bodes a poor therapeutic response. Another indicator of a poor response is the presence of anuria and advanced renal failure at initial presentation.

The serum levels of anti-glomerular basement membrane antibodies gradually diminish in most patients. The absolute levels or their persistence is not correlated with the ultimate outcome. Some patients with recurrence of measurable serum antibody levels have been reported, but the significance of this observation is not clear because it does not appear to be related to relapses of the syndrome. Relapses of the syndrome have been reported after bacterial or viral infections. As before, the ultimate outcome depends on the extent of the injury and the response to therapy.

SELECTED READING

1. Wilson CB, Dixon FJ: Antiglomerular basement membrane antibody-induced glomerulonephritis. Kidney Int 3:74, 1974

HENOCH-SCHÖNLEIN PURPURA

Henoch-Schönlein purpura, or anaphylactoid purpura, is a clinical syndrome that has also been called Schönlein-Henoch syndrome or purpura. This syndrome predominately affects children but has also been reported in adults. The characteristic findings include skin rash, arthralgias, hematuria, and gastrointestinal involvement.

The incidence of nephropathy in this disease, although quite high, varies widely (from 22 to 66%) between different reports.

During the past few decades, some confusion has been introduced into the literature since the discovery that glomerular IgA deposits were universally present in patients with Henoch-Schönlein purpura. The pattern of glomerular immune deposits is similar to that in IgA glomerulonephritis, leading some investigators to conclude that there are a group of nephropathies linked by the common finding of IgA deposits in the glomeruli. Henoch-Schönlein purpura and IgA nephropathy might therefore represent variants of a similar underlying disorder. Whether this represents an oversimplification or whether there are common pathogenetic factors remains to be proved. There clearly are immunologic abnormalities resulting in glomerular IgA deposits in both disorders, and in occasional reports both diseases have been expressed in family members within a short time frame. The main argument against a common pathogenetic process is that the two glomerular lesions have a strikingly dissimilar prognosis. The clinical course in IgA nephropathy is one of a slowly progressive loss of renal function in more than one-third of the patients, and it is the most common cause of end-stage renal disease due to glomerulonephritis in the Western world. This course of events contrasts sharply with the nephritis in Henoch-Schönlein purpura, in which the overwhelming majority of patients have no long-term renal sequelae. Those who eventually develop end-stage renal failure most often have evidence of severe renal disease at the onset of the clinical syndrome and represent a very small number of those with Henoch-Schönlein purpura.

Pathogenesis

Henoch-Schönlein purpura is often considered a hypersensitivity or leukocytoclastic vasculitis based on the presence of fibrinoid necrosis in the wall of capillaries of the skin and several other organs. The role of IgA complexes in the causation of this disease has been extensively investigated and has provided the most compelling evidence for a link between Henoch-Schönlein purpura and IgA nephropathy. IgA complexes are present in the peripheral circulation in both IgA nephropathy and Henoch-Schönlein purpura. In addition, both diseases tend to be found in the same geographic areas and affect the same types of patients.

The pathogenesis of the nephritis is unknown, although most investigators agree that the renal disease is somehow related to the presence of circulating IgA complexes. Elevated IgA levels are present in approximately one-half of the patients. As in IgA nephropathy, it has been proposed that the patients have a defect in the handling of antigens presented to the gastrointestinal mucosa and pulmonary epithelium. It has been suggested that this is the reason for the common association of acute respiratory and gastrointestinal complaints, including allergic responses, in these patients.

The role of genetic factors has yet to be determined.

Patient Presentation

The first signs of renal disease usually appear after an upper respiratory tract infection but may follow immunizations, drug ingestion, and apparent gastrointestinal viral infections. Hematuria is invariably present and may be macroscopic. Proteinuria, in contrast, is most often moderate. When the nephrotic syndrome is present, the underlying renal lesions are frequently severe and the few patients thus affected follow a rapidly progressive course to renal failure.

Serum complement levels are usually normal, although circulating immune complexes are a common feature of the acute phase of the disease.

Hypertension may be present.

Interestingly, patients may have multiple episodes of the syndrome, with each episode having the same benign outcome.

Histology

Light Microscopy

The lesions are variable but most often consist of very minor changes. To a large extent, the initial glomerular lesions appear to be a reasonable indicator of the long-term outlook, unlike that in IgA nephropathy. The International Study of Kidney Disease in Children suggested a means to classify the lesions into different grades based on the renal biopsy findings. However, renal biopsies are not routinely performed on these patients, because of the well-known benign outcome of the renal disease. Thus, the reports on the renal findings in Henoch-Schönlein purpura must be interpreted in light of the fact that rather than evaluating the entire spectrum of the renal disease, one is only viewing renal biopsy specimens of patients in whom there is a strong suspicion of the existence of lesions that are severe and unusual.

The classic description of the glomerular changes in Henoch-Schönlein purpura is focal and segmental glomerulonephritis, often associated with tiny foci of fibrin deposition (so-called necrotic areas) (Fig. 6–21). These findings are present in only a small number of patients, and the most frequent change is mild to moderate mesangial proliferation. Even this finding has been called into question because it has not been subjected to rigorous analysis by morphometric techniques. Thus, one is often left with the impression that there is mild proliferation as the principal lesion. Neutrophils may occasionally be present in small numbers. The mesangial accentuation has led some authors to append the designation mesangial arborization to the description of the glomeruli.

The glomerular changes in patients with more severe lesions may reveal areas of widespread necrosis of the glomerular tufts with the formation of thrombi, karyorrhexis, nuclear debris, and crescents in the adjacent Bowman's spaces (Fig. 6–22). These changes are most often seen in nephrotic patients with macroscopic hematuria. The proportion of glomeruli with crescents has been proposed to be a good indicator of the outcome, with crescent formation in large numbers of glomeruli representing a poor prognosis. In such cases, unlike that in IgA nephropathy, the mesangial proliferation is diffuse and the peripheral glomerular basement membranes may be duplicated, giving them an appearance resembling that of type I membranoproliferative glomerulonephritis. This has been called pseudo-membranoproliferative glomerulonephritis. More rarely, there may be diffuse circumferential crescents. Even in these cases, however, the underlying mesangial proliferation is still apparent.

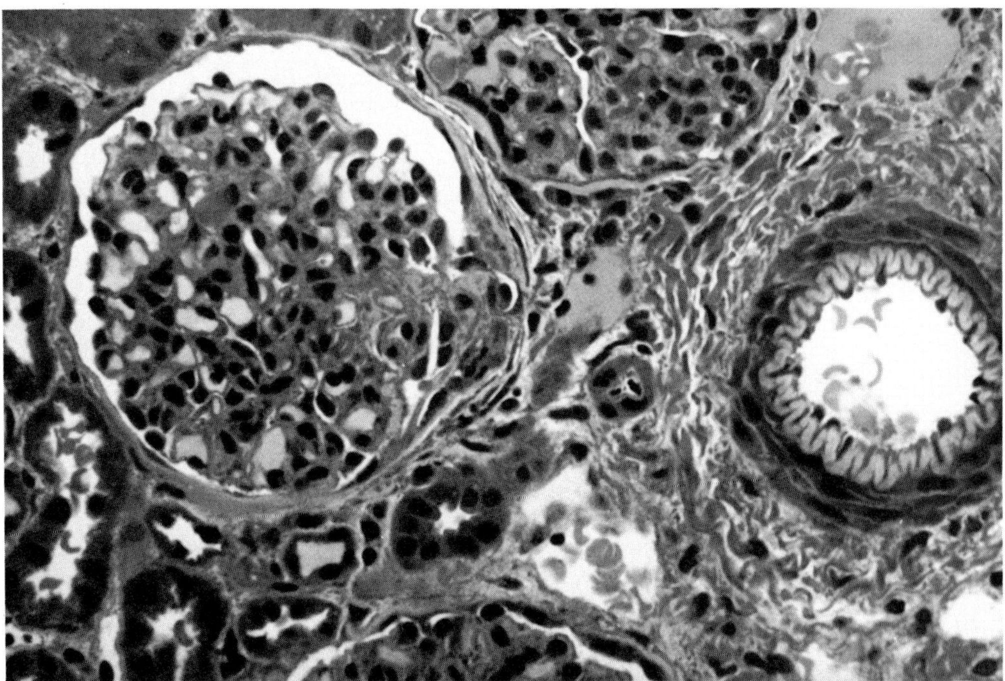

Figure 6–21. The glomerulus has a synechia in the right mid-quadrant, and the hypercellularity is accentuated in this area. The interstitium and tubules are relatively unaffected. The connective tissue surrounding the blood vessel is normal in amount. (H&E, ×300.)

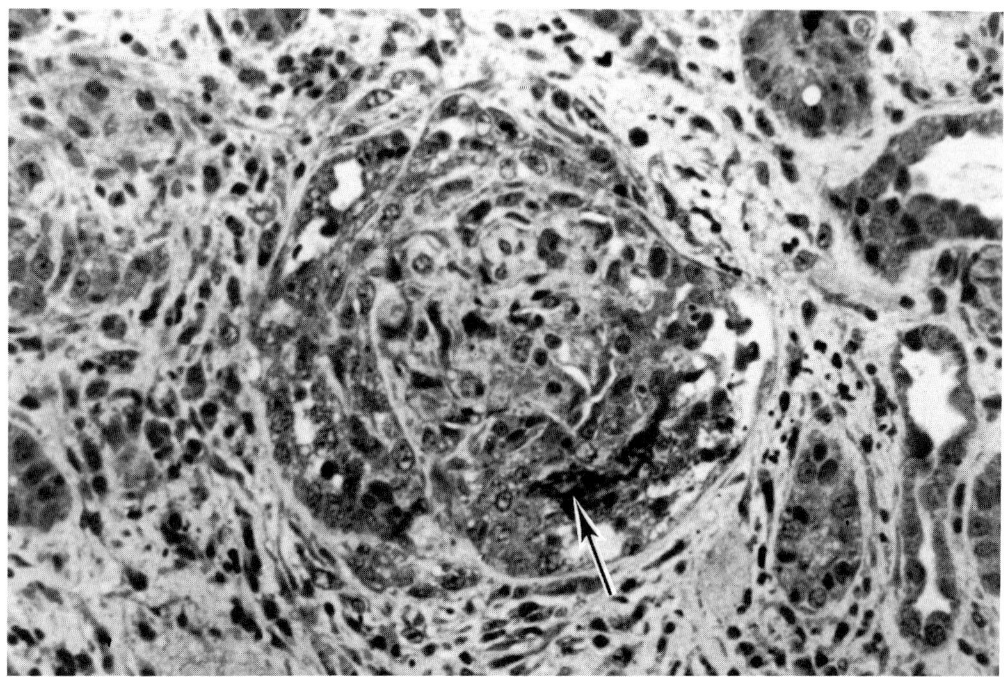

Figure 6–22. A large crescent occupies Bowman's space, and the underlying glomerulus is collapsed. Fibrin deposits (arrow) are found between the cells of the crescent. (Masson's trichrome, ×300.)

In long-standing disease, areas of glomerular sclerosis replace the necrotic foci, and localized crescents are replaced by fibrous synechiae (Fig. 6–23). The glomeruli ultimately become obsolescent. The tubulo-interstitial and vascular lesions parallel the glomerular lesions in the sclerotic stages.

The proposed classification is as follows:

Grade I: Minimal alterations
Grade II: Pure mesangial proliferation
Grade III: Less than 50% crescents
  a. Focal mesangial proliferation
  b. Diffuse mesangial proliferation
Grade IV: 50 to 75% crescents.
  Focal mesangial proliferation
  Diffuse mesangial proliferation
Grade V: More than 75% crescents
  a. Focal mesangial proliferation
  b. Diffuse mesangial proliferation
Grade VI: Pseudo-membranoproliferative glomerulonephritis

Immunofluorescence Microscopy

There are diffuse deposits of IgA in each mesangial region, even in those cases in which the glomeruli are essentially normal by light microscopy. The deposits contain IgA in a granular pattern. IgG and C3 codistribute with IgA, and there are small amounts of IgM (Fig. 6–24). There have been several reports on the presence of fibrin/fibrinogen antigens in the mesangial regions, even when there is no evidence of necrosis by light microscopy. Areas of necrosis, of course, contain large masses of material containing fibrin/fibrinogen antigens. In the presence of severe glomerular lesions, large and coarsely granular deposits of IgA and C3 extend along the peripheral glomerular basement membranes (Fig. 6–25). C1q, C4, and other complement components are not often present, although some have reported that $beta_1$-H and properdin may be present in the mesangium. Extraglomerular deposits are not frequent, but there are reports of IgA and C3 along interstitial capillary walls.

Electron Microscopy

The mesangial regions contain electron-dense deposits in the extracellular matrix; these are concentrated in the paramesangial areas. In patients with crescents, "gaps" may be seen. Occasional biopsies reveal subepithelial, electron-dense deposits (Fig. 6–26).

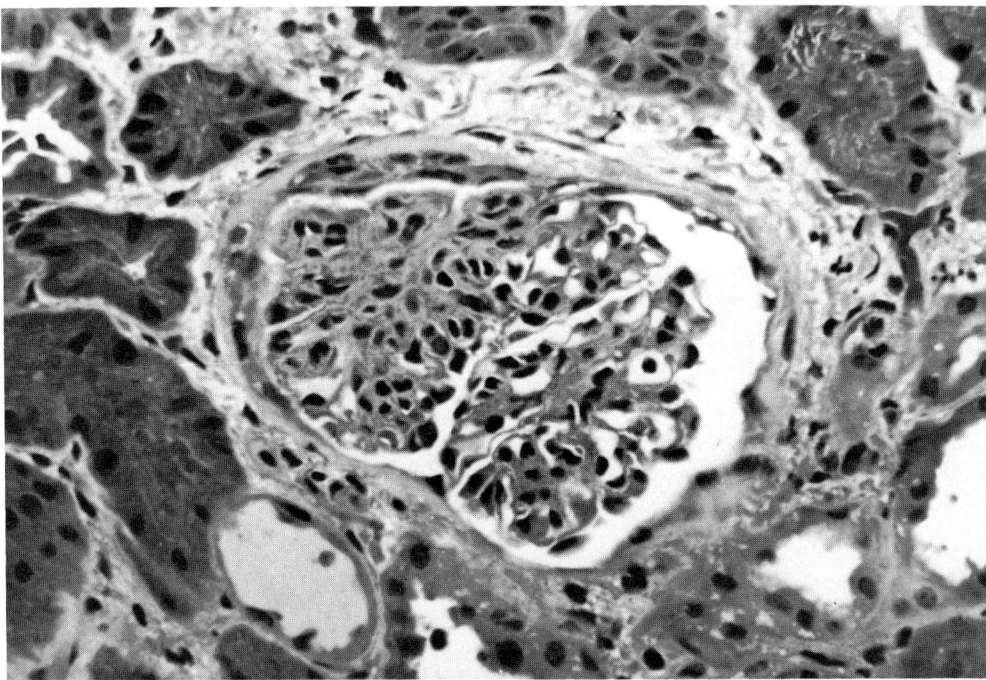

Figure 6–23. Almost one-half of the glomerulus is occupied by mesangial sclerosis and proliferation. The rest of the glomerulus is much less affected. The interstitium adjacent to the synechia (top mid-portion) is widened, and Bowman's capsule is thickened and duplicated. (H&E, ×300.)

Figure 6–24. Immunofluorescence micrograph, anti-IgG. Each mesangial region contains large deposits. (×100.)

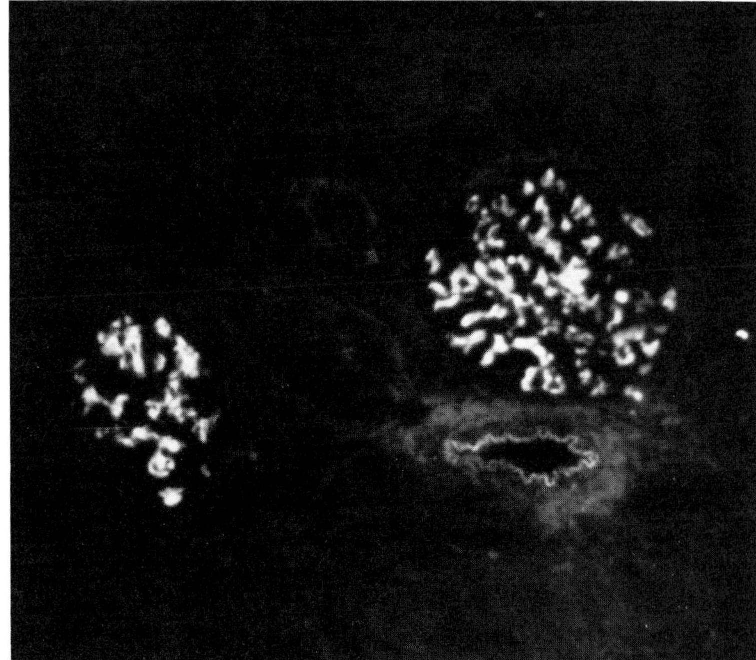

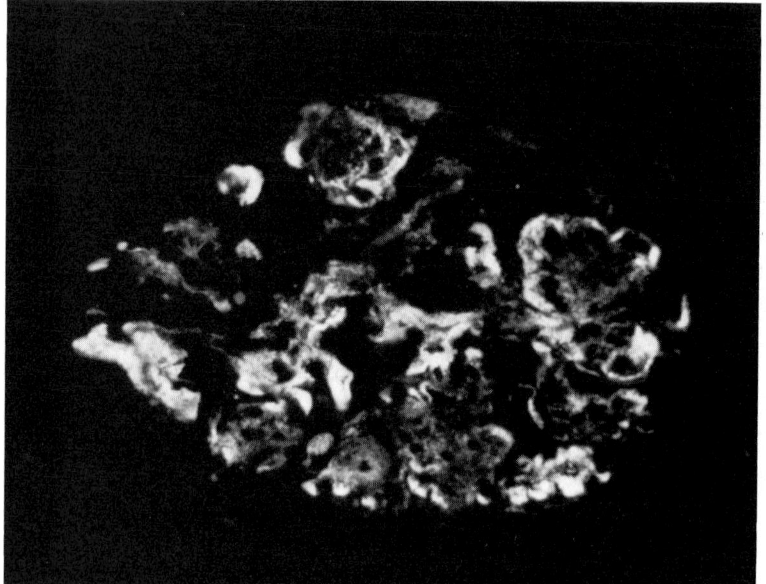

Figure 6–25. Immunofluorescence micrograph, anti-IgA. Note that these deposits occupy both the subendothelial and mesangial regions. (×250.)

Prognosis

As noted earlier, most patients with Henoch-Schönlein purpura have some hematuria and thus have a glomerular lesion. However, in the overwhelming majority of such patients, there are no long-term sequelae. Even in patients with focal areas of necrosis or crescents, the prognosis for complete resolution remains excellent. These comments also apply to patients with multiple exacerbations and remissions. Those who have the nephrotic syndrome and impaired renal function at the outset seem to have a poor prognosis, despite attempts to modify the course with various types of immunosuppressive regimens.

SELECTED READINGS

1. Fogazzi GB, Pasquali S, Moriggi M, et al: Long-term outcome of Schönlein-Henoch nephritis in the adult. Clin Nephrol 31:60, 1989.
2. Levy M, Broyer M, Arsan A, et al: Anaphylactoid purpura nephritis in childhood: Natural history and immunopathology. *In* Hamburger J, Crosnier J, Maxwell MH (eds): Advances in Nephrology. Yearbook Medical Publishers, Chicago, 1976, p 183.
3. Meadow SR, Glasgow EF, White RHR, et al: Schönlein-Henoch nephritis Q J Med 41:241, 1972.
4. Yoshikawa N, Ito H, Yoshiya K, et al: Henoch-Schönlein nephritis and IgA nephropathy in children: A comparison of clinical course. Clin Nephrol 27:233, 1987.

THROMBOTIC MICROANGIOPATHY

There are a group of diseases of the microvasculature that are characterized by endothelial injury and activation of the coagulation cascade. Syndromes in which these lesions occur include the hemolytic-uremic syndrome, thrombocytopenic purpura, and post-partum renal failure. The development of thrombi is directly correlated with the severity of the injury and is inversely correlated with the outcome. In addition, the outcome depends on the site of renal vascular involvement. The least severe lesions involve only the glomeruli, and the outlook worsens as progressively large blood vessels manifest injury. The vascular lesions that characterize thrombotic microangiopathy may be present as part of a systemic disease (thrombotic thrombocytopenic purpura) or may be restricted to the kidneys (hemolytic-uremic syndrome). The condition has been observed in acute post-partum renal failure (see Chapter 10) and has been reported as a consequence of mitomycin C and cyclosporine A toxicity.

Pathogenesis

Although the pathogenesis is far from completely elucidated, abnormalities of the coagulation system resulting in an endothelial lesion are believed to be the initiating factors leading to these syndromes. The similarity of the lesions, in the diverse syndromes mentioned earlier, has led to the concept that the glomerular and arteriolar abnormalities result from the same pathogenic events. Several hypotheses have been offered to explain the development of microthrombi in the glomeruli. Most investigators agree that endothelial damage is the key event in the pathogenesis of the glomerular and arteriolar lesions. Although the etiology of the vascular damage is not clear, multiple stimuli, including endotoxin, tumor necrosis factor, and immune complexes can induce endothelial damage in experimental animals. Platelets adhere to the damaged endothelium, and after release of various peptides and enzymes, fibrin thrombi form in the glomerular and/or arteriolar lumina. It has been proposed that patients with this disease lack a plasma factor that regulates the production of prostaglandin PGI-2 by the blood vessels. It has also been shown that the endothelial cells normally produce plasminogen activating factor and that this activity is depressed in patients with microangiopathy.

It is likely that the various syndromes associated with thrombotic microangiopathy have diverse etiologies and that the thrombocytopenia and renal lesions are the end result of the disease process. The rationale to consider these diseases together is that they show comparable lesions, and all appear to be linked to endothelial damage.

The diseases associated with thrombotic microangiopathy are as follows:

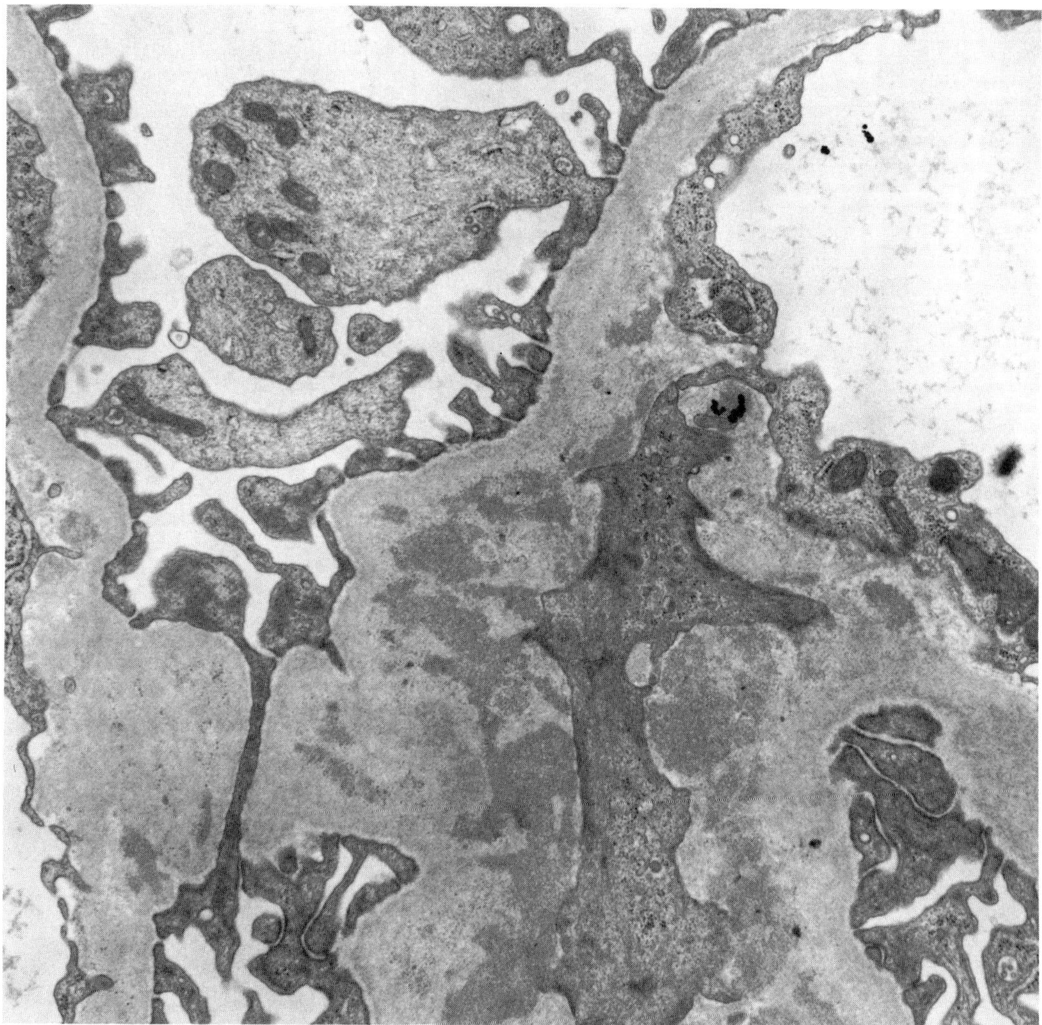

Figure 6–26. The subendothelial space is irregularly widened. The mesangium contains large, electron-dense deposits. (×5000.)

Thrombotic thrombocytopenic purpura
Hemolytic-uremic syndrome
Acute post-partum renal failure
Drug intoxication
 Mitomycin C
 Cyclosporine A
 Oral contraceptive agents

Patient Presentation

The frequency of these syndromes is difficult to estimate. Thrombotic thrombocytopenic purpura primarily affects young adults, with a female predominance. The disease is characterized by fever, hemolytic anemia, and acute renal failure. Significant hypertension is present in many patients.

The hemolytic-uremic syndrome is most commonly found in children or infants, although it may afflict adults. It may occasionally occur in the absence of hematologic involvement.

These diseases can be triggered by various viral or bacterial infections. A prodrome phase of diarrhea often precedes the renal symptoms. Anemia is always present and is often associated with signs of hemolysis and a decline in haptoglobin levels, the so-called microangiopathic anemia. Schistocytosis is almost constant, and fragmented erythrocytes may be found in glomeruli and arterioles.

Histology

Light Microscopy

There are two varieties of thrombotic microangiopathy: that in which the glomerular lesion predominates and that in which the microvascular lesions also include the arterioles. Although the lesions constitute a continuous spectrum of renal disease, this approach provides for more consistent evaluation and some prognostic information.

The glomerular loops appear large and fill the urinary space. The most conspicuous abnormality is swelling of the glomerular endothelium, resulting in a marked decrease in the lumen (Figs. 6–27 and 6–28). The glomerular basement membranes are multilaminated by silver stain, whereas they have a fluffy appearance with indistinct margins by H&E. Fibrin thrombi are often present and contribute to the severe reduction in the size of the vascular lumen (Fig. 6–29). Fragmented red blood cells may be observed in the lumen. There is a modest increase in the number of mesangial cell nuclei in occasional patients (Fig. 6–30). The mesangial spaces often appear fibrillar (mesangiolysis), but in patients who have arteriolar lesions this change is not so marked and is replaced by thickening and wrinkling of the glomerular basement membranes identical to that observed in chronic ischemic lesions.

Neutrophils and macrophages are never found in these glomeruli, in our experience.

As the lesions become chronic, the capillary loop widening decreases, to be replaced by areas of segmental collapse with sclerosis of the loops and thickening of Bowman's capsules. This progressive glomerular ischemia is accompanied by an increase in Bowman's space. This lesion is essentially only seen in patients with arteriolar and/or arterial changes.

The interstitium appears widened by diffuse edema, and there are occasional areas of sclerosis. If the lesions progress and renal failure develops, the interstitial fibrosis may become a major component.

Tubular necrosis is a common finding when biopsies are performed on anuric patients. Mitotic figures may be present in regenerating tubular epithelial cells (Fig. 6–31). Profiles of dilated tubular lumina containing fragmented erythrocytes are occasionally noted.

The degree of vascular involvement is well

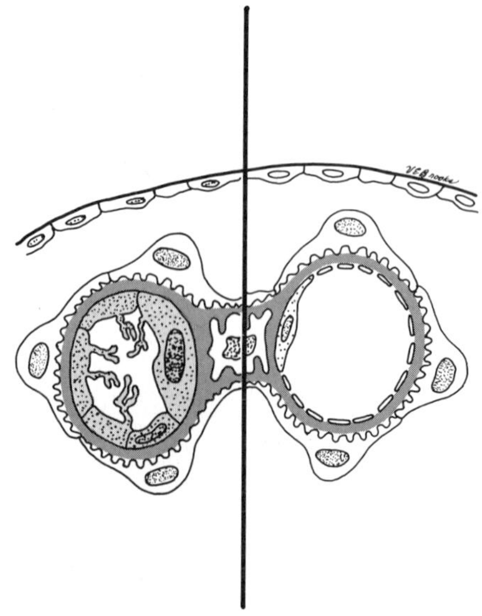

Figure 6–27. Diagram of endothelial swelling.

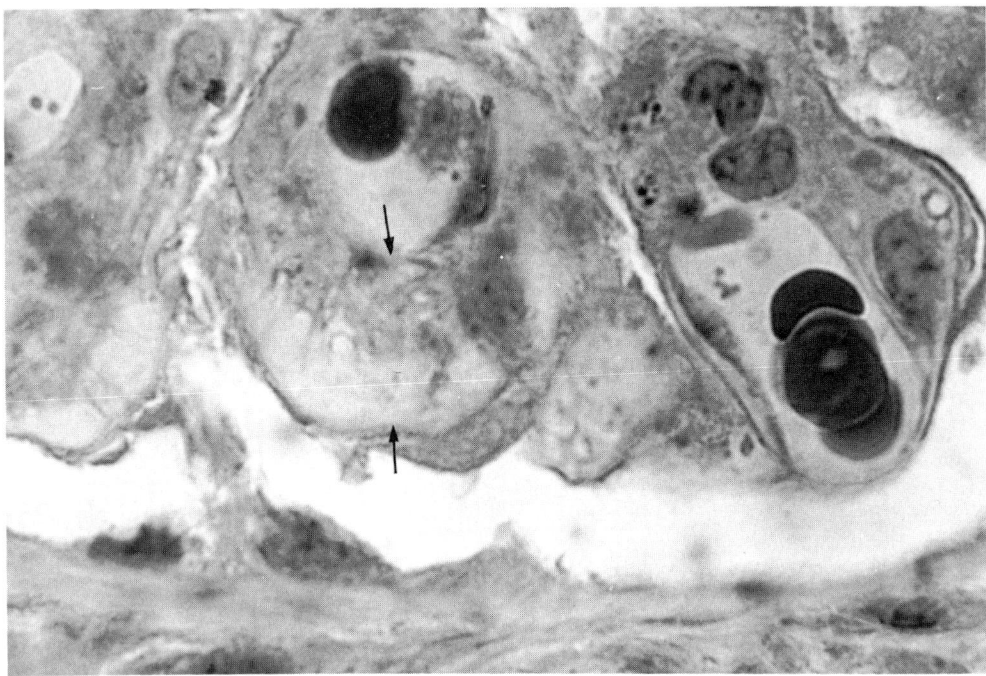

Figure 6–28. The endothelial cells are diffusely swollen (arrow), resulting in a diminution in the size of the vascular space. No inflammatory cells are present. (H&E, ×1200.)

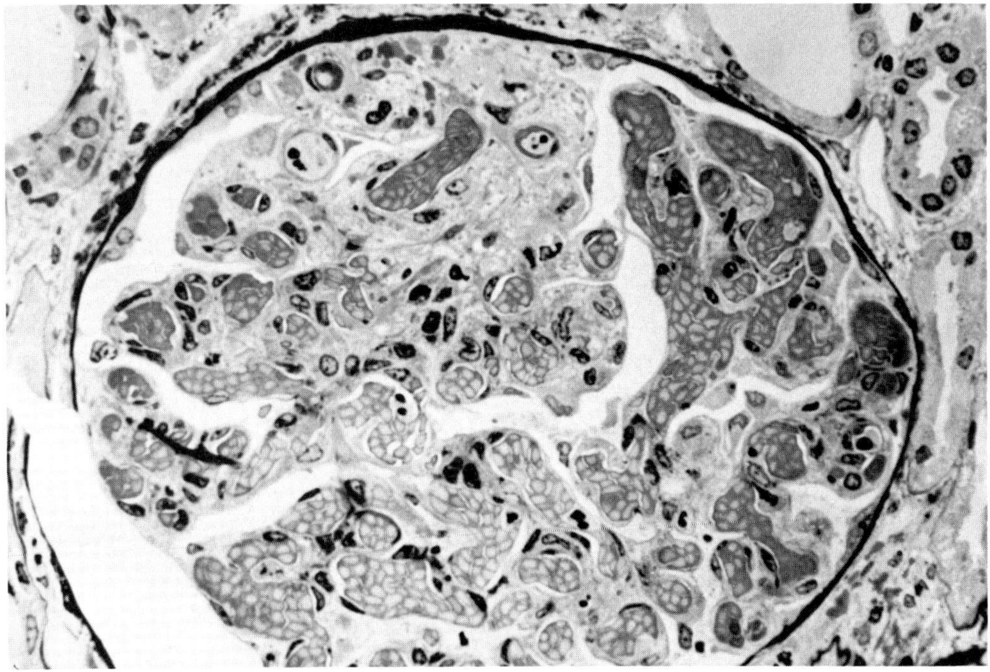

Figure 6–29. This glomerulus is ischemic. The cellular details are obscured, and there are many red blood cells within the vascular spaces. A synechia is still visible at the top of the glomerulus. (PASM, ×300.)

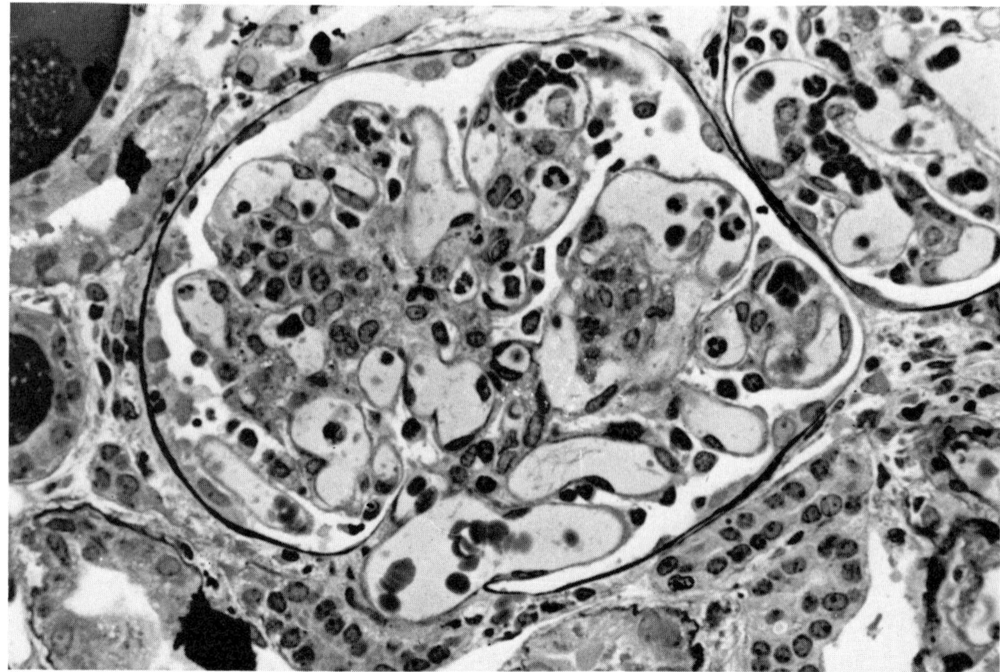

Figure 6–30. The diffuse distribution of the lesion is apparent. The vascular spaces are widely dilated, and many red blood cells and occasional neutrophils are present. (PASM, ×300.)

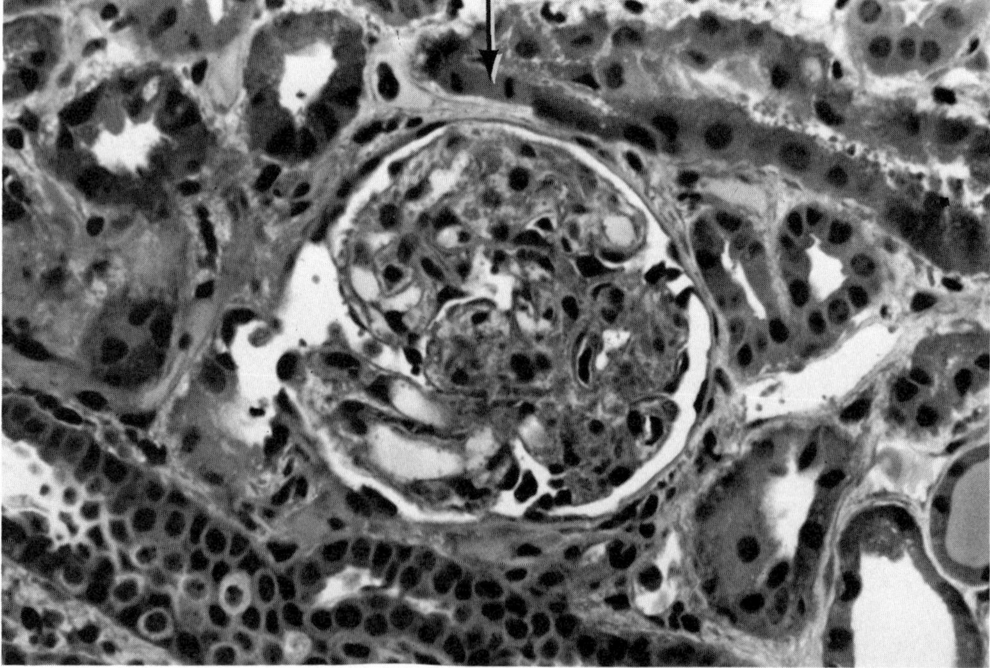

Figure 6–31. The tubules are often affected. The proximal tubule immediatedly above the glomerulus shows a dividing cell (arrow). The brush border is altered, appearing rather granular. The tubular epithelium appears thin in many areas. Many casts are present in this biopsy specimen. (H&E, ×300.)

correlated with the ultimate prognosis. The lesions in patients with little or no arterial damage are much more likely to heal completely than those with prominent arteriolopathy.

The arterioles may show thrombosis, endothelial swelling, necrosis of their walls, and intimal proliferation (Fig. 6–32). In the medium-sized arteries, intimal thickening, necrosis, and thrombosis may be observed (Figs. 6–33 and 6–34). These more severe lesions are predominately found in adult patients.

Immunofluorescence Microscopy

The immunofluorescence microscopic findings are consistent with the underlying pathogenesis of this group of diseases: Immunoglobulins are seldom found, but fibrin/fibrinogen antigens are consistently present in the glomeruli and arterioles (Fig. 6–35). These antigens outline the endothelial lining of the glomeruli and arterioles. This staining pattern affects most glomeruli and all of their segments.

C3 and IgM deposits are occasionally found in the sclerotic areas of advanced cases. These deposits may also be present in the arteries, but these findings have little specificity.

Electron Microscopy

The most characteristic lesion is hypertrophy and swelling of the glomerular endothelium with accumulation of a lucent, fluffy material in both the subendothelial and mesangial regions (Fig. 6–36). The lucent material located between the basement membrane and the endothelium often contains fibrin, fragments of red blood cells, and platelet aggregates or cellular debris. In patients with chronic or persistent changes, a new layer of basement membrane forms on the inner aspect of the original basement membrane, the layers being separated by fluffy, lucent material. The architecture of the basement membrane may thus be severely distorted.

The glomerular vascular loops contain fibrin thrombi and cell debris (Fig. 6–37). Local disruption of the basement membrane with denudation of the endothelium may result in localized aneurysms with dilated vascular loops. The mesangial areas may contain swollen cells with numerous organelles, but proliferation is uncommon. The podo-

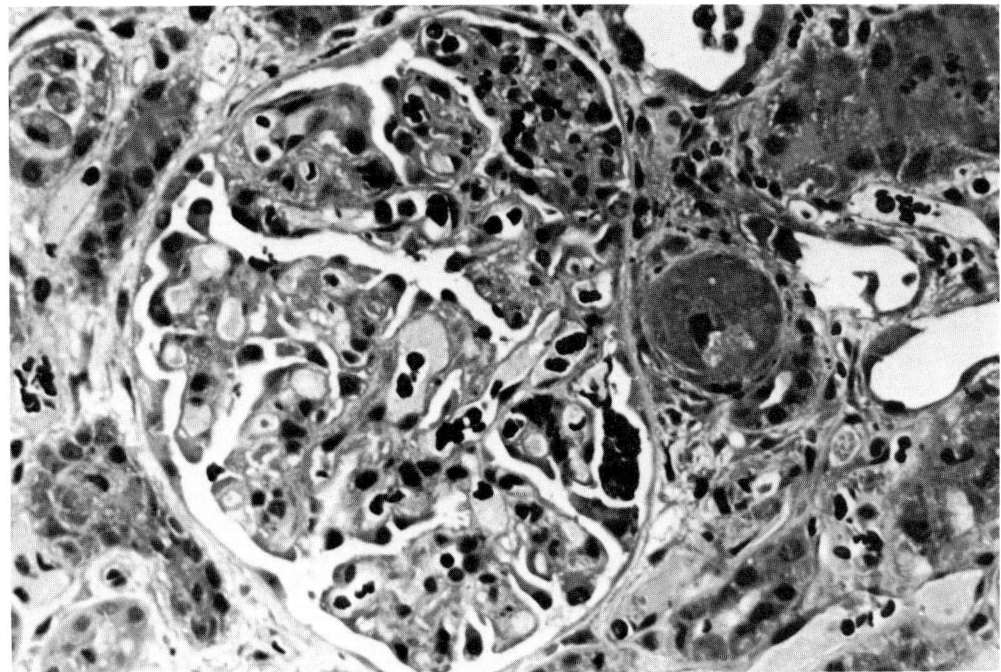

Figure 6–32. The afferent arteriole is almost completely occluded by a thrombus. The glomerulus contains inflammatory cells and a focus of necrosis in the upper right quadrant, and the vascular spaces are sharply diminished in size. The surrounding interstitium is edematous and contains many inflammatory cells. (H&E, ×300.)

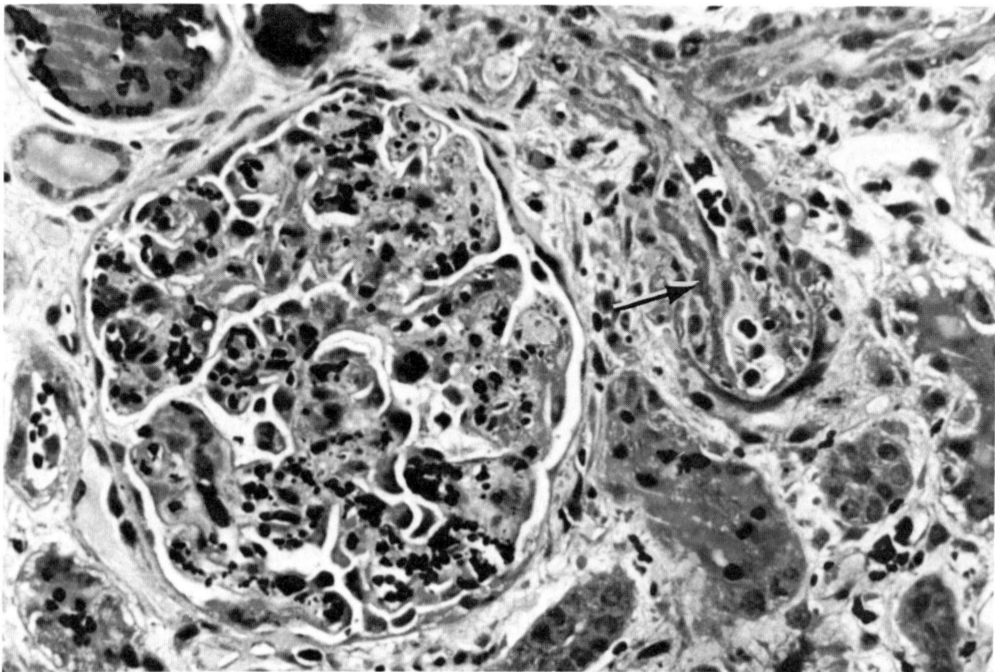

Figure 6–33. The arteriole (right center) shows disruption of the media by inflammatory cells and plasma protein deposits (arrow). The lumen is patent, but there are adherent inflammatory cells and the endothelium is swollen. The adjacent glomerulus contains many degenerating cells, aggregates of red blood cells, and the vascular spaces are small. (H&E, ×300.)

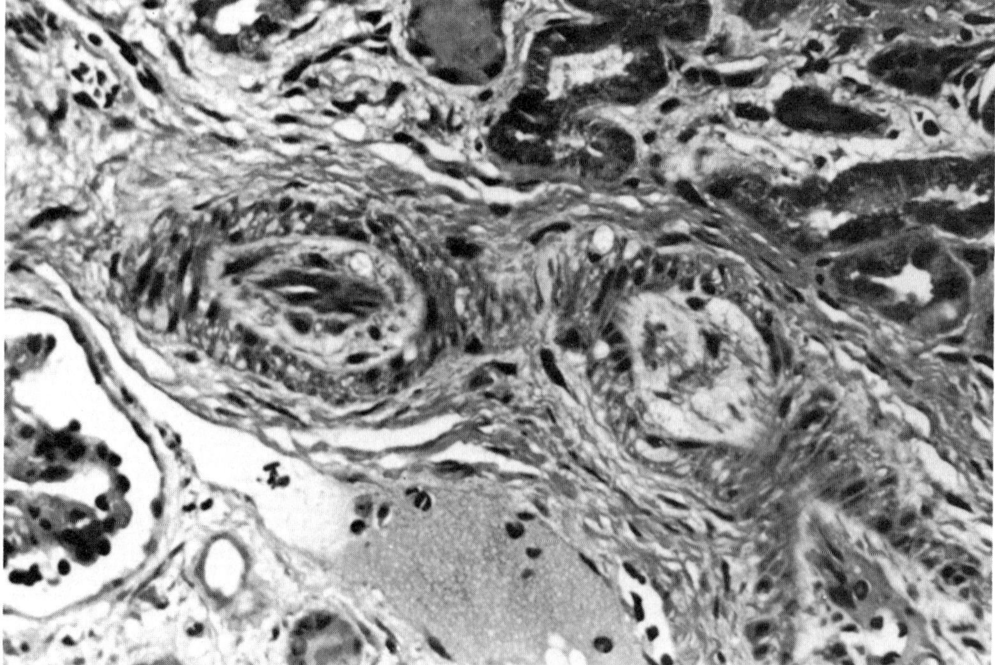

Figure 6–34. The subintimal region is widened by an increase in the number of cells and by a lightly stained extracellular matrix material. The endothelium is swollen. (H&E, ×300.)

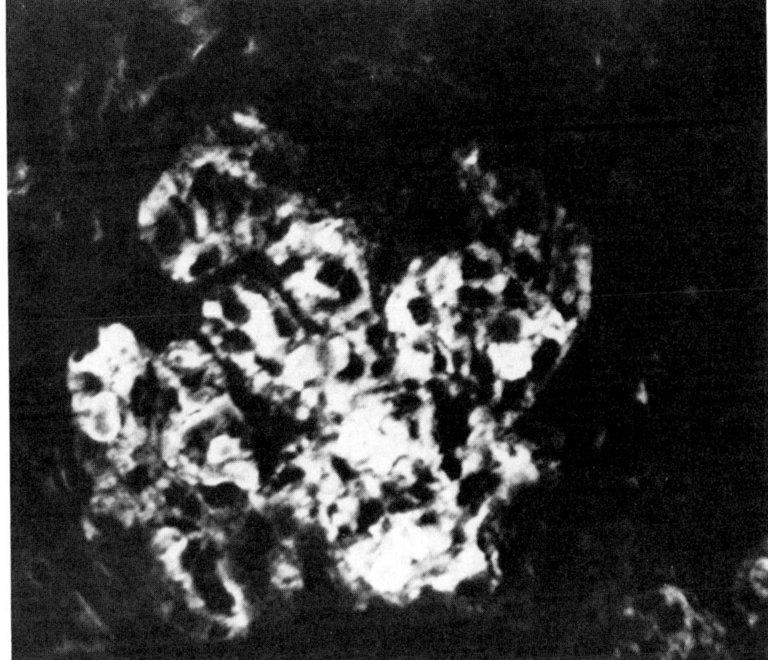

Figure 6–35. Immunofluorescence micrograph, anti-fibrin/fibrinogen. Large, irregular deposits lie along the endothelium and occlude some of the lumen. (×250.)

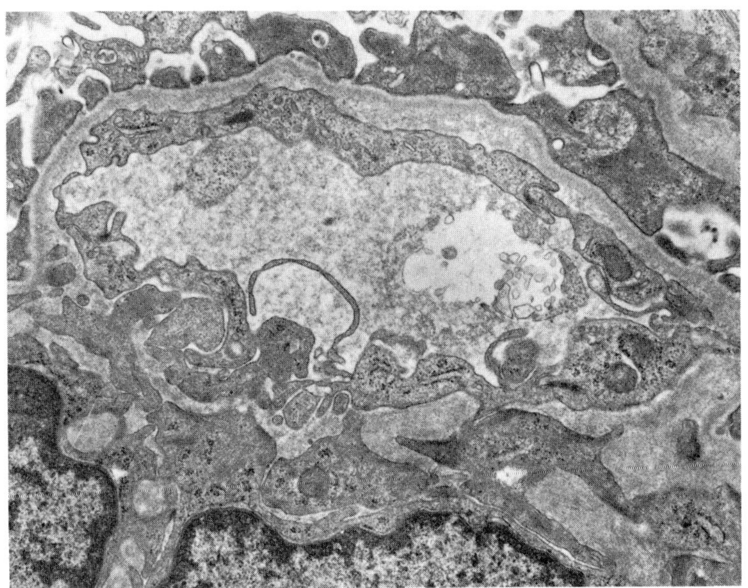

Figure 6–36. The thickened endothelium with loss of fenestrae is shown. The subendothelial space is widened and contains a lucent, flocculent material. (×1500.)

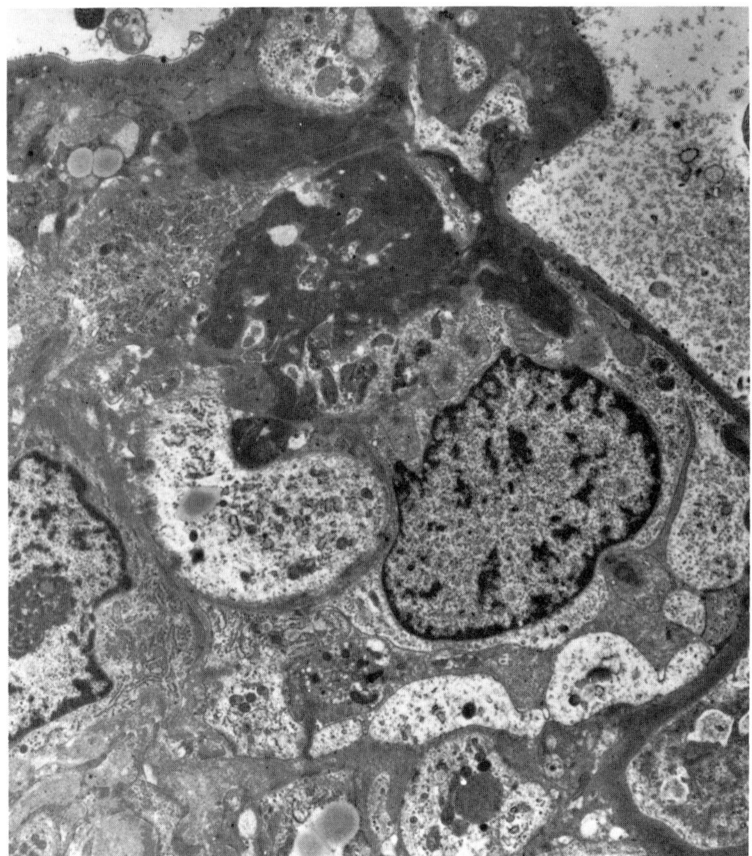

Figure 6–37. The debris found within some vascular loops consists of precipitated plasma proteins (some of which is fibrin) and fragments of degenerating cells. (×6000.)

cytes show spreading of the pedicels. The arterioles may show lesions mirroring those of the glomeruli—endothelial swelling, lucent material in the subintimal spaces, and intraluminal fibrin thrombi.

Prognosis

The renal outcome is related to the extent of arterial and arteriolar damage rather than to injury to the glomeruli. Endothelial lesions that are restricted to the glomeruli appear to be much more reversible, usually without residual damage, than those in the arterioles or arteries. When arteriolar damage is widespread, severe chronic vascular damage rapidly develops and is often accompanied by significant hypertension.

New therapies proposed in the past few years aim at the interruption of the coagulation cascade and the inhibition of platelet aggregation. Their effectiveness remains to be established.

SELECTED READINGS

1. Loirat C, Sonsino E, Varga-Moreno A, et al: Hemolytic-uremic syndrome: An analysis of the natural history and prognostic features. Acta Paediatr Scand 73:505, 1984.
2. Morel-Maroger L: Adult hemolytic-uremic syndrome. Kidney Int 18:125, 1980.
3. Morel-Maroger L, Kanfer A, Solez K, et al: The prognostic importance of vascular lesions in acute renal failure with microangiopathic hemolytic anemia (hemolytic-uremic syndrome). A clinico-pathologic study in 20 adults. Kidney Int 15:548, 1979.
4. Riella MC, Hickman RO, Striker GE, et al: The renal microangiopathy of the hemolytic-uremic syndrome in childhood. Proc Clin Dialysis Transplant Forum 4:112, 1974.

SYSTEMIC SCLEROSIS

The synonyms for progressive systemic sclerosis include *systemic sclerosis* and *scleroderma*. This multisystemic disorder belongs to the category of connective tissue disorders. The disease involves multiple organs in a process consisting of disseminated sclerosis affecting all compartments. Prominent vascular lesions typify the renal lesions. They have a major impact on the overall prognosis and are the underlying cause of the progressive loss of renal function. Systemic sclerosis is not rare and has been found in every race.

Pathogenesis

Although the pathogenesis is poorly understood, the most widely accepted postulate is that immunologic mechanisms are involved in the medial smooth muscle and endothelial cell proliferation, the increase in the synthesis of extracellular matrix, and the appearance of inflammatory cells in arteriolar walls. Also in favor of a role for immunologic disturbances is the almost universal presence of plasma anti-nuclear antibodies and immune complexes as well as a circulating substance that is toxic for endothelial cells in vitro. It is not known whether the plasma components are markers for the disease or play some role in the pathogenesis of the syndrome.

The vascular lesions result in marked narrowing of the arteriolar lumina. The clinical presentation resembles that of malignant hypertension.

The fact that women are more frequently affected than men and that similar vascular lesions may be found in the post-partum period have led to the speculation that the syndrome may have a hormonal component.

Patient Presentation

The most common presentation is scleroderma (dermal thickening). Renal disease is one of the most serious complications of systemic sclerosis and is reflective of the general state of the vasculature. Thus, renal involvement severe enough to result in an impairment of function indicates advanced and generalized vascular disease. One variety of systemic sclerosis, the CREST syndrome, does not involve the renal vasculature.

Kidney lesions most often become manifest within the first 5 years of the disease. Renal involvement ranges from mild arteriolosclerosis with minimal proteinuria to a malignant hypertensive lesion with glomerular necrosis. The latter presentation, referred to as scleroderma crisis, is associated with thrombotic microangiopathy.

Renal biopsy is not often used in the diagnosis or management of these patients because the course is now well established, and in addition, most patients have malignant hypertension. Thus, renal biopsy may be complicated by severe bleeding.

Histology

Light Microscopy

The glomerular changes are those of endothelial injury resulting in ischemia. The appearance of the lesion varies with the stage of the disease. In the acute form, the glomeruli are enlarged and the individual vascular spaces are distended with red blood cells (Fig. 6–38). The number of glomerular cells is not increased, but endothelial swelling is noted (Fig. 6–39). The peripheral basement membranes appear thickened and have indistinct margins, similar to that observed in other disorders associated with thrombotic microangiopathy (Fig. 6–40). One exquisitely acute form, scleroderma crisis, is associated with thrombotic microangiopathy and is characterized by severe necrotizing arteriolar lesions. The glomeruli are often infarcted. The juxtaglomerular apparatus may occasionally be hyperplastic.

At later stages, the glomerular basement membranes become progressively wrinkled and thickened and the vascular spaces gradually shrink. At obsolescence, the glomeruli cannot be distinguished from those due to other ischemic diseases.

The tubulo-interstitial lesions parallel those in the blood vessels. When the lesions become chronic, wrinkling and thickening of the tubular basement membranes mirror that in the glomeruli.

The vascular lesions are characteristically most prominent in the arcuate and interlobular arteries. They consist of marked thickening of the intima due to proliferation of the endothelial cells and the presence of "mucoid" extracellular matrix substances (Fig. 6–41). The elastic laminae may be duplicated. The medial and adventitial layers are thickened as a result of proliferation of the medial smooth muscle cells and the deposition of extracellular matrix.

The arterioles may also be prominently affected, including necrosis of the wall and

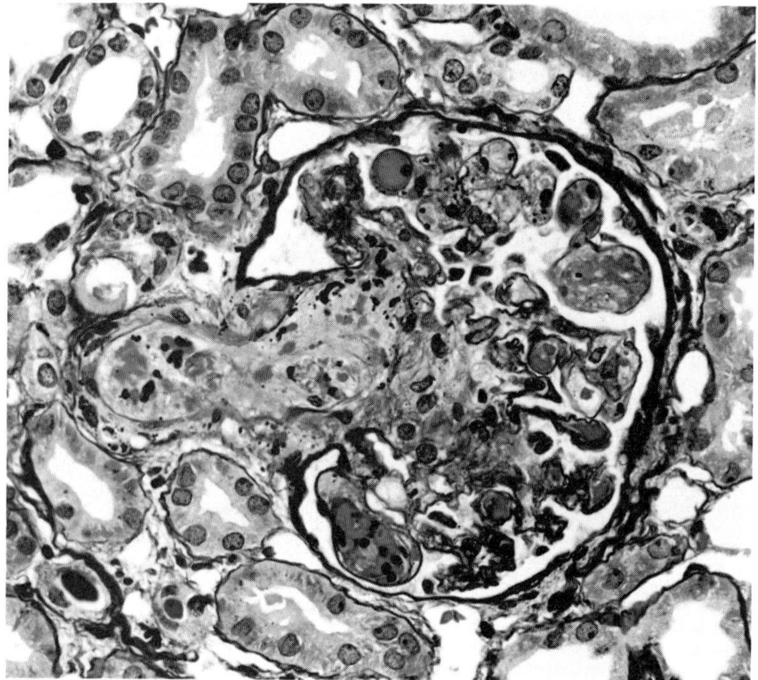

Figure 6–38. The glomerular vascular spaces are almost completely occluded. However, the tufts appear to be shrunken and some basement membranes collapsed (upper quadrant). The interstitium is widened, containing inflammatory cells and edema fluid. The afferent arteriole is filled with a thrombus. (PAS, ×300.)

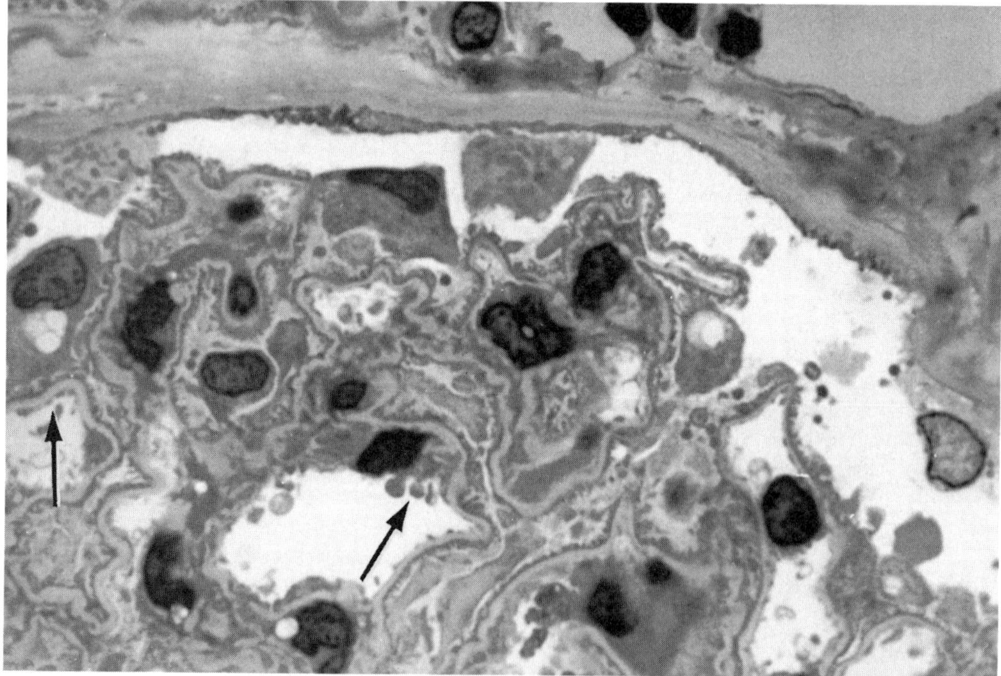

Figure 6–39. The endothelial cell cytoplasm is widened, and there are many cytoplasmic blebs (arrows). The glomerular basement membranes are shrunken in many areas. (H&E, ×600.)

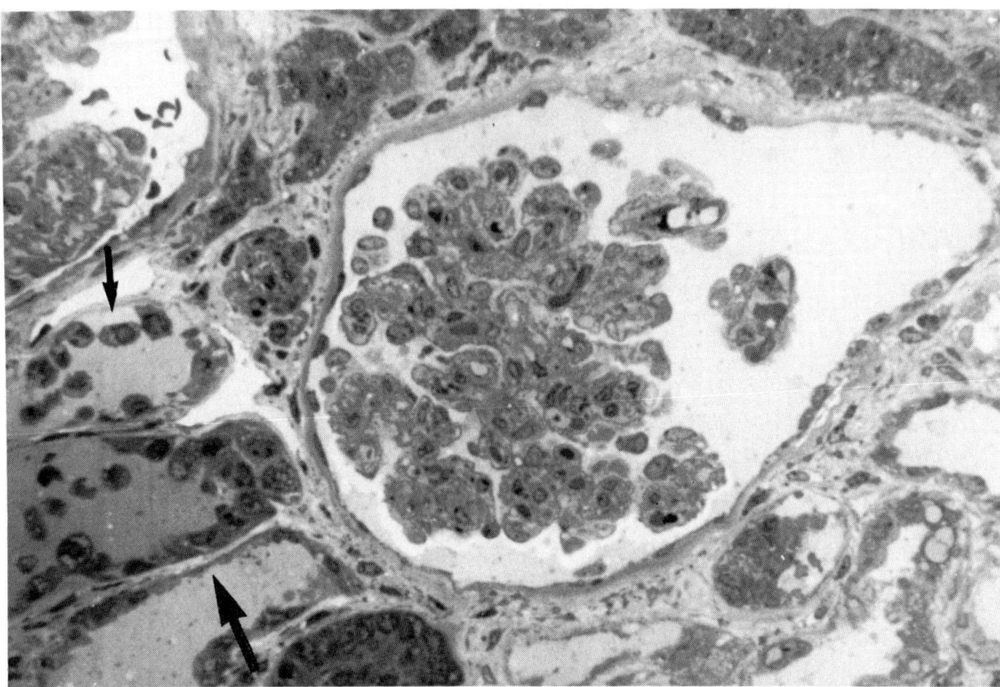

Figure 6–40. This glomerulus is small and ischemic. The vascular spaces are not evident. The tubular epithelial cells have changes varying from loss of cytoplasmic substance (heavy arrow) to complete detachment (light arrow). (H&E, ×300.)

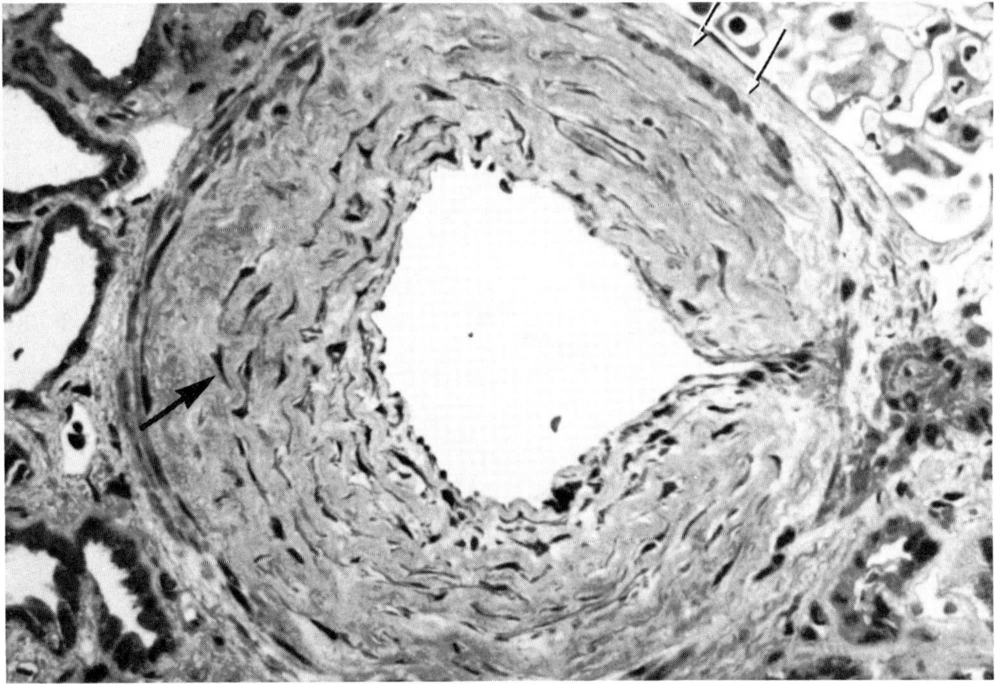

Figure 6–41. Medium-sized artery with a branch at the right quadrant. The intima and media are markedly expanded by smooth muscle proliferation (dark arrow) and concentric lamellae of extracellular matrix and mucoid material. The residual smooth muscle cells are visible at the periphery (double light arrows). (H&E, ×300.)

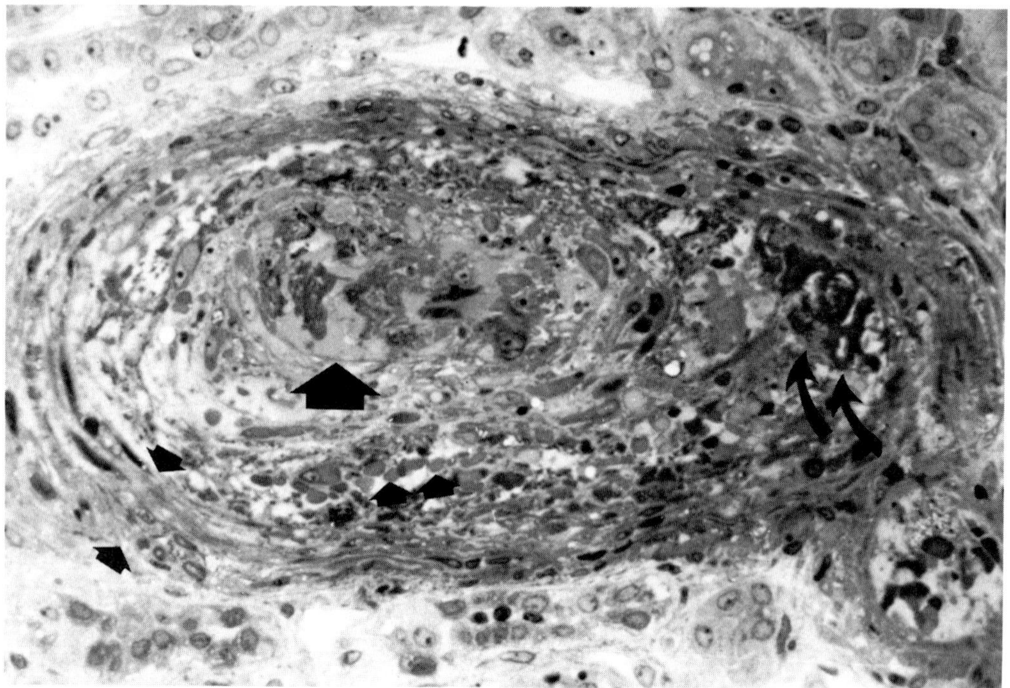

Figure 6–42. This artery has a small lumen which is filled with a thrombus (heavy arrow). The endothelium is detached. The subendothelium contains fibrin (curved arrows), degenerating cells (double heavy arrows), and a mucoid extracellular matrix material. The residual media lies at the periphery of this process (two dark, opposing arrows). (H&E, ×300.)

proliferation of intimal and medial cells (Fig. 6–42). In scleroderma crisis, the arterioles may be thrombosed. Those patients with chronic, slowly progressive disease may have arteriolar sclerosis that is not distinguishable from that of essential hypertension.

Immunofluorescence Microscopy

Fibrin/fibrinogen antigens may be present in the glomerular vascular spaces, but immune reactants are not present. The arteries and arterioles may also contain fibrin/fibrinogen antigens in their walls, but IgG, IgA, IgM, IgA, C3, and other plasma proteins may also be trapped within the thrombi. IgM and C3 are most often restricted to the sclerotic zones.

Electron Microscopy

Ultrastructural examination contributes little additional information. The glomerular basement membranes show subendothelial deposits of an amorphous lucent material. The mucoid material in the arteriolar subintimal spaces is electron lucent and may contain profiles of myointimal cells. The small arterioles show concentric layers of basement membranes that are separated by dense granular material.

Prognosis

The course is one of relentless progression of the renal disease to end stage.

SELECTED READINGS

1. Evans DJ, Cashman SJ, Walport M: Progressive systemic sclerosis: Autoimmune arteriopathy. Lancet 1:480, 1987.
2. Kahaleh MB, Sherer GK, Leroy EC: Endothelial injury in scleroderma. J Exp Med 149:1326, 1979.
3. Lapenas D, Rodman GP, Cavallo T: Immunopathology of the renal vascular lesion of progressive systemic sclerosis (scleroderma). Am J Pathol 91:243, 1978.
4. McCoy RC, Tisher CC, Pepe PF, et al: The kidney in progressive systemic sclerosis. Lab Invest 35:124, 1976.
5. Salyer WR, Salyer DC, Heptinstall RH: Scleroderma and microangiopathic hemolytic anemia. Ann Intern Med 78:895, 1973.

VASCULITIS

Systemic vasculitis comprises a group of diseases characterized by the presence of fibrinoid necrosis and/or acute inflammatory lesions principally affecting the vessel walls. It therefore encompasses a number of disorders that have multisystem involvement (Table 6–3). The definition of these diseases is based solely on an aggregation of clinical and pathologic abnormalities, because there currently is no diagnostic laboratory test. It should be remembered that in many immune-mediated glomerular diseases (such as systemic lupus erythematosus, Henoch-Schönlein purpura, or mixed cryoglobulinemia), small arterioles in the kidneys show occasional inflammatory or necrotizing lesions. The presence of these vascular lesions, when they exist as a part of other entities, does not result in their inclusion in the category of vasculitides. The designation *vasculitis* should be reserved for those vascular lesions that include a prominent inflammatory cell component.

Thus the presence of vascular lesions is not sufficient to establish the diagnosis of a vasculitis. This diagnosis is reserved for syndromes in which a vascular lesion is the primary or only lesion in a patient with a multisystem disorder. The kidneys are preferentially affected in these vasculitic disorders and may be the organs that are the main determinant of the overall prognosis. The association between vasculitis and renal disease has been known for several decades, but renewed interest in the early diagnosis and categorization of the renal lesions has been stimulated by the development of effective new therapeutic strategies.

Table 6–3. Vasculitides Affecting the Kidneys

Polyarteritis nodosa group
Macroscopic (Kussmaul-Maier)
Microscopic
Relapsing polychondritis
Overlap syndrome
Wegener's granulomatosis
Allergic angiitis and granulomatous disease (Churg-Strauss)
Lymphomatoid granulomatosis
Hypersensitivity vasculitis
Drug-induced
Systemic diseases (Henoch-Schönlein, systemic lupus erythematosus, mixed cryoglobulinemia)
Idiopathic
Hypocomplementemic (McDuffie)
Giant cell arteritis
Takayasu's disease
Temporal arteritis
Behçet's disease

This section is devoted to the renal lesions occurring in the primary systemic vasculitides. These diseases share certain general characteristics:

Unknown pathogenesis
Involvement of several organs
Frequent glomerular involvement
Rapid course if untreated.

The principal diseases described in this section are polyarteritis nodosa (and its variants) and Wegener's granulomatosis. These diseases are often characterized by the occurrence of necrosis and crescents in the glomeruli and acute inflammatory lesions in the intrarenal vessel walls. A brief description of the other systemic vasculitides is included, as they may occasionally be associated with renal lesions, although much less frequently.

Pathogenesis

It is generally accepted that the systemic vasculitides are caused by immunologic disturbances, but the exact nature and sequence of events leading to the lesions are largely unknown. The lack of identifiable immune reactants and the presence of macrophages in the lesions have led many investigators to the conclusion that cell-mediated immunity plays an important part in the development of the lesions.

Experimental vasculitis can be induced by antigen-antibody complexes in serum sickness. However, in humans, a role for immune complexes in systemic vasculitis has never been satisfactorily proved. Patients with a vasculitis rarely show immunoreactants in their glomeruli, and their plasma complement levels are in the normal range. In contrast, the role of cell-mediated immunity has received more support because of the abundance of macrophages in both glomerular crescents and the vascular wall lesions. This macrophage infiltrate may be so significant that granulomatous lesions may be seen.

Although the pathogenesis of the vasculitides remains unknown, a few observations may be significant. Several viral infectious agents have been incriminated in the development of polyarteritis nodosa, especially hepatitis B and cytomegalovirus. In addition, recent studies show that antibodies to neutrophil cytoplasmic components are present in the sera of patients with Wegener's syndrome. This observation may be of help in defining the disease process as well as providing a clue to the pathogenesis of the disease. Finally, several investigators believe that nonimmune crescentic glomerulonephritis is a form of vasculitis limited to the kidneys, based on the similarity of the glomerular lesions in these two disorders.

Polyarteritis Nodosa

General clinical manifestations of polyarteritis nodosa include fatigue, fever, weight loss, myalgias, and arthralgias. Pulmonary disease is not a feature, and its presence constitutes one of the major criteria used to define a separate disease spectrum called the overlap syndrome.

Macroscopic Form of Polyarteritis Nodosa

The macroscopic form of polyarteritis nodosa was originally described by Kussmaul and Maier. There may be few signs of renal disease other than those produced by renal ischemia, except for hypertension, which is an almost universal accompaniment. Acute renal failure in this disease is almost always due to cortical necrosis secondary to widespread involvement of large renal vessels.

Histology

LIGHT MICROSCOPY

The likelihood of making a diagnosis of this condition by renal biopsy is small, and biopsy is therefore not indicated except for evaluation of cortical necrosis in the few patients who present with acute renal failure. Nonetheless, if a renal biopsy is performed on a patient who is clinically suspected of having this condition, the sample must be serially sectioned in the search for vascular involvement, because the blood vessel lesions are very segmental and focal in distribution. The lesions are most commonly found in medium-sized arteries (i.e., arcuate, interlobar, and intralobular). The arterial and arteriolar walls contain either localized or circumferential lesions consisting of necrosis and an inflammatory infiltrate (Figs. 6–43 and 6–44). The composition of the infiltrate is most often mixed, but large numbers of neutrophils, macrophages, and lymphocytes are seen. Eosinophils are present in small numbers or are absent. The lesions may be limited to the intima but are seldom restricted to the media or adventitia. The extracellular matrix, including the elastic laminae, may be disrupted in the areas of necrosis. The endothelium often has adherent neutrophils and fibrin thrombi.

Microscopic Form of Polyarteritis Nodosa

Almost all patients with the microscopic form of periarteritis nodosa have glomerular involvement. The general presenting clinical features are similar to those of the macroscopic form of the disease, except for those related to large vessel occlusion. The renal disease is heralded by signs of an acute, severe glomerular disease. The patients almost always present with hematuria, and the presence of rapidly progressive glomerulonephritis may be the first evidence of the syndrome.

Histology

LIGHT MICROSCOPY

The renal lesions in the microscopic form of periarteritis nodosa are diffuse, in contrast to the focal involvement of the kidney occurring in the macroscopic form. The most common glomerular lesion is fibrinoid necrosis of glomerular tufts. This lesion is usually focal and segmental (Fig. 6–45). The extent of the areas of necrosis varies widely within

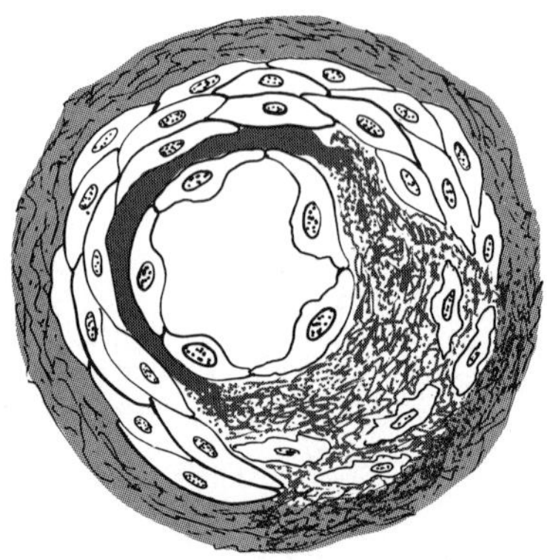

Figure 6–43. Diagram of an artery with segmental necrosis of the wall.

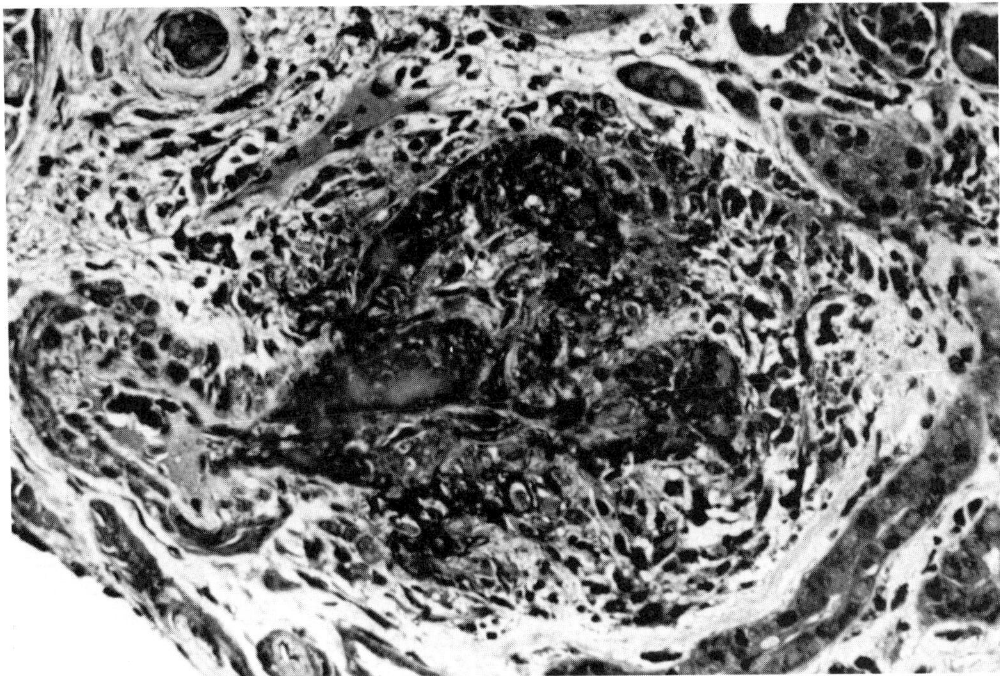

Figure 6–44. The irregularity and the focal nature of the vascular lesion are visible in this small artery that has two severely affected branches (right center). Both branches demonstrate diffuse infiltration of the entire thickness of the wall by inflammatory cells, fibrin deposition, and thrombi within their lumen. The inflammatory process extends to involve the adventitia. (Masson's trichrome, ×100.)

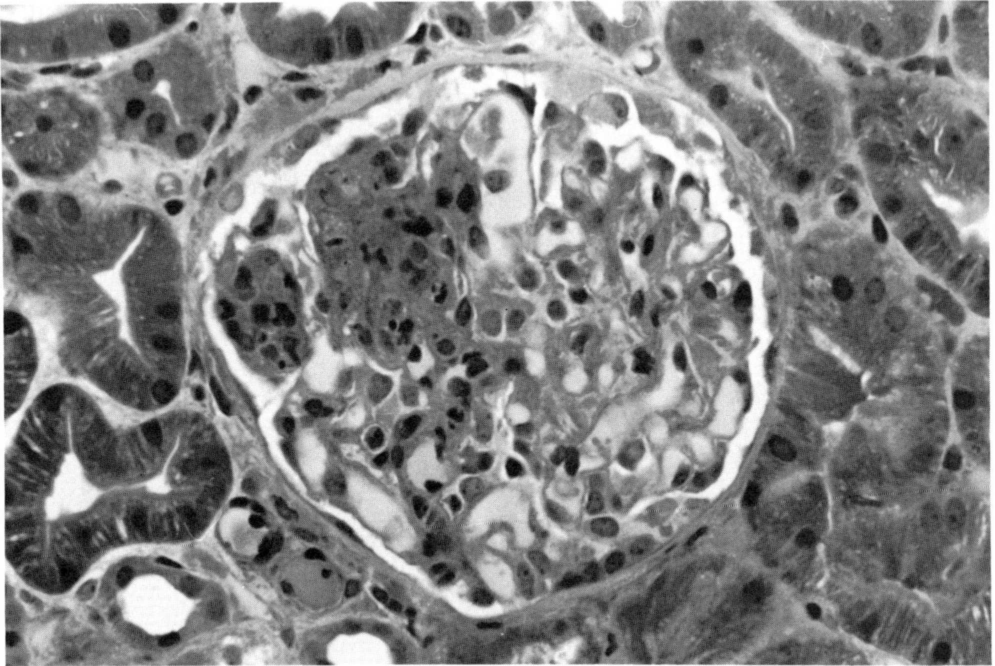

Figure 6–45. The left portion of this glomerulus contains a focus of necrosis, inflammatory cell infiltrate, and cellular proliferation. (H&E, ×300.)

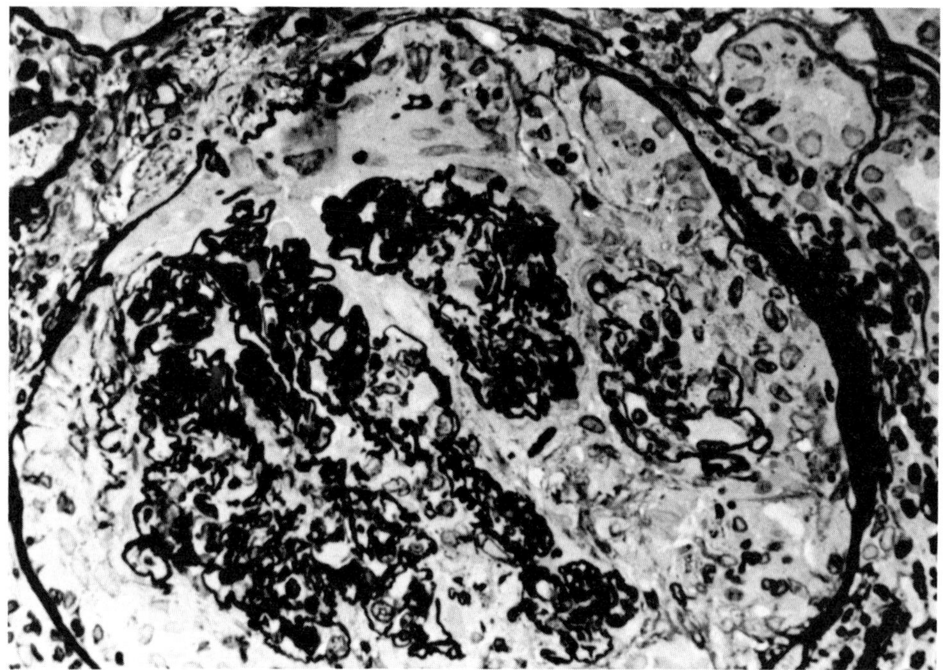

Figure 6–46. Bowman's space is filled with a crescent, which is undergoing partial organization as evidenced by the appearance of extracellular matrix between cells of the crescent. Note that the basement membrane of Bowman's capsule is interrupted (top left). The glomerulus is collapsed. (PASM, ×300.)

a biopsy specimen and between patients. Crescents are often associated with areas of necrosis, and their number and size parallel that of the necrotic foci (Fig. 6–46). Bowman's capsule may be interrupted, in which case the urinary space is invaded by interstitial cells and a fibrous crescent rapidly forms. Lesions of diverse age coexist in the biopsy material: Along with the florid crescentic glomerulonephritis may be focal areas of intraglomerular sclerosis and organized synechiae (Fig. 6–47). Intraglomerular proliferation is seldom a conspicuous feature and when pronounced should suggest a search for another cause.

The interstitial infiltrate and edema parallel the degree of epithelial cell proliferation, although no specific tubular changes are seen. Later in the disease, tubular atrophy and interstitial fibrosis accompany the glomerulosclerosis.

The general assumption is that middle-sized arteries are not affected in the microscopic form of periarteritis nodosa; however, our experience is that they may be affected. This is seldom a major feature, but in four of our patients with a necrotizing, crescentic glomerulonephritis an associated inflammatory vascular wall lesion involved the medium-sized arteries (Figs. 6–48 and 6–49). The arterioles may also be affected by the acute inflammatory process, which consists of necrosis of the wall, endothelial cell injury, and a dense infiltrate of inflammatory cells (Fig. 6–50).

Immunofluorescence Microscopy

Fibrin is almost invariably found in early lesions. It is localized to circumscribed masses corresponding to the areas of necrosis and crescent formation. Immunoglobulins and complement components are not prominent and when present appear to be a component of the other plasma proteins trapped in the areas of necrosis. They may also be present in small amounts in the areas of sclerosis, but here again, this is a feature common to all sclerosing diseases, rather than to the vasculitides. There is no convincing evidence of specific deposits in glomeruli or in segments of glomeruli that do not have necrotic foci (Fig. 6–51). Fibrin may be found in the vessel walls as well (Fig. 6–52).

Electron Microscopy

No additional information is obtained by electron microscopy, except for the fact that it confirms the absence of electron-dense de-

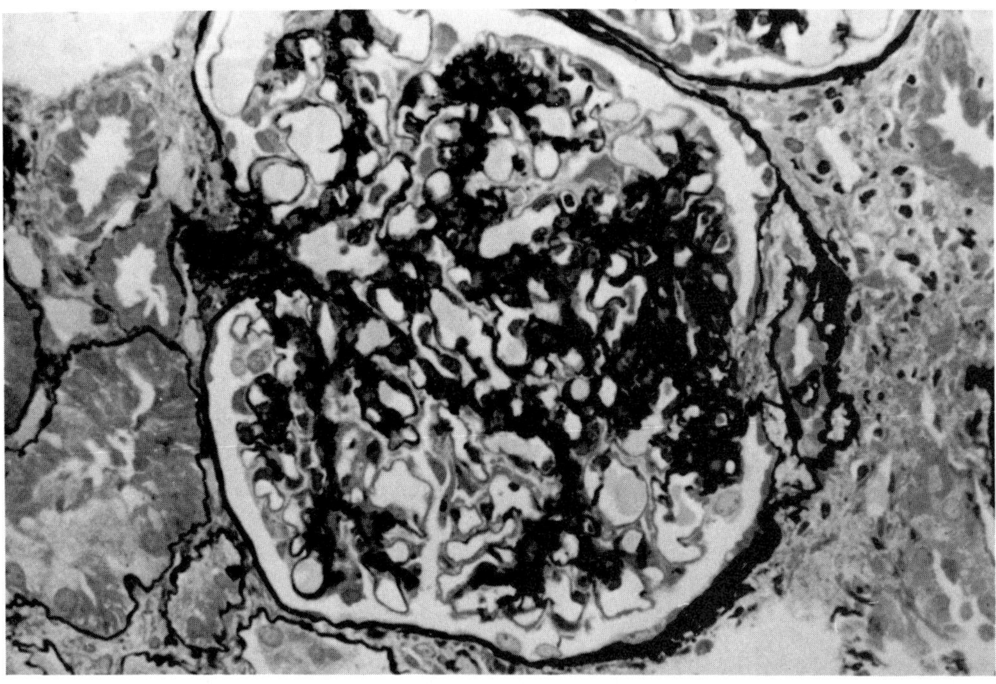

Figure 6–47. The mesangial matrix is diffusely increased in amount, and there is an organized synechia (right center). (PASM, ×300.)

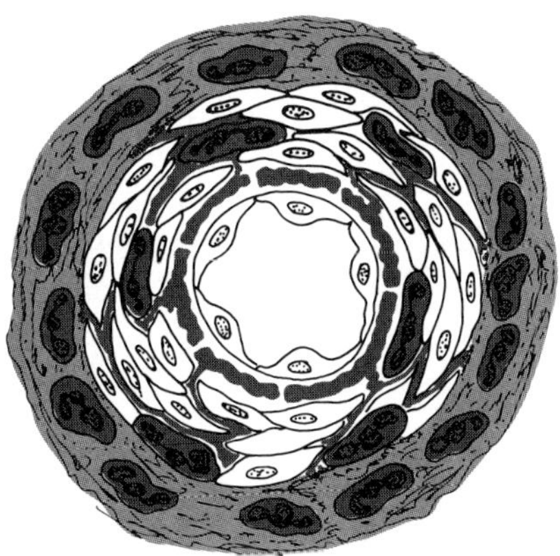

Figure 6–48. Diagram of an artery with infiltration of the wall by neutrophils.

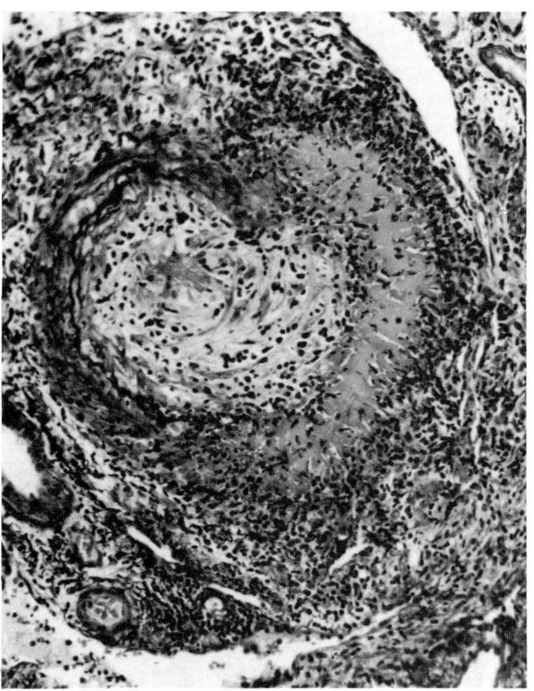

Figure 6–49. The wall of this medium-sized artery is invaded by a dense inflammatory cell infiltrate that extends into the perivascular areas. The lumen is severely compromised. The inflammatory cells consist of mononuclear cells and neutrophils. (H&E, ×100.)

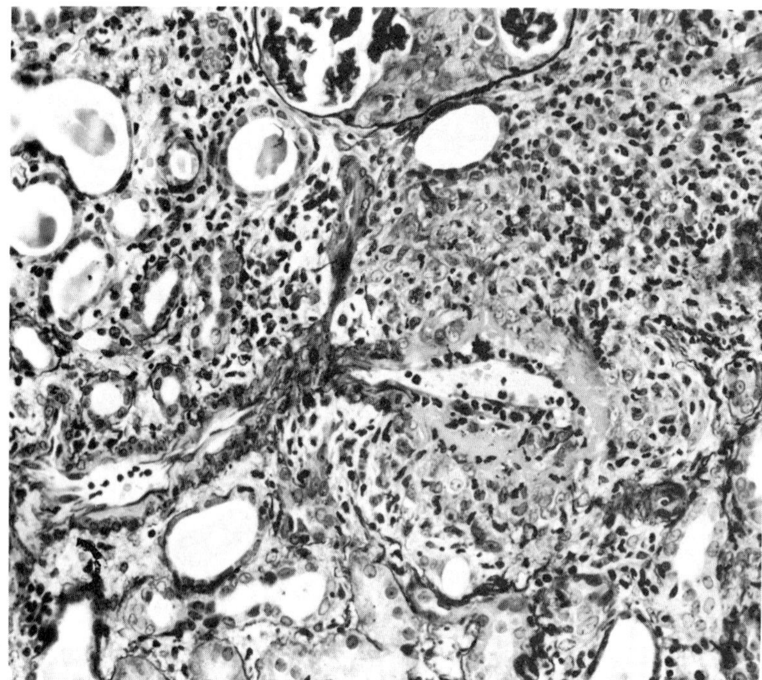

Figure 6–50. One arteriolar branch of this small artery is obliterated by an inflammatory cell infiltrate (right, lower). (Masson's trichrome, ×250.)

posits, allowing one to differentiate this lesion from an immune complex glomerulonephritis.

Overlap Syndrome

Overlap syndrome encompasses a process characterized by a collection of features found in polyarteritis nodosa and in some of the allergic and granulomatous diseases. The renal lesions resemble those of the microscopic form of polyarteritis nodosa—a nonimmune crescentic glomerulonephritis. The pulmonary lesions overshadow those in the kidney, and thus the clinical presentation is different from that of the usual patient with the microscopic form of polyarteritis nodosa. This difference has led to some confusion in the literature, and its resolution awaits better definition of the pathogenesis and etiology of these syndromes.

Prognosis

The outcome is as variable as the underlying histologic lesions. In the macroscopic form, only a minority of the patients develop end-stage renal disease, whereas this is much more common in the microscopic form.

Treatment regimens including steroids and/or cyclophosphamide have resulted in a marked improvement of the overall survival in polyarteritis nodosa. However, the renal prognosis in the diffuse crescentic forms of glomerulonephritis remains bleak. The majority of such lesions result in rapid scarring and obliteration of the glomeruli. The small number of such patients has made the performance of clinical trials difficult.

Wegener's Granulomatosis

Wegener's granulomatosis consists of a necrotizing small vessel vasculitis, with characteristic involvement of the respiratory tract, accompanied by a necrotizing focal glomerulonephritis. The clinical presentation resembles that of other types of vasculitis and includes fever, anorexia, and weight loss. These symptoms may precede and overshadow those referable to the respiratory tract or the kidneys. This syndrome has been reported in all age-groups, including children.

Pathogenesis and Patient Presentation

The renal manifestations may occur at any stage of the disease. Asymptomatic hematuria and proteinuria are the most common labo-

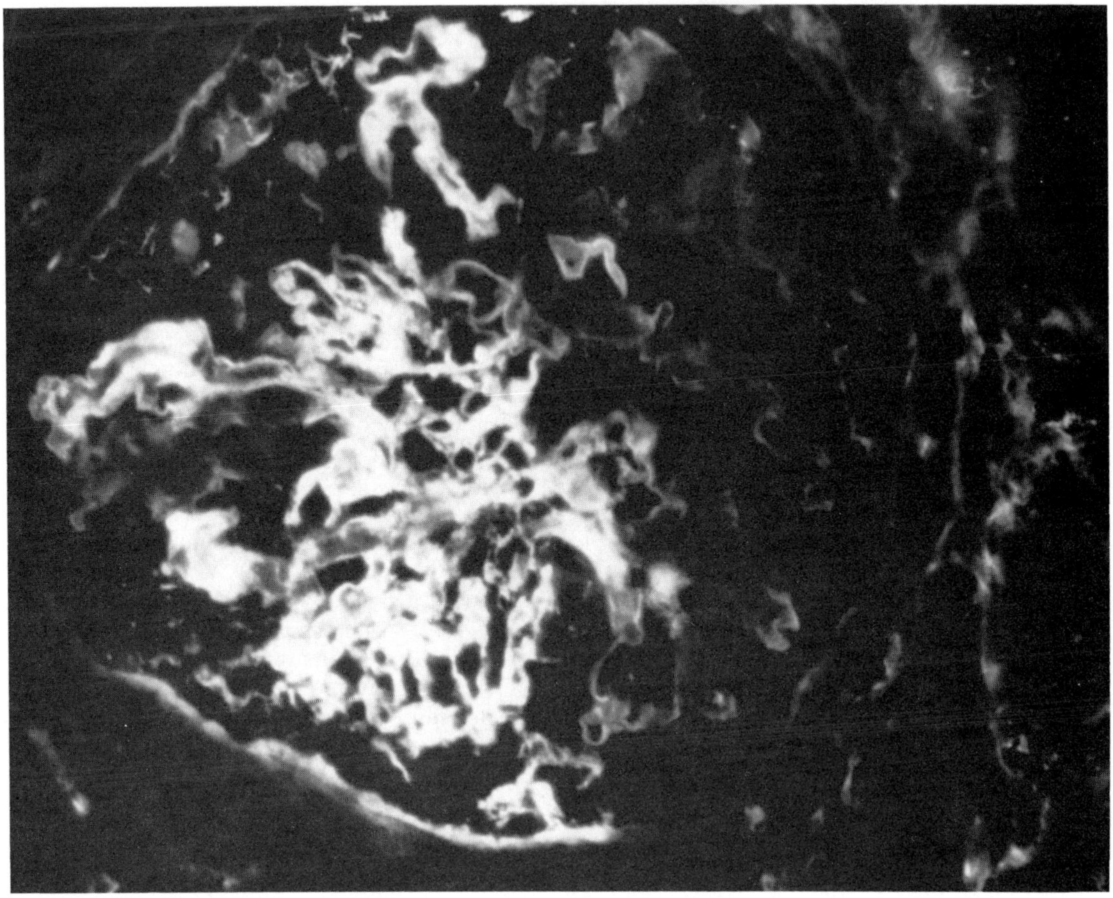

Figure 6–51. Immunofluorescence micrograph, anti-fibrin/fibrinogen. Deposits lie within Bowman's space and along the glomerular basement membranes. (×250.)

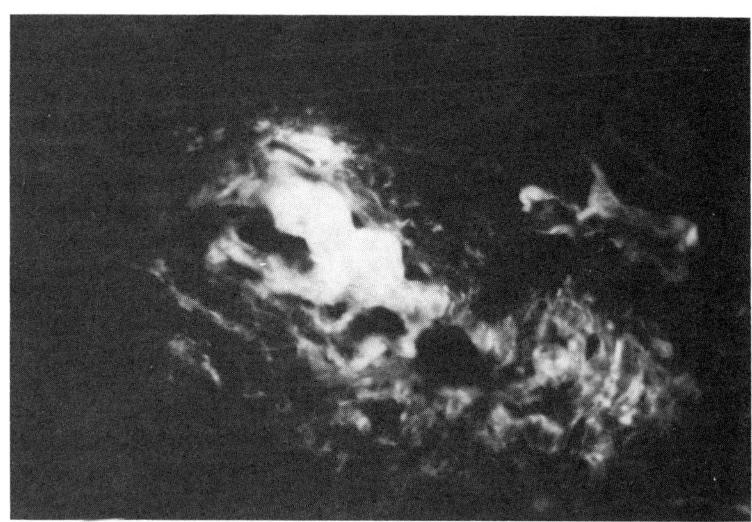

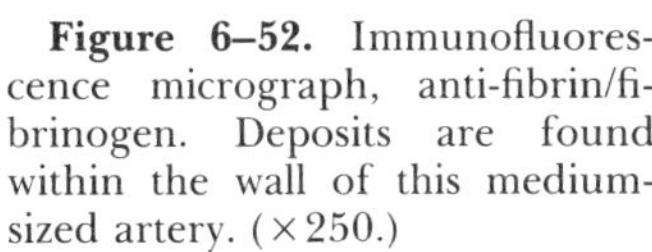

Figure 6–52. Immunofluorescence micrograph, anti-fibrin/fibrinogen. Deposits are found within the wall of this medium-sized artery. (×250.)

ratory findings, but patients may present with rapidly progressive renal failure.

There are no specific serologic findings. C-reactive protein levels may be elevated, and circulating immune complexes may be elevated, but serum complement levels are almost always normal. These changes are shared with other forms of vasculitis. However, it has recently been observed that the sera of these patients contain antibodies to neutrophil cytoplasmic components. If this observation can be confirmed and is specific and/or consistent, it will be of considerable use in establishing the diagnosis of this syndrome.

Histology

Light Microscopy

As in polyarteritis nodosa, a necrotizing glomerulonephritis with crescents is noted. The lesions are focal and segmental in the mild forms, and limited areas of necrosis are seen in the tufts (Fig. 6–53). In the unaffected glomerular segments, the mesangial and vascular spaces appear normal. It is often necessary to obtain serial sections of the biopsy material in mild forms of the disease, because of its focal nature.

When the lesions are diffuse and severe, most glomeruli are affected and circumferential crescents and extensive necrosis may be seen (Fig. 6–54). In these cases, the vascular tufts are compressed and collapsed. Bowman's capsule may be interrupted or even completely effaced by the inflammatory cells, which constitute the major cell type of the crescent at this stage of the disease (Fig. 6–55). In these cases, the periglomerular macrophage inflammatory cell process merges with that of the adjacent interstitium, forming what appears to be a periglomerular granuloma. This has been called granulomatous glomerulonephritis. As noted with other forms of crescentic glomerulonephritis in which Bowman's capsule is disrupted, the periglomerular space becomes rapidly replaced with interstitial connective tissue, and the result is an obsolescent glomerulus.

This disease is characterized by exacerbations and remissions. One may therefore find sclerotic lesions and areas of acute inflammation with necrosis occupying the same or adjacent glomeruli.

The interstitium may contain large numbers of inflammatory cells in the regions of glomerular crescents and vascular lesions. In such cases, it is often necessary to apply PAS or silver stains to recognize the underlying normal structures. Granulomatous lesions

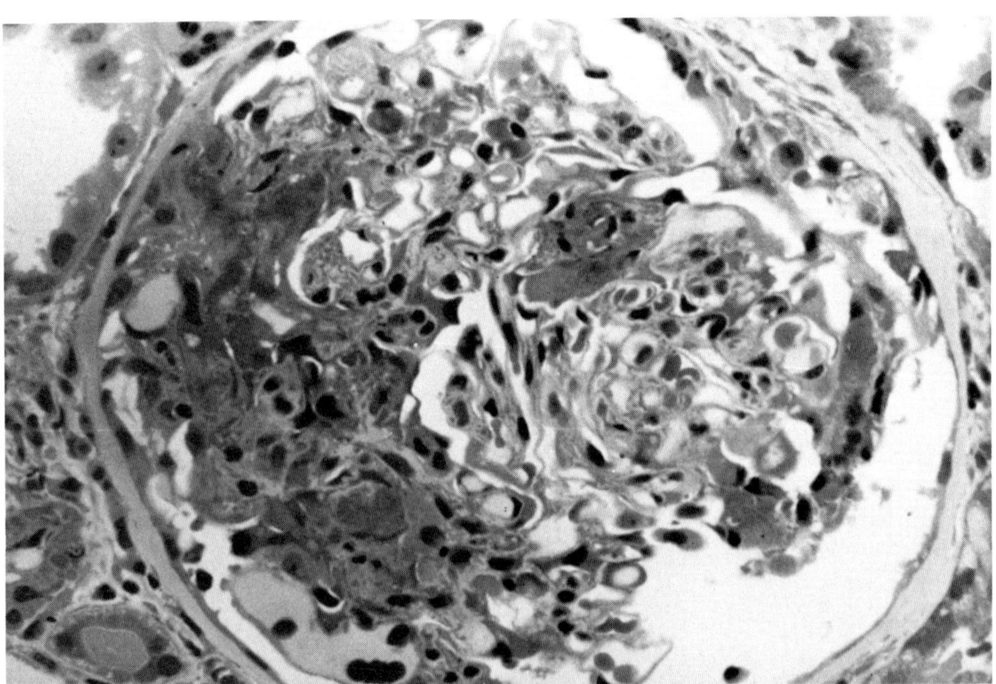

Figure 6–53. Note the irregular involvement of this glomerulus by proliferation of epithelial and intraglomerular cells. The vascular spaces contain a few neutrophils as well as fibrin aggregates. (H&E, ×300.)

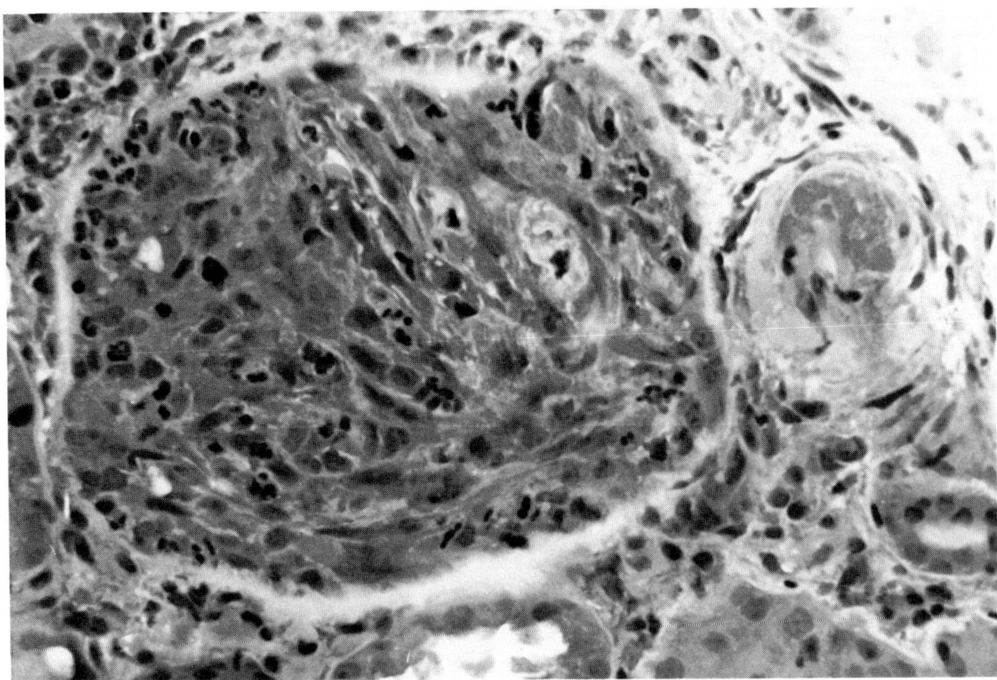

Figure 6–54. The large crescent is filled with neutrophils. The glomerular basement membranes are collapsed and visible as only one small zone of refractile material (right center quadrant). The adjacent interstitium contains many inflammatory cells. (H&E, ×300.)

Figure 6–55. Bowman's capsule is interrupted, and the adjacent interstitium contains many inflammatory cells. (PASM, ×250.)

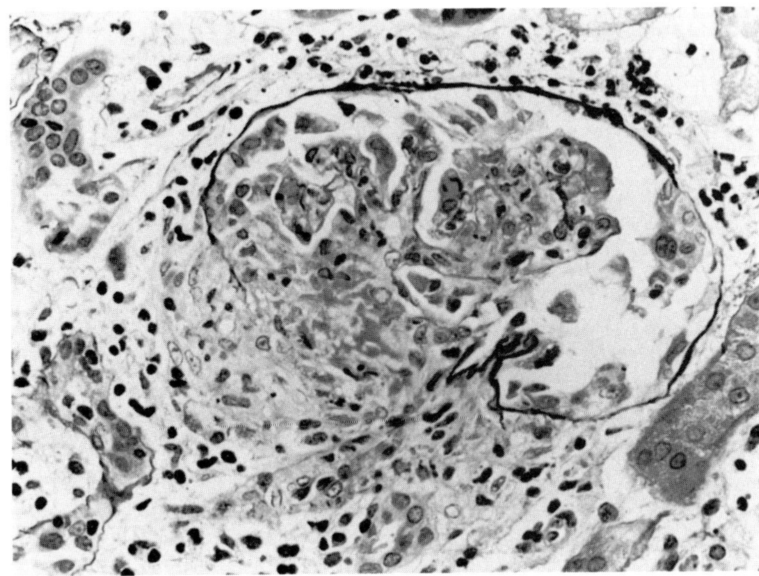

are seldom seen in the interstitium unless they are contiguous with a similar process involving the blood vessels.

The characteristic vascular lesion of Wegener's vasculitis is a granuloma involving the medial layer of an artery (Fig. 6–56). This is a very focal and segmental lesion, and thus many biopsies may miss such a lesion. Serial sections should be obtained when this diagnosis is entertained.

Immunofluorescence Microscopy

The areas of necrosis always contain fibrin/fibrinogen related antigens. The glomeruli as a rule contain no immunoreactants, except in localized areas of necrosis and/or sclerosis. In these instances, they most likely represent passive trapping rather than deposition as part of a pathogenetic process. Small deposits of IgM in the mesangium have occasionally been reported.

Electron Microscopy

The electron microscopic appearance of the lesions does not add significant new information to that found by light or immunofluorescence microscopy.

Prognosis

The introduction of an effective therapy by Fauci's group at the National Institutes of Health has completely transformed the prognosis in patients with Wegener's granulomatosis. Approximately 80% of the patients respond to therapy with cyclophosphamide and have a prolonged survival time. The glomerular lesions heal rapidly, forming local sclerotic areas. Thus, the ultimate prognosis for renal function depends on the severity and extent of the initial lesions. For this reason, early diagnosis and an aggressive therapeutic posture seem well justified.

Other Vasculitides

Several other vasculitides may affect the kidneys. Each group comprises only a small number of patients, but each has been proposed as a separate category in the classification of the vasculitides because they do not fit in the described schema. These will be mentioned very briefly.

Kawasaki's Disease

Kawasaki's disease, also known as mucocutaneous lymph node syndrome, is an acute

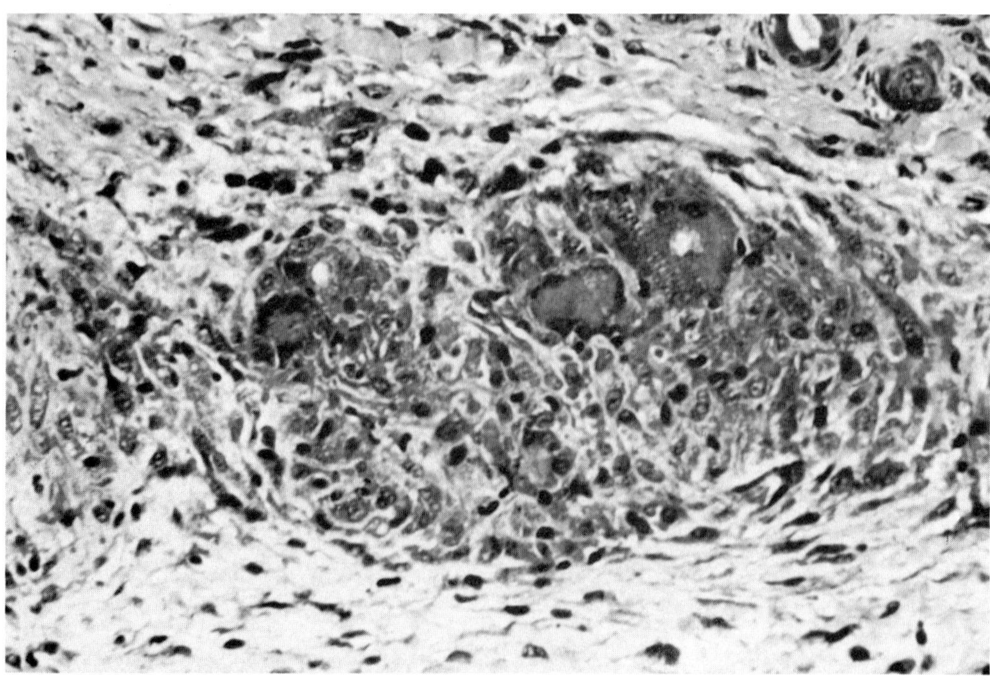

Figure 6–56. The artery is effaced by an inflammatory cell infiltrate that contains several multinucleated giant cells. (Masson's trichrome, ×300.)

multisystemic illness occurring in children. The coronary arteries are the most frequent site of vascular involvement. The vasculature of the kidneys is less commonly involved, but when present, the most prominent lesions are in the mid-sized arteries. Glomerular disease has been described, but it is not clear whether the observed changes are due to vascular lesions affecting the medium-sized arteries or are due to circulating immune complexes. Mild glomerular cell proliferation has been reported, accompanied by granular deposits of C3 and IgM in the mesangium.

Relapsing Polychondritis

Several patients have been described who have a relapsing polychondritis and an associated crescentic glomerulonephritis that is indistinguishable from that in patients with polyarteritis nodosa.

Churg's Allergic Granulomatosis

A very small number of patients have been reported to have glomerular lesions similar to those in periarteritis nodosa, along with the additional feature of interstitial granulomas that contain many eosinophils. These patients may also have inflammatory lesions of the small arteries and arterioles.

Takayasu's Disease

Few renal biopsies have been performed in patients with Takayasu's disease. However, in those studied, the findings consist of mild mesangial prominence with scattered small deposits of immune reactants.

Hypocomplementemic Vasculitis

Only a few cases of hypocomplementemic vasculitis have been reported. The clinical and laboratory findings include urticaria and hypocomplementemia. Membranoproliferative glomerulonephritis has been a rare accompaniment.

Lymphomatoid Granulomatous Disease

Neither laboratory nor renal biopsy evidence of renal disease is common in lymphoid granulomatous disease, but nodular interstitial infiltrates may be seen with the newer imaging techniques.

Temporal Arteritis

Only one case of renal disease has been reported in temporal arteritis, a relatively common, benign form of arteritis. This patient had membranous glomerulonephritis, and the relation of the glomerulonephritis to the vasculitis remains conjectural.

Behçet's Disease

Few systematic studies of the kidneys have been performed in patients with Behçet's disease. In the several case reports, sufficient consistency has been observed in the nature of the renal lesions to suggest that there may be an associated renal defect. The most common finding has been mild mesangial hypercellularity with small deposits of IgG and C3 in the mesangial and subendothelial regions. A few cases with crescentic glomerular lesions and a clinical syndrome of rapidly progressive renal failure have also been reported.

The question of a common pathogenesis between non-immune crescentic glomerulonephritis and vasculitis remains open.

SELECTED READINGS

1. Croker BP, Lee T, Gunnells JC: Clinical and pathologic features of polyarteritis nodosa and its renal-limited variant: Primary crescentic and necrotizing glomerulonephritis. Hum Pathol 18:38, 1987.
2. Cupps TR, Fauci AS: The vasculitides. *In* Smith LH (ed): Major Problems in Internal Medicine. WB Saunders, Philadelphia, 1981, pp 173–202.
3. Fauci AS, Wolff SM: Wegener's granulomatosis: Studies in eighteen patients and a review of the literature. Medicine 52:535, 1973.
4. Horn RH, Fauci AJ, Rosenthal AJ, et al: Renal biopsy pathology in Wegener's granulomatosis. Am J Pathol 74:423, 1974.
5. Lockwood CM, Jones S, Moss DW, et al: Association of alkaline phosphatase with an autoantigen recognized by circulating anti-neutrophil antibodies in systemic vasculitis. Lancet 1:716, 1987.
6. Ronco P, Verroust P, Mignon F, et al: Immunopathological studies of polyarteritis nodosa and Wegener's granulomatosis: A report of 43 patients with 51 renal biopsies. Q J Med 206:212, 1983.
7. Yoshimura M, Kida H, Saito Y, et al: Peculiar glomerular lesions in Takayasu's arteritis. Clin Nephrol 24:120, 1985.

GLOMERULAR LESIONS IN CHRONIC HYPOXEMIC CONDITIONS

Glomerular lesions have been reported in a number of diseases associated with chronic hypoxemia. The spectrum of diseases is large, but cardiac and pulmonary diseases are most commonly associated with this glomerular lesion. Polycythemia may be present, although the renal lesion does not seem to be related to this finding.

Pathogenesis

The pathogenesis of the glomerular lesion is unknown, but the presence of glomerulosclerosis has led some researchers to speculate that the lesions are due to an increase in glomerular vascular hydrostatic pressure.

Patient Presentation

The lesions are most often incidentally noted at autopsy, but some patients may have overt proteinuria. The list of conditions associated with glomerular lesions includes the following:

- Cyanotic heart diseases (especially tetralogy of Fallot)
- Cor pulmonale
- Mitral stenosis
- Severe pulmonary emphysema
- Extreme obesity
- Chronic hemosiderosis
- Polycythemia vera
- Thalassemia

The natural history of the glomerular diseases, their frequency, and their detailed characteristics are not well established. We will only provide those clues that may be useful in suspecting or establishing the diagnosis of these conditions.

Histology

Light Microscopy

The glomeruli appear to be large and congested, and the vascular loops are distended with erythrocytes. This feature is particularly striking because of the fact that the glomeruli do not contain many red blood cells in either normals or in most parenchymal diseases. The mesangial matrix may be increased in amount, and less frequently, the number of mesangial cells may be increased. The peripheral glomerular basement membranes and Bowman's capsule frequently appear thickened and wrinkled.

Inflammatory cells are not evident.

The tubular basement membranes may also be modestly thickened.

Arterial and arteriolar sclerosis may be found.

Immunofluorescence Microscopy

No deposits of immune reactants are found.

Electron Microscopy

The glomerulosclerosis consists of increased mesangial matrix and irregular thickening of the lamina densa of the peripheral glomerular basement membrane.

Prognosis

This is most often an incidental finding; thus the glomerular lesion adds nothing to the patient's course.

SELECTED READINGS

1. Ingelfinger JR, Kissane JM, Robson AM: Glomerulomegaly in a patient with cyanotic congenital heart disease. Am J Dis Child 120:69, 1970.
2. Spear GS: The glomerulus in cyanotic congenital heart disease and primary pulmonary hypertension: A review. Nephron 1:238, 1970.

Chapter

7

HERITABLE DISEASES, PRIMARY GLOMERULAR

CONGENITAL NEPHROTIC SYNDROME

The appearance of the nephrotic syndrome during the first few months of life is relatively uncommon and has been called the congenital nephrotic syndrome. It is most often evident shortly after birth, and to fit into this pathogenetic category it must become apparent within the first 6 months of life. The type of underlying histologic lesion in the Western world depends on the patient's genetic background. Patients with a strong genetic linkage are of Finnish extraction and have a macrocystic cortical renal lesion. The others are of various European extractions and have glomerular lesions of two types. The first is restricted to the mesangial regions and, like the microcystic variety, is evident shortly after birth. The second, non-heritable variety consists of the general types of inflammatory or toxic lesions found in older age-groups and thus can usually be placed into one of the conventional histologic categories of kidney diseases.

In addition to these types of the nephrotic syndrome presenting at birth, another type of nephropathy is associated with Wilms' tumor and pseudohermaphroditism. The glomerular lesions consist of severe membranoproliferative glomerulonephritis. This disorder has been called the Drash syndrome.

Pathogenesis

Essentially nothing is known of the pathogenesis of the Finnish type of the nephrotic syndrome. The glomerular basement membranes have been shown to have a decrease in negatively charged sites, and the proteinuria is glomerular in origin at the outset. The urine protein composition changes to include evidence of a tubular origin, as the renal cysts appear and become the dominant renal abnormality.

Patient Presentation

The mode of inheritance of the Finnish type is autosomal recessive. The diagnosis can be suspected at birth because of an increased placental size and weight, skeletal abnormalities, and the presence of proteinuria. Afflicted infants are susceptible to infections and have all of the serologic abnormalities typical of the nephrotic syndrome. In addition, renal functional impairment becomes evident within the first few weeks and progressively worsens.

The other forms of the nephrotic syndrome that present in the first 6 months of life do not differ in their signs, symptoms, or outcome from those of similar lesions in older children.

Histology

Light Microscopy

Finnish Type, Early. Detailed studies have been made of the renal lesions in these patients. As early as 16 to 24 weeks of gestation, slight dilation of tubules has been noted. This lesion remains the most useful histologic finding in renal biopsies of newborns (Figs. 7–1 and 7–2). Microdissection studies reveal that both proximal and distal segments may be involved. A note of caution with respect to this finding is that cystic lesions have been reported in 67 to 75% of most large series, and occasional dilated tubular segments may be seen in other forms of glomerular disease that occur in infants (and adults, of course). Thus, the overall histologic pattern must be evaluated before a diagnosis of the presence or absence of the Finnish type of congenital nephrotic syndrome is made when the lesions are examined during the first few weeks of life. Mesangial proliferation has been described at this stage, but the glomerular changes are usually quite modest and are overshadowed by those in the tubular compartment.

Finnish Type, Late. The cystic lesions progress to involve the entire cortex (see Figs. 7–1 and 7–2). The interstitium becomes increasingly fibrotic, and a mononuclear infiltrate is often seen. Again, the glomeruli do not appear to be the primary site of the renal disease, although they may show segmental mesangial proliferation and sclerosis (see Fig. 7–2). The lesions in all compartments increase in severity as the syndrome evolves. Because afflicted children are particularly prone to infection, it may be difficult to separate the secondary effects of the patients' overall condition from those due to the underlying genetic defect at this late stage.

Other Types of Renal Disease. This is not a homogeneous group, and the recent epidemic of intravenous drug use in child-bearing women and its accompaniment with human immunodeficiency virus (HIV) even further complicates this picture. However, it is important to differentiate these forms of renal disease from the Finnish type of the nephrotic syndrome in childhood. The his-

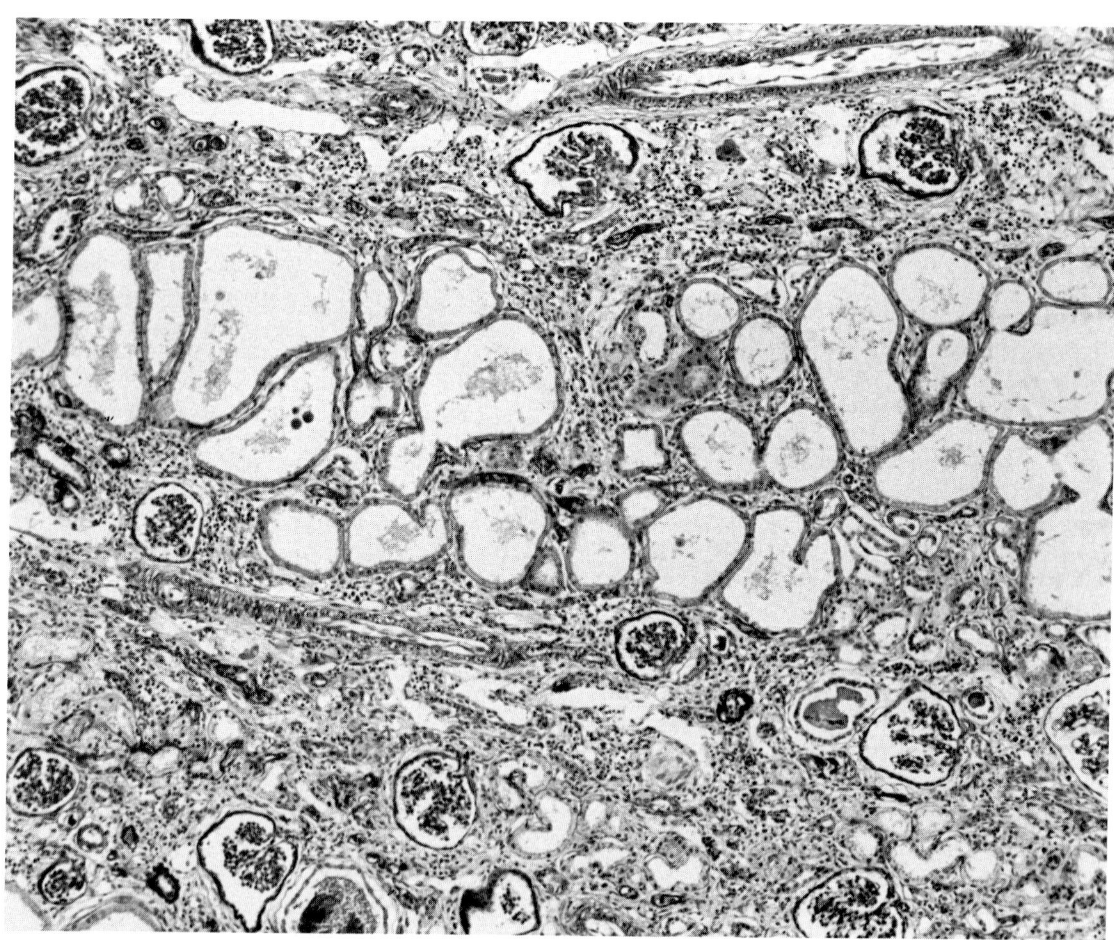

Figure 7–1. In this section from an autopsy specimen, the principal abnormality at low power is marked dilation of the tubules and interstitial fibrosis and infiltration. (H&E, ×75.)

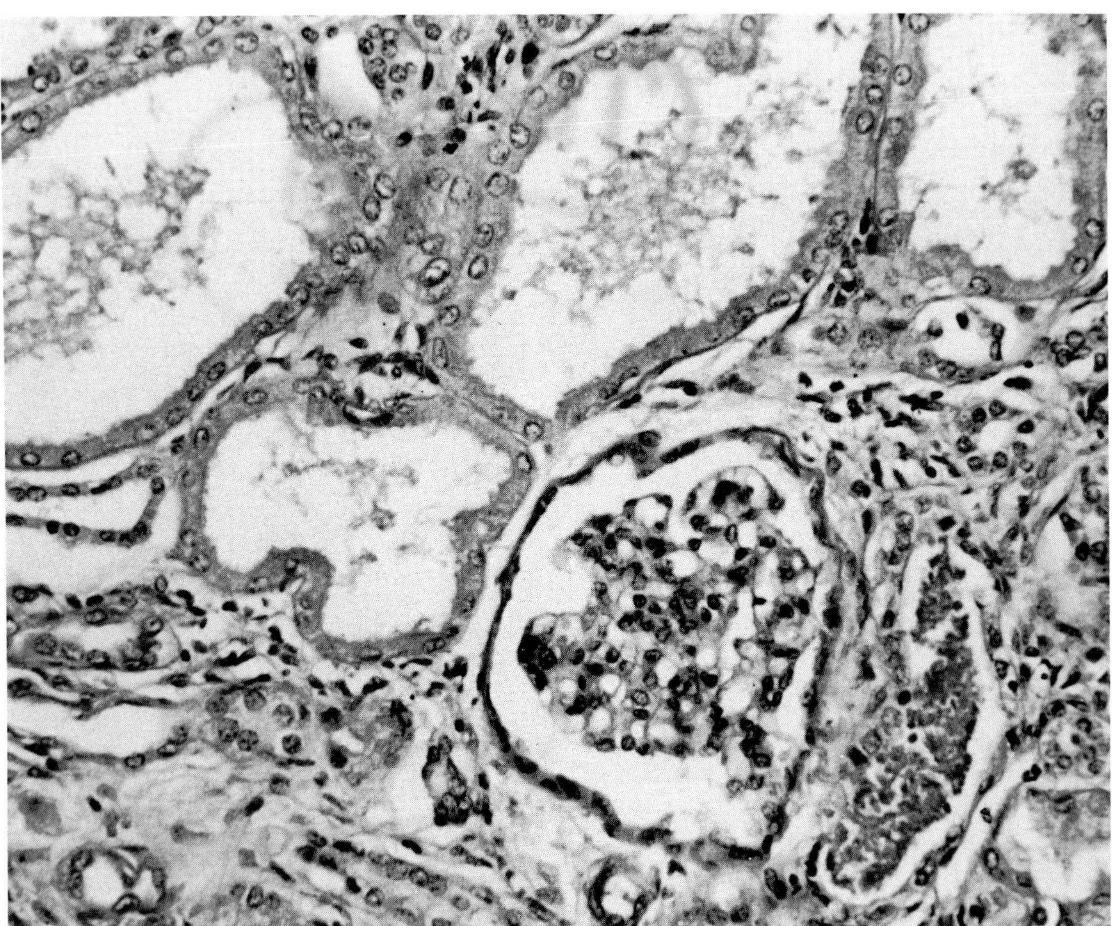

Figure 7–2. At higher magnification, the glomerulus is normal, but the tubules have low-lying epithelium and are dilated. The interstitial fibrosis and infiltration are apparent. (H&E, ×300.)

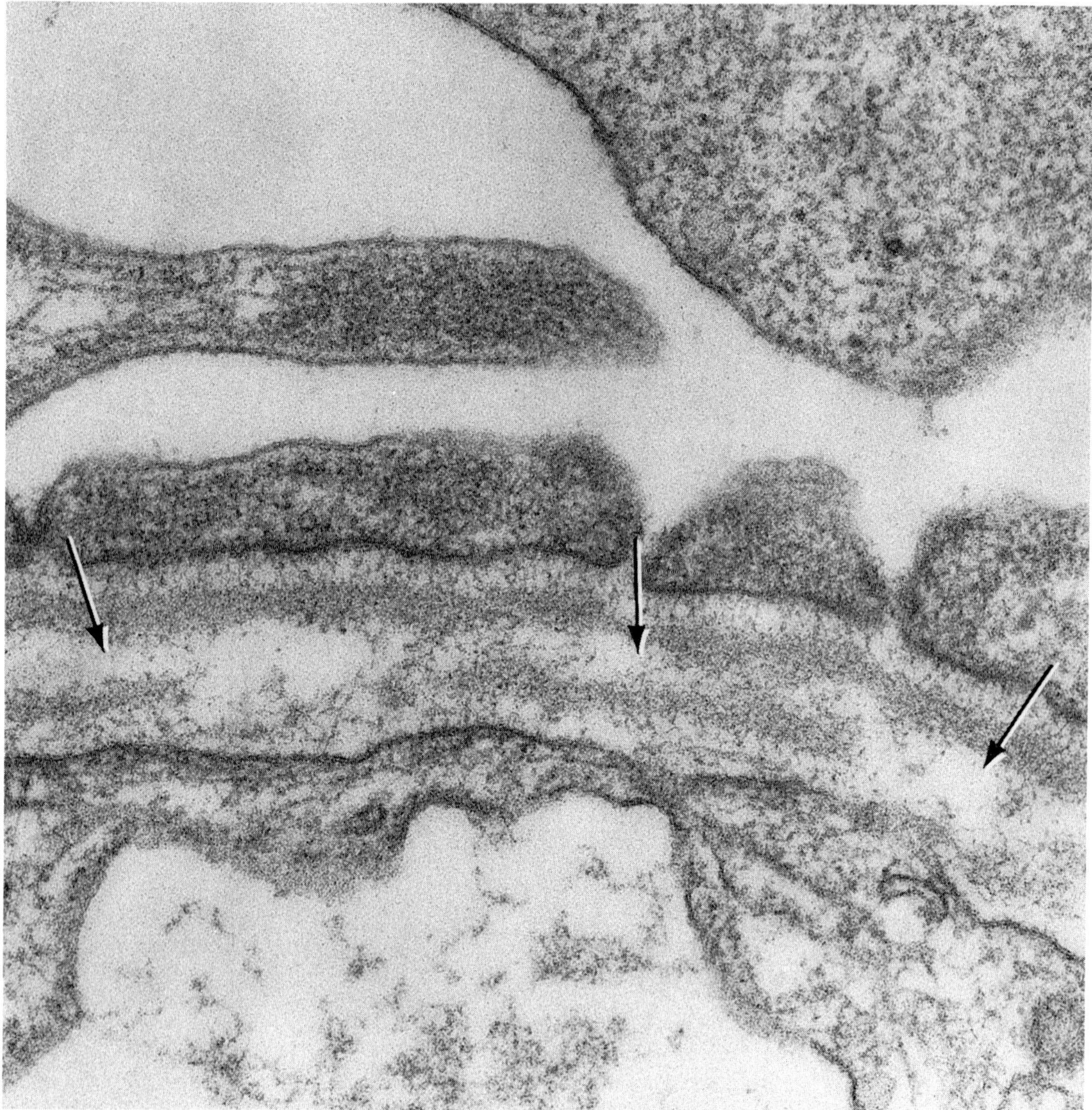

Figure 7–3. A small fraction of the peripheral glomerular basement membranes are irregularly duplicated. The space between the laminae is filled with a flocculent material. The podocytes are normal in configuration. The endothelial cell cytoplasm is thickened. (×30,000.)

tologic lesions in these cases are not different from the expression of the diseases in adults, except for the fact that they are occurring in an infant's kidneys. The main problem in the differential diagnosis is that most observers are unfamiliar with the normal structure of a neonate's kidney. For instance, the glomeruli are normally small, the glomerular basement membranes are thinner than those of adults, the proximal tubules are much shorter than in adults, and so on. Therefore, it may be useful to obtain pediatric consultation in evaluating these lesions.

Immunofluorescence Microscopy

Finnish Type. There is no evidence that an immune component exists in the pathogenesis of this disease. Thus, there are no immune reactants in the kidneys of these patients. Of course, such deposits may develop after infections, but they are not part of the underlying defect. At the late stages, the sclerotic glomerular lesions may also contain C3 deposits. However, this finding is identical to that in other diseases, irrespective of age or disease etiology.

Other Types of Renal Disease. Immune reactants are often found in the glomeruli of these patients. As noted by the light microscopy, they correspond to that expected for the associated clinical and histologic disease.

Electron Microscopy

Finnish Type. At the earliest times of fetal life studied, the glomerular basement membranes have been shown to be prominently altered. The glomerular basement membrane lesion consists of focal splitting of the lamina densa, which is thinner than normal (Fig. 7–3). The overall thickness of the peripheral glomerular wall remains almost normal because of widening of the lamina rara interna and the lamina rara externa. Extensive changes are also noted in the visceral cells, consisting of effacement of the pedicels, microvillus formation, and an increased number of cytoplasmic vacuoles. The mesangial regions are also abnormal, containing an increased amount of extracellular matrix. As the lesions advance, the mesangial sclerosis may become more prominent.

Other Types of Renal Disease. The changes are not homogeneous, reflecting the nature of the glomerular process present. These are described in other chapters. No special features are added by the young age of the patients.

Prognosis

Finnish Type. The nephrotic syndrome appears shortly after birth, and renal function progressively deteriorates to end-stage renal disease within the first 3 to 4 years. The most life-threatening complication is sepsis. The nephrotic syndrome is unremitting, and afflicted children are at continuous risk of infections of the body cavities (e.g., pleura, peritoneum, dura). No effective therapy for the nephrotic syndrome has been found, but patients can be managed with renal transplantation.

Other Types of Renal Disease. The prognosis depends on the cause. If the cause is HIV infection, the outlook is quite poor. On the other hand, if the offending agent can be removed, the prognosis may be quite good. We found that almost two-thirds of the patients reach maturity without evidence of significant renal failure. Others report a less optimistic view, but the ultimate prognosis depends on the particular cause of the underlying disease; therefore, it is difficult to make meaningful comparisons between patients or series of patients.

SELECTED READINGS

1. George CRP, Hickman RO, Striker GE: Infantile nephrotic syndrome. Clin Nephrol 5:20, 1976.
2. Habib R, Bois E: Congenital and infantile nephrotic syndrome. Pediatr Nephrol 2:335, 1976.
3. Hallman N, Norio R, Rapola J: Congenital nephrotic syndrome. Nephron 11:101, 1973.
4. Huttunen NP: Congenital nephrotic syndrome of Finnish type: Study of 75 patients. Arch Dis Child 41:344, 1976.
5. Mahan JD, Mauer SM, Sibley RK, et al: Congenital nephrotic syndrome. Evolution of medical management and results of renal transplantation. J Pediatr (Paris) 105:549, 1984.
6. Norio R: Heredity in the congenital nephrotic syndrome. Ann Paediatr Fenn (Suppl) 27:1, 1966.
7. Oliver J: Microcystic renal disease and its relation to "infantile nephrosis." Am J Dis Child 100:312, 1960.
8. Sibley RK, Mahan J, Mauer SM, et al: A clinicopathologic study of forty-eight infants with nephrotic syndrome. Kidney Int 27:544, 1985.

BENIGN FAMILIAL HEMATURIA

Benign familial hematuria is a recently described disease in which the lesion is limited to thinning of the glomerular basement membranes. The presence of a renal disease is signaled by the presence of chronic hematuria, which may be either macroscopic or microscopic or may consist of intermittent periods of gross and microscopic hematuria. It has a completely benign course. One report described some patients who progressed to end stage, but this outcome must be considered to be very exceptional.

Patient Presentation and Pathogenesis

In a large prospective study of Netherlands patients with persistent hematuria but without azotemia, 17 of 54 patients (31%) had thin basement membranes. This frequency was approximately the same as in IgA nephropathy. In this recently published study, the measured glomerular basement membrane thickness in normal persons was 361 ± 69 nm and in those with thin basement membranes was 191 ± 28 nm. In agreement with others, these researchers found that patients with this lesion have persistent microscopic hematuria, and only 1 of 18 had macroscopic hematuria. A feature previously noted and thought to predict a poor outcome was that 6 of 17 patients had more than 500 mg of urine protein per 24 hours and an additional 5 had 180 to 500 mg of urine protein per 24 hours. These data suggest that the presence of proteinuria, at least in this population in the Netherlands, was not predictive of the underlying lesion. They noted that 6 of 17 patients had a family history of microscopic hematuria. The mean duration of follow-up was 50 months.

The mode of inheritance is autosomal dominant, for the most part. However, in some kindreds the mode seems to be autosomal recessive inheritance.

Histology

Light Microscopy

The typical finding is that the biopsy material is essentially completely normal by light microscopy. A few erythrocytes may be seen within tubule lumina. The only other changes are those consistent with the patient's age.

Fluorescence Microscopy

Most investigators report that no immune reactants are present, but as noted earlier, in the Netherlands study, 7 of 18 patients with thin basement membranes had diffuse mesangial staining for C3.

Electron Microscopy

The thickness of the glomerular basement membranes in normal subjects has been well studied by the Minnesota and Netherlands groups, who are in agreement that it is 354 ± 55 nm. Patients in the group with thin basement membranes were very distinct from the normals and from patients with various diseases, measuring 191 ± 28 nm (Fig. 7–4). There was no overlap between the latter and either of the former groups. It should be emphasized, however, that the width of the

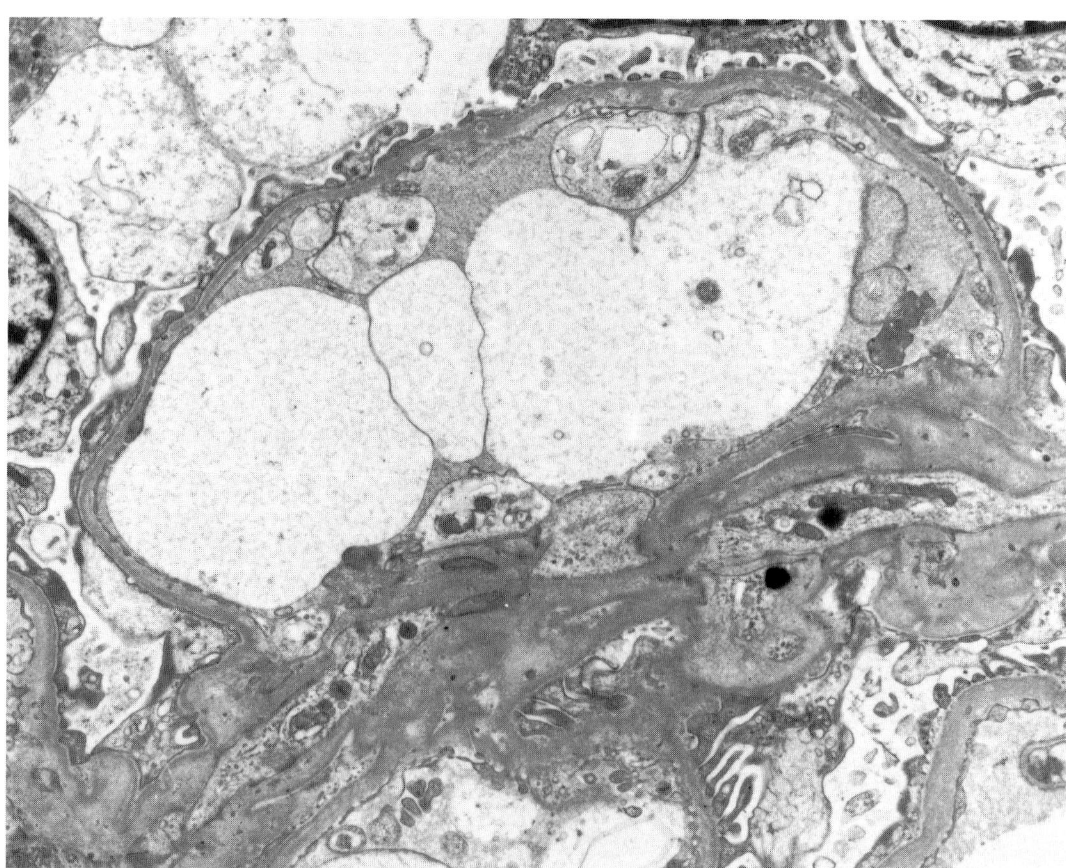

Figure 7–4. The peripheral glomerular basement membranes are uniformly thinned. The pedicels of the epithelial cells are focally spread. (×7800.)

glomerular basement membranes in children slowly increases as a function of age. Thus, caution must be used to match the biopsy specimen in question very carefully to the appropriate controls.

Other lesions have been described in these patients, including mesangial thickening. However, lesions have not been demonstrated in the prospective, long-term studies.

Prognosis

Most reports state that the prognosis is excellent. This option has recently been challenged on the basis of the finding that patients with glomerular basement membranes of 206 to 301 nm may have hypertension and azotemia. However, because the exact thickness of the glomerular basement membranes had not previously been well characterized, some of these reports may have to be reevaluated. Similarly, the significance of proteinuria in these patients needs to be subjected to long-term study before the true significance of this observation can be established.

SELECTED READINGS

1. Fujigaki Y, Mitsumasa N, Kobayashi S, et al: Alterations of glomerular basement membrane relevant to haematuria. Virchow's Arch [A] 413:159, 1988.
2. Gubler MC, Levy M, Naizot C, et al: Glomerular basement membrane changes in hereditary glomerular disease. Renal Physiol 3:405, 1980.
3. Piel CF, Biava CG, Goodman JR: Glomerular basement membrane attenuation in familial nephritis and "benign" hematuria. J Pediatr 101:358, 1982.
4. Seymour A, Canny A, Spargo B: Thickening of glomerular capillary walls: A guide to differential diagnosis by electron microscopy. Ultrastruct Pathol 4:123, 1983.
5. Tiebosch T, Van Breda Vriesman P, Mooy J, et al: Thin-basement-membrane nephropathy in adults with persistent hematuria. N Engl J Med 320:14, 1989.
6. Tina L, Jenis E, Jose P, et al: The glomerular basement membrane in benign familial hematuria. Clin Nephrol 17:1, 1982.

ALPORT'S SYNDROME

Alport's syndrome was first recognized in 1902 and then fully described in 1927 as a clinical syndrome consisting of a hereditary form of progressive renal disease associated with high-frequency deafness. The syndrome was found to affect males more severely than females. The first family described had deaf members without renal disease, and although the males died of renal disease, the females did not. This syndrome is not geographically restricted, and the gene frequency estimates range from 1:5,000 to 1:10,000 in the United States.

Pathogenesis

It was initially thought that the mode of inheritance was autosomal dominant transmission. However, the observations of the unequal severity between affected males and females and a decreased proportion of affected males born of affected fathers now make this hypothesis less tenable. As more studies have been performed, it has become clear that the mode of inheritance is heterogeneous, with both autosomal dominant and recessive modes as well as X-linked forms reported. Support for an X-linked mode comes from two independent sources: (1) The gene-linkage studies of Utah patients show a common linkage to the long arm of the X chromosome. (2) The observations by electron microscopy and immunochemistry reveal that the basement membranes of males are more altered than those of females.

The nature of the biochemical defect is unknown, but it has recently been shown that the glomerular basement membranes of certain kindreds lack an epitope recognized by Goodpasture's serum. This has been found to localize to the non-collagenous domain of the amino terminal end of the type IV collagen molecules of the glomerular basement membranes. An interesting but unexplained finding is that the amyloid P component of the glomerular basement membranes is also missing in these patients.

Patient Presentation

The first indication of the renal aspects of this syndrome is microscopic hematuria. It may be apparent at birth and is most often apparent before school age. The hematuria may on occasion be macroscopic in males, but microscopic hematuria is continuous. Females seldom have continuous microscopic hematuria, and some carriers never have red blood cells in their urine. Proteinuria, often absent during the first few years, slowly in-

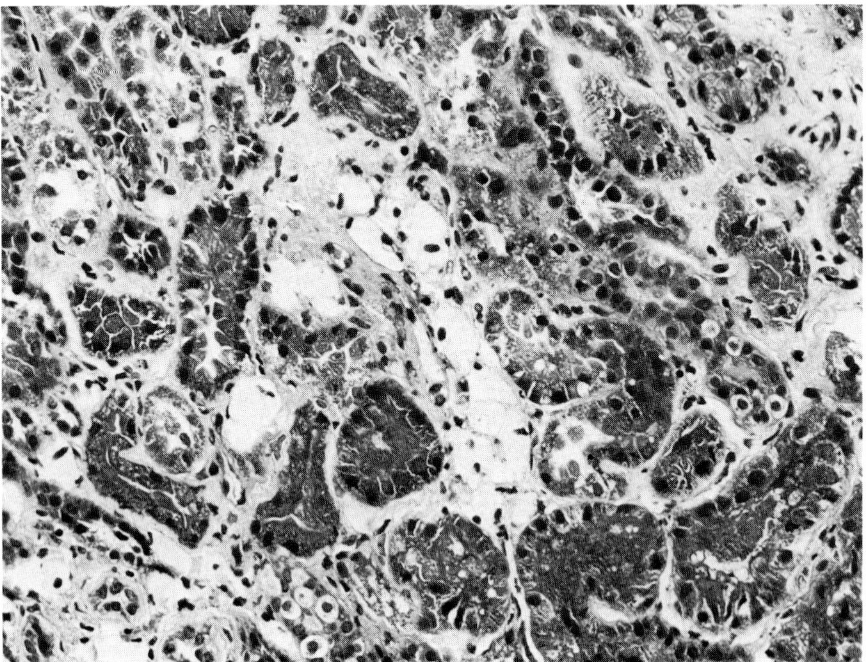

Figure 7–5. There is a mild, generalized increase in the amount of interstitial connective tissue. Foam cells are also found within the interstitium. (H&E, ×300.)

creases in amount in males. When renal failure and hypertension are present, the nephrotic syndrome may also be manifest. Because females seldom develop renal failure, it is not surprising that they seldom have proteinuria.

The most common extrarenal lesion is a progressive cochlear defect that is apparent in males by age 15. Some families without a hearing defect have been described. In affected females, the hearing defect is usually not as severe as in males, except in those women who are destined to develop severe renal lesions. Ocular defects may afflict 15 to 30% of patients, with anterior lenticonus being the most common form. Other defects have also been reported, but their frequency is low.

Histology

Light Microscopy

The morphology by light microscopy depends entirely on the stage of the disease at which the biopsy is performed. Early, the only lesion is a slight, irregular increase in the amount of extracellular matrix in the mesangium and Bowman's capsule. Later, the glomerular changes become slightly more diffuse and evident. At this stage, the principal lesion may appear to be in the interstitium, which may be quite prominently fibrotic and contain foam cells (Fig. 7–5). This observation led previous investigators to the conclusion that foam cells in a fibrotic interstitium were the hallmarks of this disease. It was not until much later that it was shown that interstitial foam cells could be found in many proteinuric states and thus were not a useful diagnostic indicator for hereditary nephritides.

The glomerular changes at late stages consist of a marked increase in all aspects of the basement membranes and mesangium, ultimately resulting in complete sclerosis. The interstitial lesions progress, and tubular atrophy appears.

Immunofluorescence Microscopy

No immune reactants are found at early stages. As sclerosis appears, IgM and complement components (especially C3) may be noted.

Electron Microscopy

The lamina densa of the peripheral glomerular basement membrane is multilami-

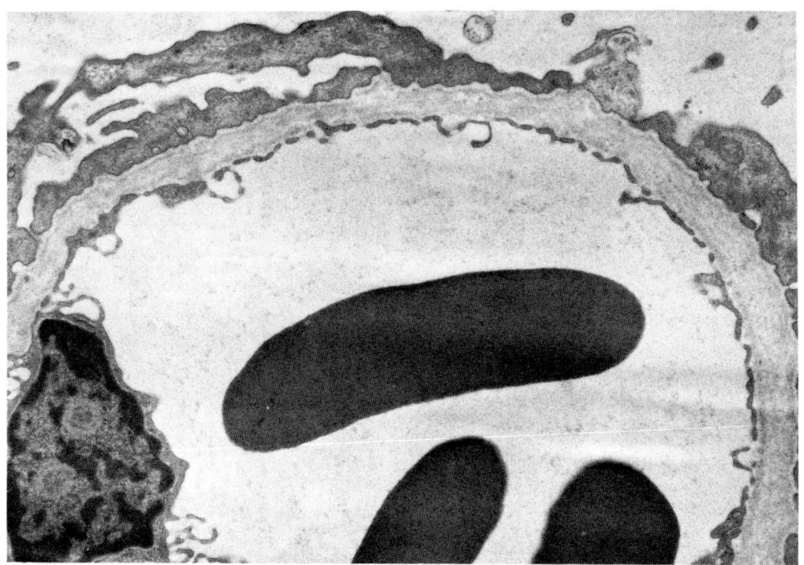

Figure 7–6. The glomerular basement membranes show diffuse multilamination and fragmentation. (×4000.)

nated, and the individual laminae are quite irregular in contour, continuity, and thickness (Fig. 7–6). The clear areas between the laminae are of variable width and are filled with a granular, mottled material. These changes are irregularly distributed within and between glomerular loops, but all glomeruli are affected. The lamina densa alterations in affected females are much less severe and often consist mainly of thinning and irregularity in thickness. The basement membranes of Bowman's capsule and the tubules often show similar lesions.

Prognosis

As noted earlier, the lesions appear in boys before the age of 10 years. If signs of renal disease are not present by this time, it is quite unlikely that the patient will be affected. Affected males practically always progress to renal failure. There are kindreds in which renal failure occurs in the third decade and others in which it presents at a much later time. Females seldom have significant evidence of renal functional impairment.

SELECTED READINGS

1. Alport SC: Hereditary familial congenital hemorrhagic nephritis. Br Med J 1:50, 1927.
2. Butkowski RJ, Wieslander J, Wisdom BJ, et al: Properties of the globular domain of type IV collagen and its relationship to Goodpasture's antigen. J Biol Chem 260:3739, 1985.
3. Coleman M, Haynes WD, Dimopoulos P, et al: Glomerular basement membrane abnormalities associated with apparently idiopathic hematuria. Hum Pathol 17:1022, 1986.
4. Habib R, Gubler MC, Hinglais N, et al: Alport's syndrome: Experience at Hospital Necker. Kidney Int 21:S20, 1982.
5. Savage COS, Pusey CD, Kershaw MJ, et al: The Goodpasture antigen in Alport's syndrome: Studies with a monoclonal antibody. Kidney Int 30:100, 1986.
6. Shaw RF, Kallen RJ: Population genetics of Alport's syndrome: Hypothesis of abnormal segregation and the necessary existence of mutation. Nephron 16:427, 1976.
7. Spear GS, Slusser RJ: Alport's syndrome. Emphasizing electron microscopic studies of the glomerulus. Am J Pathol 69:213, 1972.
8. Yoshikawa N, Cameron AH, White RHR: The glomerular basal lamina in hereditary nephritis. J Pathol 135:199, 1981.

NAIL-PATELLA SYNDROME

The nail-patella syndrome has been recognized as an entity since the end of the 19th century, but it was not until the early 1970s that the presence of a renal lesion was clearly documented. It has an autosomal dominant mode of inheritance, and the gene frequency in the population is approximately 2:100,000. There is a strong linkage to the ABO blood group locus on chromosome 9. The multiple associated skeletal abnormalities include absence or subluxation of the patella, subluxation of the radial head, iliac spurs, and fingernail changes.

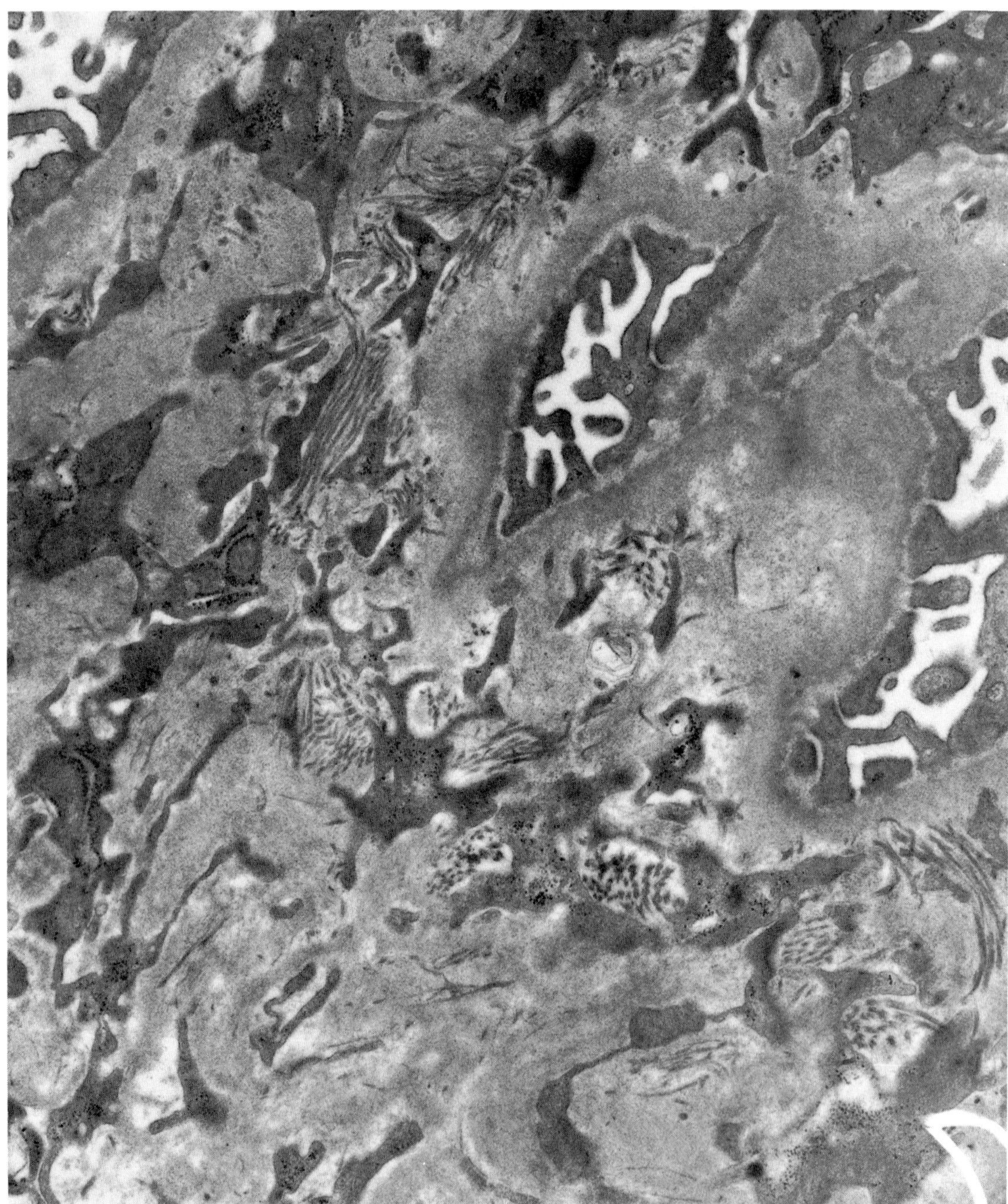

Figure 7–7. Multiple banded fibrils are found within the mesangial matrix and the substance of the peripheral glomerular basement membranes. (×6300.)

Pathogenesis

Essentially nothing is known about the genesis of the renal lesion in this rare condition. The fact that a disproportionate number of other congenital malformations of the skeleton and urinary tract are concomitant suggests that the lesion is generalized, but there are few studies of the extrarenal abnormalities.

Patient Presentation

The presence of renal disease can be the first sign of the syndrome, although somewhat less than one-half of affected patients have detectable kidney involvement. Hematuria is seldom present, and the nephrotic syndrome is exceptional.

Histology

Light Microscopy

The renal tissue most often appears normal at early stages of the disease. As the disease progresses, glomerulosclerosis appears. It is in the form of diffuse, regular thickening of the basement membranes and mesangial sclerosis. The extraglomerular connective tissue components are also affected, resulting in interstitial fibrosis and tubular basement membrane thickening.

Immunofluorescence Microscopy

No deposits are seen, because there is no evidence of an immune pathogenesis. The trapping of complement components and immunoglobulins in areas of sclerosis is observed in late lesions.

Electron Microscopy

The lesions can only be appreciated at the ultrastructural level. They consist of multiple lucent areas within basement membranes, which contain debris and regularly banded fibrils (Fig. 7–7). The fibrils resemble interstitial collagen and are best seen after phosphotungstic acid staining. They are not seen in all lacunae and may be present in patients without proteinuria. Although most glomeruli are affected, the distribution of the lesions between individual loops or glomeruli may be very irregular.

Prognosis

It appears that less than 10% of affected patients develop significant renal failure, and less than 50% have proteinuria. The basement membrane lesions do not recur in transplanted kidneys.

SELECTED READINGS

1. Ben-Bassat M, Cohen L, Rosenfeld J: The glomerular basement membrane in the nail-patella syndrome. Arch Pathol 92:350, 1971.
2. Bennett WM, Musgrave JE, Campbell RA, et al: The nephropathy of the nail-patella syndrome: Clinicopathologic analysis of 11 kindreds. Am J Med 54:304, 1973.
3. Hawkins CF, Smith OE: Renal dysplasia in a family with multiple hereditary abnormalities including iliac horns. Lancet 1:803, 1950.
4. Hoyer JR, Michael AF, Vernier RL: Renal disease in nail-patella syndrome: Clinical and morphologic studies. Kidney Int 2:231, 1972.
5. Schleutermann DA, Bias WB, Murdoch JL, et al: Linkage of the loci for the nail-patella syndrome and adenylate kinase. Am J Hum Genet 21:606, 1969.

SICKLE CELL DISEASE

Renal disease may afflict patients with sickle cell disease (hemoglobin SS or SA). In most patients with sickle cell anemia, the renal abnormalities are not severe enough to warrant a renal biopsy. A concentrating defect is the most commonly reported lesion. However, proteinuria and the nephrotic syndrome have been described. In these cases, the underlying renal lesion is focal and segmental glomerulosclerosis or membranoproliferative glomerulonephritis. Renal lesions are seen most frequently in patients with hemoglobin SS and in children.

Pathogenesis

It has been generally assumed that patients with sickle cell anemia have an increased glomerular hydrostatic pressure and glomerular blood flow. The current paradigm to explain the pathogenesis of progressive glomerular lesions predicts the type of glomerulosclerotic lesion in these patients. However, this hypothesis does not explain the presence of glomerular lesions of similar intensity in patients both with and without proteinuria.

The discovery of iron deposits in the mes-

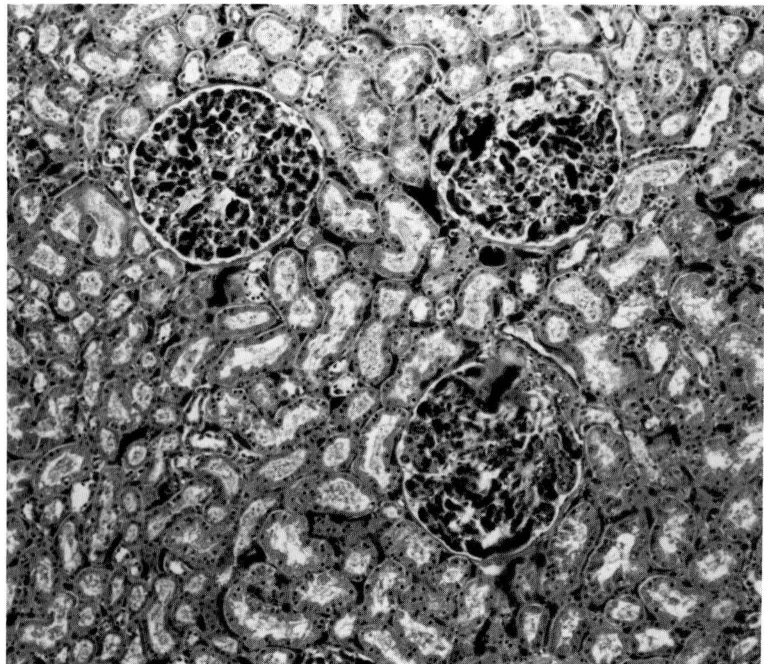

Figure 7–8. The glomeruli are large and filled with red blood cells. (H&E, ×100.)

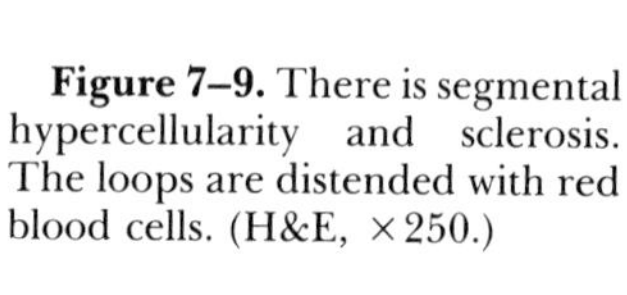

Figure 7–9. There is segmental hypercellularity and sclerosis. The loops are distended with red blood cells. (H&E, ×250.)

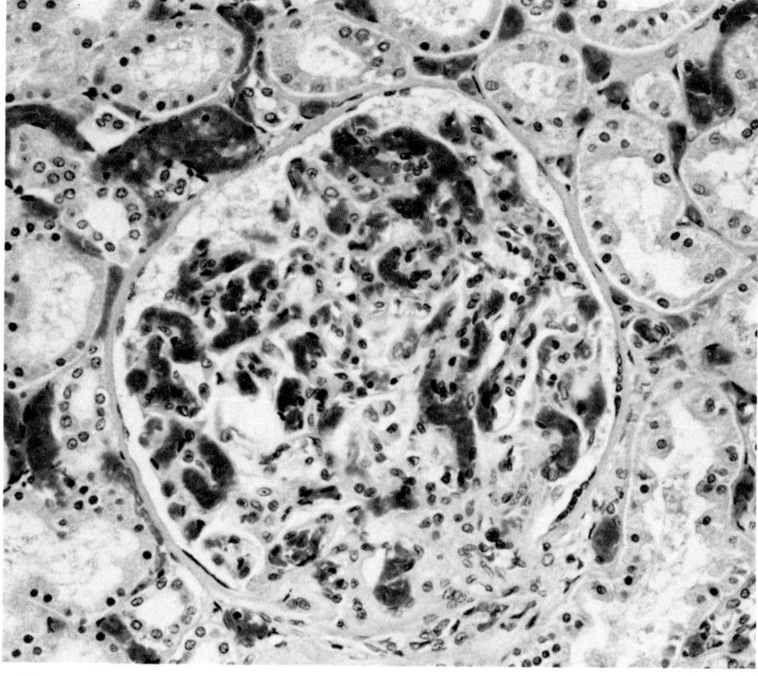

angium of some patients suggests that the chronic anemia state also contributes to the mesangial lesions. The means by which the iron arrives in the mesangium and its relation to the glomerulosclerosis are not clear. The exact relationship between the genetic defect and the occurrence of the glomerular lesion is not known, and the small number of cases makes further study difficult.

Patient Presentation

Although sickle cell trait has been described as a potential cause of renal disease, the presence of renal lesions has mainly been restricted to autopsy studies. Thus, significant proteinuria or the nephrotic syndrome with hematuria is only encountered in sickle cell anemia. Few detailed studies of renal function have been performed, but they reveal an increase in glomerular filtration rate and renal plasma flow.

Histology

Light Microscopy

The glomeruli often appear to be distended with erythrocytes, some of which may be abnormal in shape (Fig. 7–8). Some have described the glomeruli as large, but morphometric data do not exist. Deposits of iron may be revealed in glomerular and tubular cells by special stains.

Several varieties of glomerular disease have been reported, and they all share the features of mesangial sclerosis and/or hypercellularity (Fig. 7–9). The mesangium may be irregularly affected with areas of focal sclerosis. Hyalin is not detected. The glomeruli may be irregularly affected, with some being normal and some completely obsolescent (so-called global sclerosis).

The peripheral glomerular basement membranes often appear thick and wrinkled. When the glomerular basement membrane changes are marked and the mesangium is severely affected, the term *membranoproliferative glomerulonephritis* has been applied. However, the lesions are much more sclerotic than proliferative, thus the descriptor *glomerulosclerosis* seems more appropriate.

Patients with sickle cell disease may be affected by other renal diseases, but the hemoglobinopathy seems to add little to those processes.

Immunofluorescence Microscopy

There are no deposits of immune reactants due to the sickle cell disease.

Electron Microscopy

The mesangial matrix is focally increased in amount, and the glomerular basement membranes are irregularly thickened, duplicated, and wrinkled. Occasional intracellular membrane-bounded vesicles are seen to contain a granular electron-dense substance thought to represent iron-containing materials. The pedicels are irregularly effaced near areas of sclerosis.

Prognosis

Few long-term studies have been performed, but those available suggest that the prognosis in patients with glomerulosclerosis is one of slow, inexorable progression. However, this conclusion is far from established.

SELECTED READINGS

1. Buckalew VM Jr: The kidney in sickle cell disease. Kidney Int 11:11, 1978.
2. de Jong PE, Van Es LWS: Sickle cell nephropathy: New insights into its pathophysiology. Kidney Int 27:711, 1985.
3. Schlitt LE, Keitel HG: Renal manifestations of sickle cell disease: A review. Am J Med Sci 239:773, 1960.
4. Tejani A, Phadke K, Adamson O, et al: Renal lesions in sickle cell nephropathy in children. Nephron 39:352, 1985.

Chapter

8

GLOMERULAR DISEASES ASSOCIATED WITH SPECIFIC METABOLIC DISEASES

DIABETIC NEPHROPATHY (KIDNEY DISEASE OF DIABETES MELLITUS)

Diabetes mellitus is a common metabolic disorder characterized by a deficiency of insulin secretion or action resulting in hyperglycemia. Since the discovery of insulin and its availability as a therapeutic measure, the renal complications of diabetes have predominated as the chief causes of morbidity and mortality in this disease. Renal disease is a major complication of diabetes, eventually causing renal failure in approximately 40% of patients with insulin-dependent diabetes. Renal disease also complicates type II (insulin-independent) diabetes mellitus, and although its exact frequency has not been determined, most researchers now consider that renal disease is as common in type II as in type I diabetes mellitus. It is responsible for about 10% of the deaths in this population. Several forms of renal disease have been described. The most common is diabetic glomerulosclerosis, often associated with Kimmelstiel-Wilson nodules. The small blood vessels of the kidneys are particularly affected. Other changes involving the kidneys but less likely to be seen in renal biopsy specimens include papillary necrosis and pyelonephritis. Whether or not diabetic persons are more likely to develop renal infections than nondiabetics is currently controversial.

Pathogenesis

The first description of diabetic glomerulosclerosis was presented in 1936 by Kimmelstiel and Wilson. Since that time, many investigators have attempted to determine the pathogenesis of these alterations. The role of hyperglycemia has been investigated, but a causal relation remains unproven. Some researchers have suggested that close control of blood glucose decreases the incidence and severity of diabetic nephropathy. It has recently been found that many proteins are non-enzymatically glycosylated in the presence of glucose concentrations similar to those in diabetic patients. This parameter is best measured in patients by assessing the glycosylation of hemoglobin A1c. It has been suggested that glycosylation of glomerular basement membrane proteins might alter them in ways to affect their sieving characteristics, allowing the passage of high-molecular-weight substances into the urine. These include albumin and immunoglobulins. Because less than one-half of patients develop renal disease despite the fact that essentially all have plasma glucose levels high enough to result in non-enzymatic glycosylation, this remains as an interesting but still unproven association.

Another factor that may play a role in the pathogenesis of these lesions includes systemic and microvascular hypertension. Insulin-dependent diabetic patients often have an increased glomerular filtration rate at the onset of their disease. Changes in glomerular hemodynamics, in particular elevations of intraglomerular pressure, lead to glomerulosclerosis in animals, but this outcome has not yet been clearly demonstrated in humans. However, numerous uncontrolled clinical studies have suggested that lowering of systemic blood pressure slows the progression of diabetic nephropathy. Additional evidence regarding the relationship between changes in glomerular hemodynamics and the evolution of diabetic nephropathy has been gathered using streptozotocin-induced hyperglycemia in rats, a model of type I diabetes. Increased intraglomerular pressure is observed before the time that glomerular lesions are histologically recognizable. Others dispute the importance of these alterations in initiating the damage but accept their importance in progression of the injury.

There is considerable morphometric evidence of nephron hypertrophy in diabetes. Glomerular hypertrophy is present, including an increase in the mean volume of glomeruli and total mesangial volume. Mesangial expansion is inversely correlated with the total vascular area available as a filtering surface area. This may account, in part, for the decrease in renal function found in late lesions. In addition, hypertrophy may accentuate changes in intraglomerular pressure. Furthermore, through mechanisms not yet elucidated, it may reflect glomerular injury that is independent of hemodynamic changes. Considerable additional research is required in this area before the etiology of the renal lesions of diabetes mellitus will be fully understood.

The development of glomerulosclerosis in type I diabetes mellitus seems to depend on the overall duration of the disease, with the incidence of renal lesions continuing to increase for the first 20 years of diabetes mellitus. After that time, there is no further increase.

The development of sclerosing lesions is also related to the age of onset, especially in type II diabetes mellitus. In this population, in which the onset of diabetes typically occurs at a late age, the renal lesions develop at a much more accelerated rate. This accounts for the fact that the average time to onset of renal dysfunction is estimated to be approximately 10 to 15 years, that is, nearly one decade shorter than in type I diabetes.

Patient Presentation

Renal insufficiency most often becomes evident 15 to 20 years after the onset of type I diabetes mellitus and after 10 to 15 years in type II diabetes mellitus. Early, there may be an elevated glomerular filtration rate, increased renal size, and exercise-induced or resting microalbuminuria (urinary albumin excretion of greater than 50 μg/minute). Some researchers have suggested that microalbuminuria predicts the development of subsequent proteinuria and renal disease. Others have not been able to support this correlation. The onset of diabetic nephropathy is suspected by the appearance of proteinuria. However, proteinuria is a marker of renal disease, not a predictor. In other words, significant renal disease may be present in the absence of proteinuria, and microalbuminuria may be present in the absence of renal disease. It is relatively unusual for patients to present with hypertension and proteinuria in the nephrotic range. The urinary sediment is inactive, although hematuria may be present.

Diabetic patients may also have non-diabetic renal disease, alone or in addition to diabetic glomerulosclerosis. This finding has been reported to occur in as many as 10% of diabetic patients undergoing renal biopsy. The presence of another renal disease should be suspected when the clinical and laboratory findings differ from those expected in a diabetic patient with nephropathy.

Histology

Light Microscopy

The glomerular lesions are quite complex and consist of two general types: nodular and diffuse. It is not clear whether these two forms represent a continuum or whether they are two separate categories of renal disease. In any case, hypertrophy of the nephron is the earliest alteration. The enlargement may not be obvious in the presence of renal insufficiency, although hypertrophy may still be evident in isolated, less-affected glomeruli.

The characteristic glomerular alterations in the diffuse lesion include uniform thickening of glomerular basement membranes, hyalinosis, diffuse mesangial sclerosis, and mesangial proliferation (Figs. 8–1 and 8–2). Hyalinosis, also referred to as an "exudative"

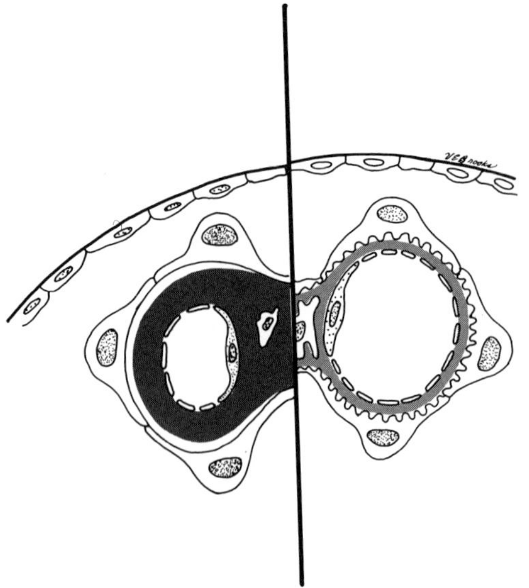

Figure 8–1. Diagram of diffuse glomerular basement membrane thickening and mesangial sclerosis.

lesion, represents an accumulation of plasma proteins in the subendothelial space (Figs. 8–2 and 8–3). The hyalin material may eventually fill the lumen. It stains bright pink with periodic acid-Schiff (PAS) stain and may contain lipid droplets or foam cells (see Fig. 8–3). This is not a specific finding because similar lesions may be seen in many glomerular diseases. Their pathogenesis is not understood.

The lesion considered to be diagnostic of diabetic renal disease is the Kimmelstiel-Wilson nodule (Figs. 8–4 and 8–5). These structures were first described by Kimmelstiel and Wilson in 1936. The nodules are randomly and irregularly spread throughout the glomeruli and may assume two forms. They most commonly appear as mesangial nodules consisting of an increase in the amount of matrix admixed with mesangial cell proliferation arranged in a concentric pattern. The nodules stain with both PAS and silver stains. Some nodules have a distinctly laminated appearance, giving rise to the postulate that the nodules represent healed microaneurysms. The nodules in light-chain systemic disease can be distinguished from those in diabetes by the fact that they are quite uniform in size and distribution in light-chain systemic disease, whereas in diabetes they are irregular in both size and distribution.

The formation of microaneurysms is thought to result from a process of mesangiolysis. This process may be seen in a variety of glomerular diseases. As these changes progress, glomerular obsolescence ensues. Although some glomeruli simply demonstrate wrinkling and collapse due to the vascular disease, other obsolescent glomeruli are

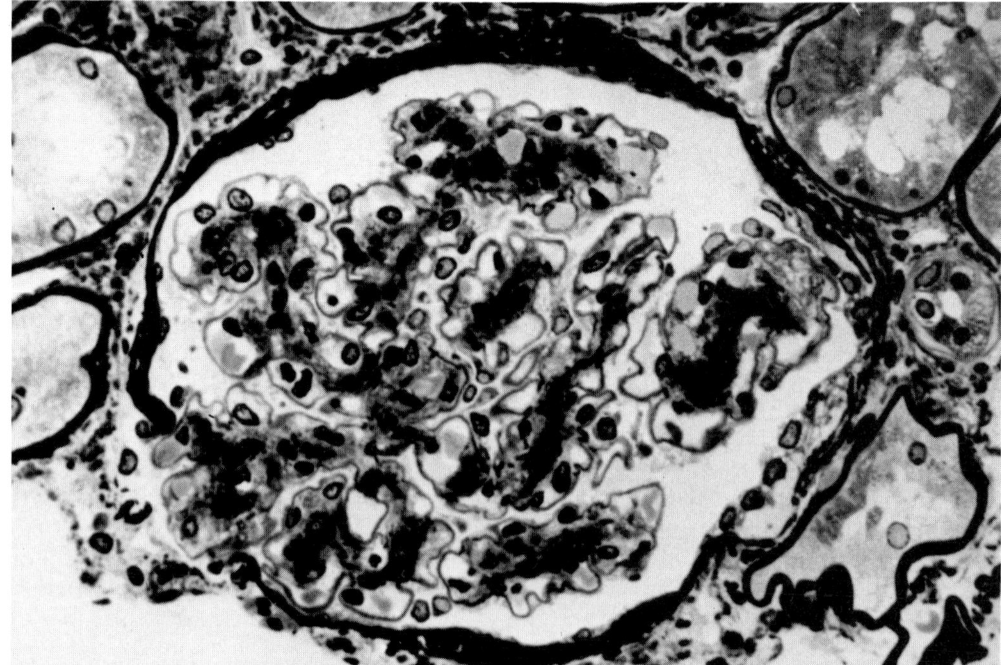

Figure 8–2. There is diffuse mesangial cell proliferation and mesangial sclerosis. The basement membranes of the glomerulus, Bowman's capsule, and the tubules are thickened. (PASM, ×300.)

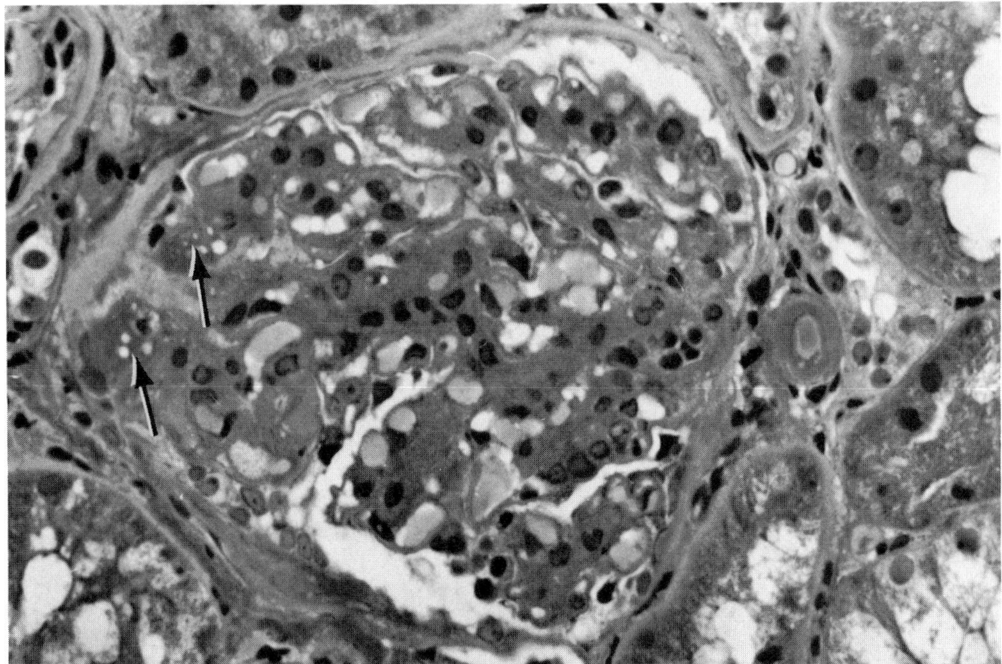

Figure 8–3. The mesangial regions are irregularly affected by the proliferative and sclerotic process. Synechiae are present in the left quadrant and contain "insudative" lesions (arrows). The afferent arteriole contains a large circular hyalin deposit (right). (H&E, ×300.)

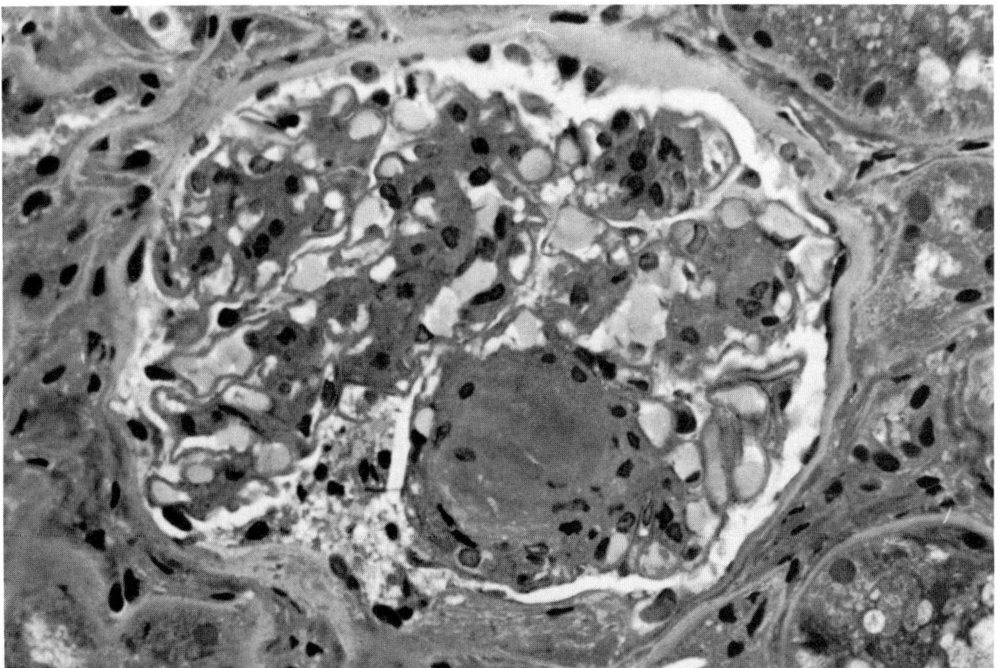

Figure 8–4. A large mesangial nodule is present in the lower, middle region. Elsewhere the mesangial matrix is also increased in amount, and there is an increase in the number of nuclei. The peripheral glomerular basement membranes are thickened. There are many vacuoles within the cytoplasm of the adjacent tubules. (H&E, ×300.)

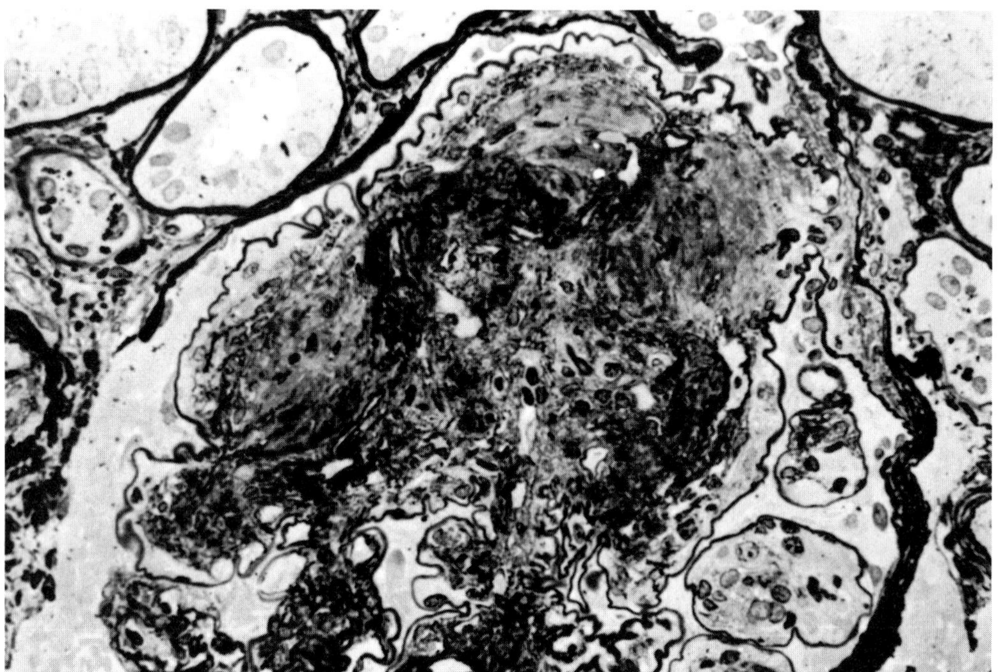

Figure 8–5. The nodules have a laminated substructure. The glomerular loops are compressed to the periphery of these large sclerotic nodules. The glomerulus is markedly increased in overall size. (PASM, ×400.)

normal or enlarged as a result of the sclerotic process. These large obsolescent glomeruli may be a helpful feature in distinguishing the end-stage kidney due to diabetes mellitus from that of other diseases.

Another lesion described by Kimmelstiel and Wilson is the capsular drop or fibrin cap (see Fig. 8–3). It consists of a mass of hyalin lying within the substance of the basement membrane of Bowman's capsule. This lesion is not seen in other types of renal diseases and thus has the same specificity for diabetic glomerular disease as the Kimmelstiel-Wilson nodule.

The glomerular alterations are accompanied by tubular atrophy with marked thickening of tubular basement membranes and interstitial fibrosis (Figs. 8–6 and 8–7).

Because diabetes mellitus is often accompanied by severe atherosclerosis, large arteries often show advanced degrees of intimal thickening and internal elastic lamina reduplication.

Hyalin arteriosclerosis is identical in appearance to that which occurs in patients with hypertension (Figs. 8–8, 8–9, and 8–10). However, in diabetic patients it may be present in both afferent and efferent arterioles, in which case it is considered to be pathognomonic for diabetes mellitus. Furthermore, the presence of numerous arterioles with hyalin deposits, particularly in young patients, should suggest the diagnosis of diabetes mellitus.

Immunofluorescence Microscopy

Diffuse linear staining of glomerular and tubular basement membranes with antibodies to IgG and albumin may be seen. Glomerular and arteriolar deposits of hyalin contain IgM and C3.

Electron Microscopy

The earliest observable alteration is uniform thickening of the glomerular basement membranes, which may have a three- to fourfold increase, measuring as much as 1200 to 1500 nm (Fig. 8–11). The glomerular visceral epithelial cells may show an irregular effacement of the pedicles, although this is not a constant finding. Hyalin deposits, recognized by their subendothelial location and uniform density, may occasionally occur within the mesangium. Lipid, either within macrophages or lying loose within the lesion, may also be seen. The mesangial matrix is increased in amount and may contain cell debris and microcalcifications. Immune depos-

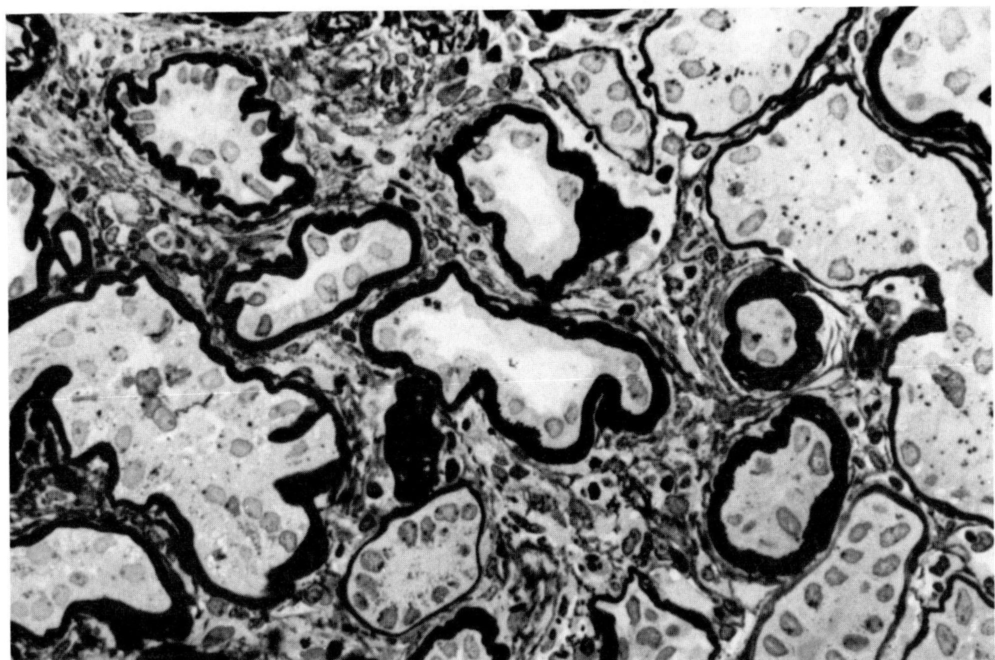

Figure 8–6. The interstitium contains an increased amount of connective tissue and scattered inflammatory cells. The tubular basement membranes are thickened, especially in the areas of interstitial fibrosis. (PASM, ×300.)

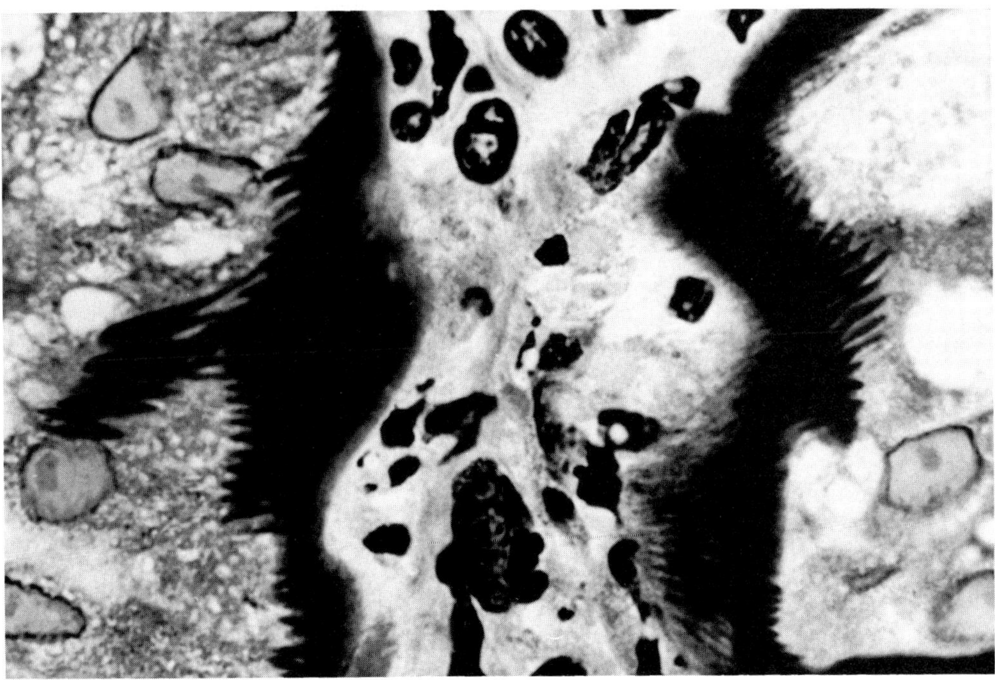

Figure 8–7. The tubular basement membrane thickening extends between the basilar interdigitations of the epithelial cells, resulting in a comblike appearance. (PASM, ×1200.)

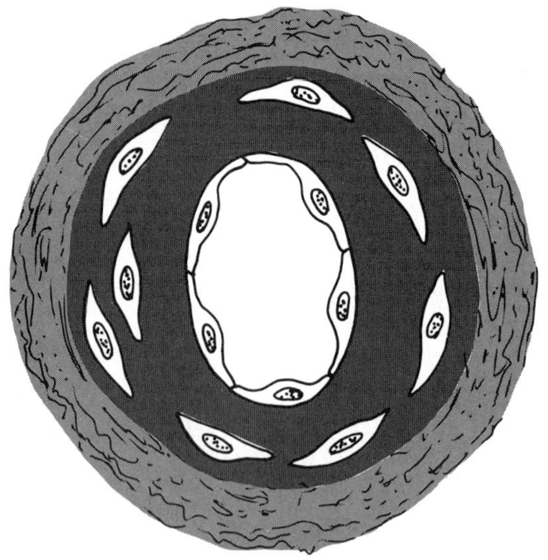

Figure 8–8. Diagram of an artery with a diffuse increase in extracellular matrix of the wall.

its are not identified unless another glomerular lesion is superimposed on the diabetic state. The tubular basement membranes are frequently duplicated.

Prognosis

Once begun, diabetic nephropathy seems to follow an inexorably progressive course of deteriorating renal function, finally ending in renal failure requiring dialysis or kidney transplantation. Diabetic nephropathy has been reported to recur in transplanted kidneys at a more rapid rate than in native kidneys. Therefore, the course may be considerably shortened from the 15 to 20 years required for the evolution of the original disease. Without renal replacement therapy, the prognosis is grim, with mean survival

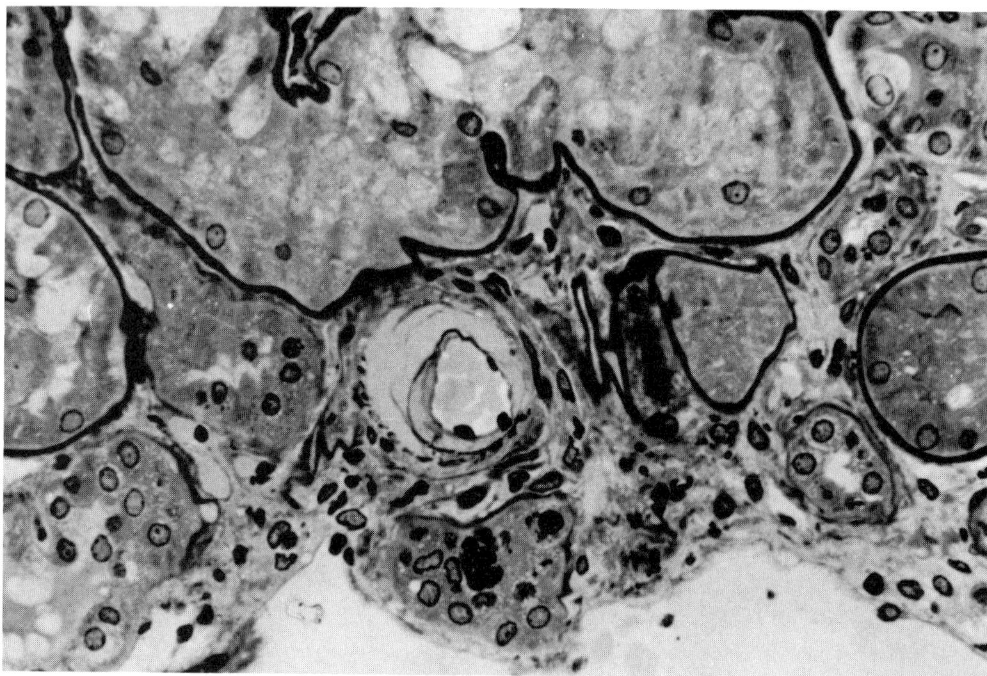

Figure 8–9. The wall of this arteriole contains large hyalin deposits, which displace the smooth muscle cells and distort the architecture of the blood vessel. (PASM, ×1200.)

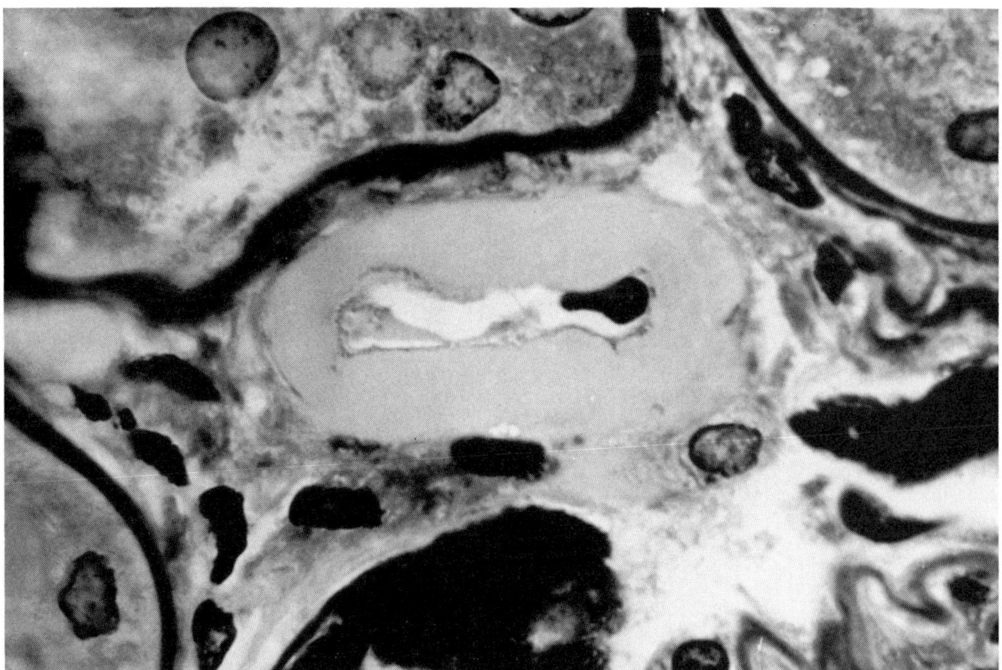

Figure 8–10. The wall of this arteriole is completely replaced by a circumferential hyalin deposit. (PASM, ×1200.)

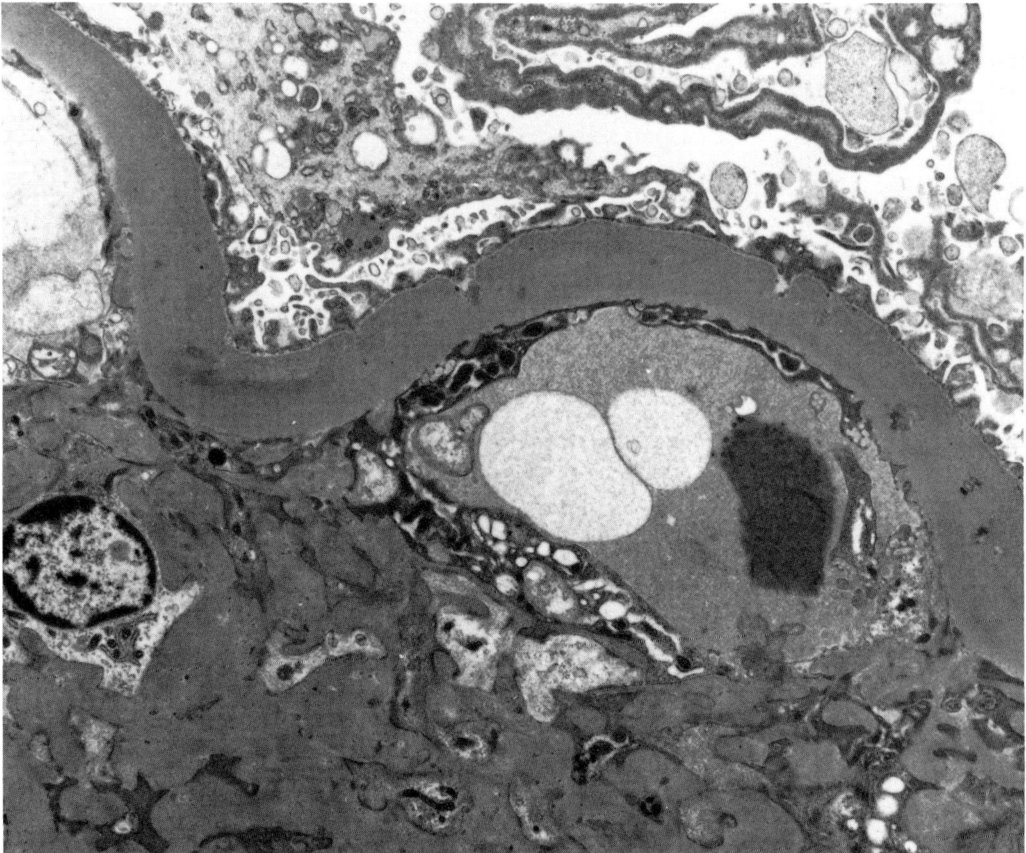

Figure 8–11. The glomerular basement membranes are uniformly and diffusely thickened. The epithelial cells show microvillous transformation, and there is irregular and focal spreading of the pedicels. Marked mesangial sclerosis is also present. (×3200.)

only 7 years after onset of clinical proteinuria.

SELECTED READINGS

1. Gundersen H, Osterby R: Glomerular size and structure in diabetes mellitus II. Late abnormalities. Diabetologia 13:43, 1977.
2. Kimmelstiel P, Wilson C: Intercapillary lesions in glomeruli of the kidney. Am J Pathol 12:83, 1936.
3. Krolewski AS, Warram JH, Christlieb AR, et al: The changing natural history of nephropathy in type I diabetes. Am J Med 78:785, 1985.
4. Kunzelman C, Pettitt D, Bennett P, et al: Incidence of nephropathy in type 2 diabetes mellitus. Am J Epidemiol 122:547, 1985.
5. Mathiesen ER, Oxenboll B, Johansen K, et al: Incipient nephropathy in type I (insulin-dependent) diabetes. Diabetologia 26:406, 1984.
6. Mauer SM, Steffes MW, Ellis EN, et al: Structural-functional relationships in diabetic nephropathy. J Clin Invest 74:1143, 1984.
7. Myers BD:, Winetz JA, Chui F, et al: Mechanisms of proteinuria in diabetic nephropathy: A study of glomerular barrier function. Kidney Int 21:633, 1982.
8. Osterby R, Gundersen H:Glomerular size and structure in diabetes mellitus. Diabetologia 11:225, 1975.
9. Salinas-Madrigal L, Pirani CL, Pollak VE: Glomerular and vascular "insudative" lesions of diabetic nephropathy. Electron microscopic observations. Am J Pathol 59:369, 1970.
10. Salomon MI: Diabetic nephropathy: Clinicopathologic correlation. A study based on renal biopsies. Metabolism 12:687, 1963.
11. Zatz R, Brenner BM: Pathogenesis of diabetic microangiopathy. Am J Med 80:443, 1986.

CYSTINOSIS

Cystinosis is a metabolic disorder, first described after the turn of the century. It is rare and is transmitted in an autosomal recessive manner. The gene frequency in the population is unknown, and the chromosomal localization has not been elucidated. The heterozygous carriers have no clinical symptoms but may be recognized by examination of the cystine content of their peripheral leukocytes.

There are three forms: nephropathic, juvenile, and adult. The nephropathic form is the most common and becomes manifest at birth by the presence of aminoaciduria. The juvenile form is much less common and appears after the age of 10 years, with renal failure developing in the second or third decades of life. The adult form is much milder and consists of mild elevations of cystine in various tissues.

The nephropathic form is associated with diffuse deposits of cystine in all organs. The deposits consist of large intracellular accumulations of cystine crystals. The kidneys are affected early in life, and renal failure is a serious complication in this syndrome.

This stands in sharp contrast to cystinuria, in which the kidneys are the only site of increased cystine accumulation. In cystinuria, the principal defect is thought to be in the proximal tubule and is due to a defective amino acid transport process involving cystine, lysine, ornithine, and arginine. The result is that these amino acids are lost in the urine and can be found within the lumen of tubules. Cystine forms crystals and eventually renal calculi.

Pathogenesis

The defect is in the intracellular metabolism of cystine. The end result is the intracellular accumulation of cystine crystals. The entire tissue eventually becomes filled with cystine crystals within the cells. The crystals eventually reach the interstitium, where they excite an inflammatory reaction. The result is considerable distortion of the indigenous cell function, as well as of the surrounding interstitium. The eyes, kidneys, and skeleton have the most obvious lesions.

Patient Presentation

The first evidence of this syndrome may appear within the first month of life, in the form of Fanconi's syndrome consisting of aminoaciduria, glycosuria, hyperphosphaturia, proximal renal tubular acidosis, and a concentrating defect. Affected infants develop this syndrome by approximately the sixth month of life. Thereafter, the maintenance of normal fluid and electrolyte balance, bone growth and maturation, and body growth become increasingly severe problems. Renal failure is first evident between 18 and 24 months. Renal function progressively declines and frequently reaches end stage by age 5 years.

Histology

Light Microscopy

The first renal lesions consist of the formation of lysosomal crystals in the epithelium

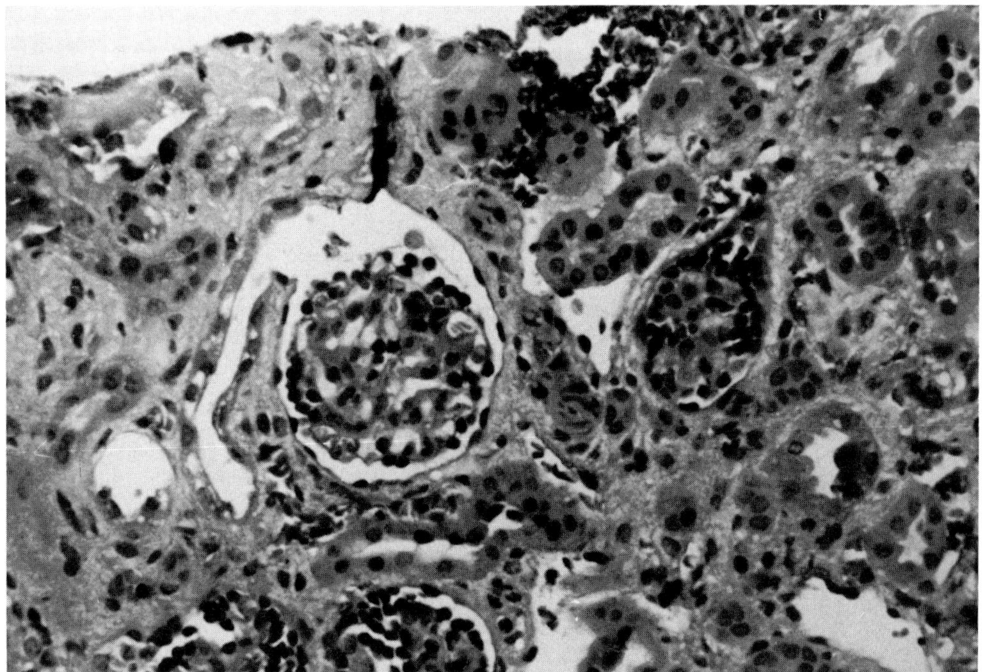

Figure 8–12. The epithelium of the first portion of the proximal tubule is atrophied, resulting in the appearance of the classic "swan neck" lesion. The glomerular epithelial cells are prominent, consistent with the frequent appearance of multinucleated cells in this location by electron microscopy. (H&E, ×300.)

of the glomeruli and the first part of the proximal convoluted tubule. The epithelium of this segment of the proximal tubule eventually atrophies, leading to the so-called swan neck lesion (Fig. 8–12). The visceral glomerular epithelial cells also have crystalline inclusions, and they may become multinucleated. As the disease progresses, the interstitium becomes more fibrotic, with the formation of interstitial infiltrates. Intracellular crystals with the typical rhomboid-shaped crystals are seen in many cells. Tubular atrophy, glomerular sclerosis, and nephron loss relentlessly progress.

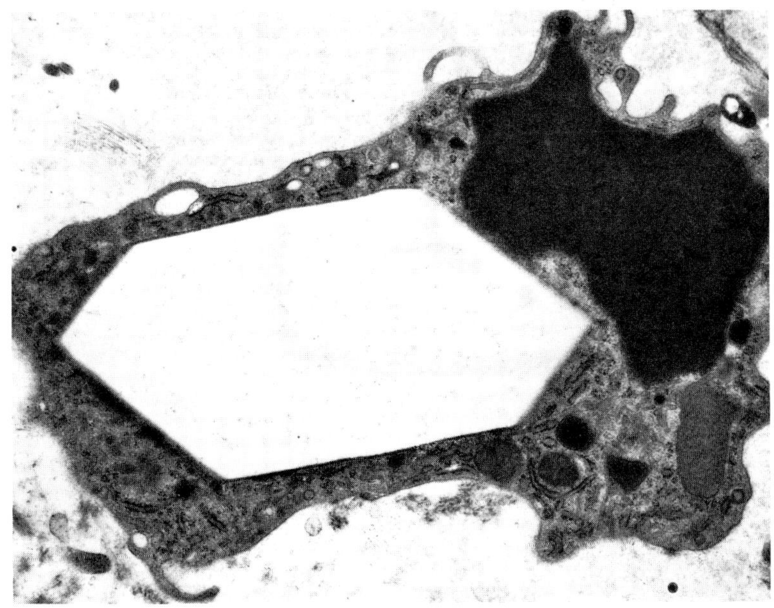

Figure 8–13. Rhomboid-shaped crystals are present in many cells within the interstitium. Similar crystals may be seen within epithelial cells, although they may have other configurations in these locations. (×5000.)

Immunofluorescence Microscopy

There are no immune reactants in these biopsy specimens.

Electron Microscopy

The first lesions are those in the podocytes and the epithelium of the S1 segment of the proximal tubule. Needle-shaped crystals are found in membrane-bounded vesicles, within the first 6 months of life (Fig. 8–13). Thereafter, the podocytes may become multinucleated, and the epithelial cells of the S1 segment of the proximal tubule are replaced by a low-lying sheet of thinned cytoplasm. Tubular, glomerular, and interstitial extracellular matrix increase in concert with mounting deposits of crystals in the kidney. The end result is complete nephron loss and renal atrophy.

Prognosis

An inexorable decline in renal function to end stage was previously the rule. Cysteamine has recently shown promise in preventing progression of the disease, but studies of this effect are not yet complete.

Renal transplantation has been used in many patients. The transplanted organs do not develop lysosomal deposits, but infiltrating recipient leukocytes contain cystine crystals, and the kidneys thus become secondarily affected.

SELECTED READINGS

1. Chesney RW: Etiology and pathogenesis of the Fanconi syndrome. Miner Electrolyte Metab 4:303, 1980.
2. Dent CE, Rose GA: Amino acid metabolism in cystinuria. Q J Med 20:205, 1951.
3. Mahoney CP, Striker GE, Manning GB, et al: Renal transplantation for childhood cystinosis. N Engl J Med 283:397, 1970.
4. Schneider JA, Schulman JD: Progress in endocrinology and metabolism. Cystinosis: A review. Metabolism 26:817, 1977.
5. Schneider JA, Schulman JD: Cystinosis. *In* Stanbury JB, Wyngaarden JB (eds): The Metabolic Basis of Inherited Disease. McGraw-Hill, New York, 1983, pp 1844–1866.

GLYCOGENOSIS I

Glycogenosis I is characterized by the pathologic accumulation of glycogen in the kidneys, liver, and gastrointestinal tract. This disease, also known as type I glycogen storage disease or glycogenosis, is accompanied by renal dysfunction in most patients.

Pathogenesis

The disease is an autosomal recessive condition. Some patients lack glucose-6-phosphatase, and others are unable to transport glucose-6-phosphate. The result of either of these defects is the inability to transport glycogen out of the cell, resulting in its accumulation in large intracellular vacuoles. The cause of the renal disease is the accumulation of glycogen in the various renal compartments. It is interesting that most patients have recently been shown to have significant hyperfiltration, which appears to be unrelated to hypertension, increased protein intake, or abnormal lipid levels.

Patient Presentation

Glycogenosis I is frequently manifest during childhood. The incidence of renal dysfunction in patients who survive past the age of 10 years is 70%. As in other lysosomal storage diseases, the first evidence of renal disease is the appearance of proteinuria. A few patients have the nephrotic syndrome as the presenting condition. Another small subset of patients have Fanconi's syndrome (i.e., glycosuria, aminoaciduria, and polyuria). The renal disease is one of continuous progressive loss of renal function leading to end stage.

Histology

Light Microscopy

The glomerular lesions are focal and segmental glomerulosclerosis with areas of hyalinosis (Fig. 8–14). They are identical to those described in Chapter 4. These lesions progressively involve more glomeruli, and eventually they all are obsolescent.

The tubular epithelium contains large intracellular PAS-positive inclusions that become progressively larger.

The interstitium is initially increased in amount and contains an inflammatory cell infiltrate in the periglomerular regions. As the glomerular lesions progress, the interstitial changes become more generalized.

There are no lesions in the vasculature.

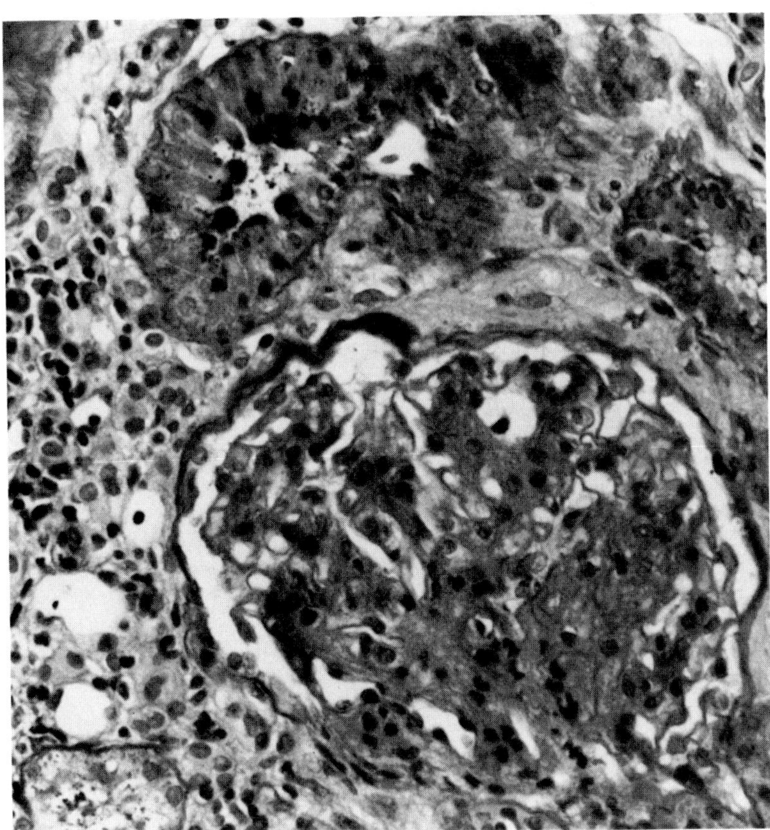

Figure 8–14. Moderately advanced focal and segmental glomerulosclerosis. Note the interstitial infiltrate and fibrosis and vacuolation of some proximal tubular cells. (PAS, ×250.)

Immunofluorescence Microscopy

There are no deposits of immune reactants except for those nonspecifically trapped within sclerotic areas.

Electron Microscopy

No additional findings are revealed by electron microscopy. The mesangial matrix is irregularly increased in amount. No deposits are seen. The glomerular basement membranes may be wrinkled and thickened near the zones of marked mesangial sclerosis but are otherwise unremarkable. Large amounts of glycogen are present in the tubular epithelium, especially in the proximal tubules.

Prognosis

Most patients develop proteinuria during the second to third decade of life. Renal failure eventually ensues.

SELECTED READINGS

1. Chen Y, Coleman RA, Scheinman JI, et al: Renal disease in Type I glycogen storage disease. N Engl J Med 318:7, 1988.

FABRY'S DISEASE

Fabry's disease represents a deficiency of the enzyme alpha-galactosidase A. This enzyme is found in lysosomes throughout the body; therefore, the manifestations of the disease occur throughout each organ system. The result of the enzyme defect is the accumulation of the glycosphingolipid galactosylceramide. Fabry's disease is an X-linked disorder that is characteristically encountered in hemizygous males.

Pathogenesis

The X-linked defective gene is located on the long arm of the X chromosome. Although there are intra- and interfamilial variations, the gene has high penetrance. Hemizygous males are severely affected. Curiously, females are less affected clinically. Identification of the exact biochemical defect makes it possible to diagnose the condition in utero and to identify carriers. The gene frequency has been estimated to be 1:40,000 in the United States. It is more frequently seen in Caucasians, but it has been reported in essentially all racial groups.

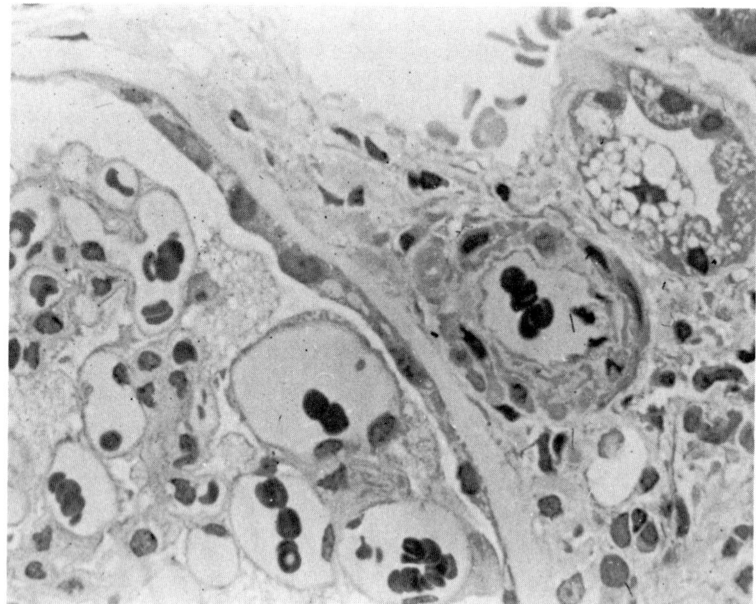

Figure 8–15. The glomerular epithelial cells are vacuolated, giving the glomerulus a honeycomb appearance. (H&E, ×400.)

Patient Presentation

The cutaneous manifestations were first recognized at the turn of the century, and the term *angiokeratoma corporis diffusum* was coined to describe the skin changes. Shortly thereafter, proteinuria and eye lesions (retinal, conjunctival, and corneal) were recognized.

The renal lesion has been the leading cause of morbidity and mortality in Fabry's disease. It most often presents as mild, asymptomatic proteinuria during early adulthood. The urine also contains oval fat bodies and occasionally a few red blood cells. Renal function gradually deteriorates during a period of 10 to 20 years, with most patients developing renal failure before the age of 50 years.

Signs and symptoms related to involvement of other organs, especially the autonomic nervous system, may develop at nearly the same time as those due to renal involvement.

Histology

Light Microscopy

The glomerular visceral epithelial cells are prominently and obviously affected. Their cytoplasm is filled with tiny, clear vacuoles giving the glomeruli a honeycomb appearance (Fig. 8–15). The endothelial and mesangial cells are not as conspicuously affected; therefore, it may be difficult to appreciate cytoplasmic vacuoles in these cells by light microscopy.

The mesangial matrix and the peripheral glomerular basement membranes are not altered in the early stages of the disease. However, as the process evolves, diffuse mesangial sclerosis with segmental or complete sclerosis develops.

The tubules are much less affected, and the epithelial cell cytoplasm contains only a few inclusions, for the most part (Fig. 8–15).

The blood vessels are often very involved, with the endothelium containing large number of lysosomes. Hyaline deposits are commonly seen in the media as the lesion advances.

Immunofluorescence Microscopy

There are no deposits of immune reactants.

Electron Microscopy

Multiple lysosomal inclusions are seen in all renal cells (Fig. 8–16). The inclusions vary in size, shape, and intracellular location. They have been variously called myelin figures, lamellated structures, osmiophilic inclusions, zebra bodies, and so on. They may have an onion-skin configuration with an array of concentric layers of electron-dense material, or the layers may consist of parallel arrays (Fig. 8–17). At high magnification,

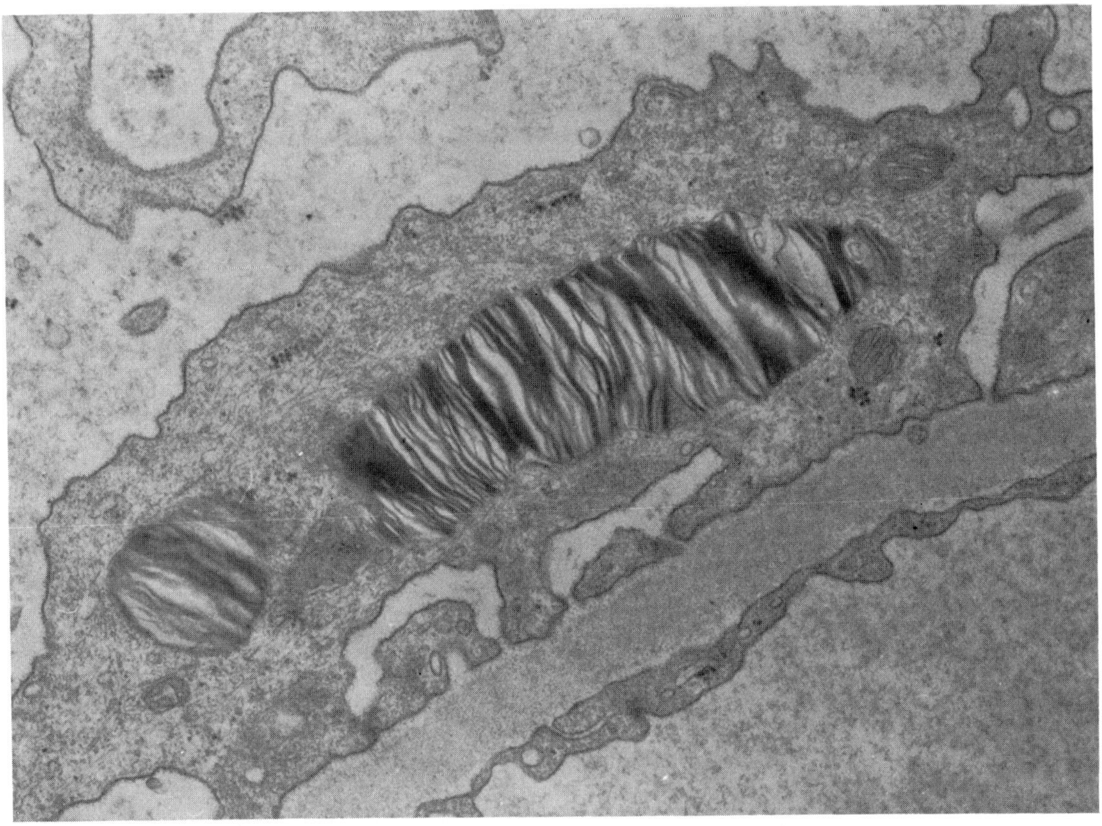

Figure 8–16. Myelin figures are present in the glomerular epithelial cells. (×10,000.)

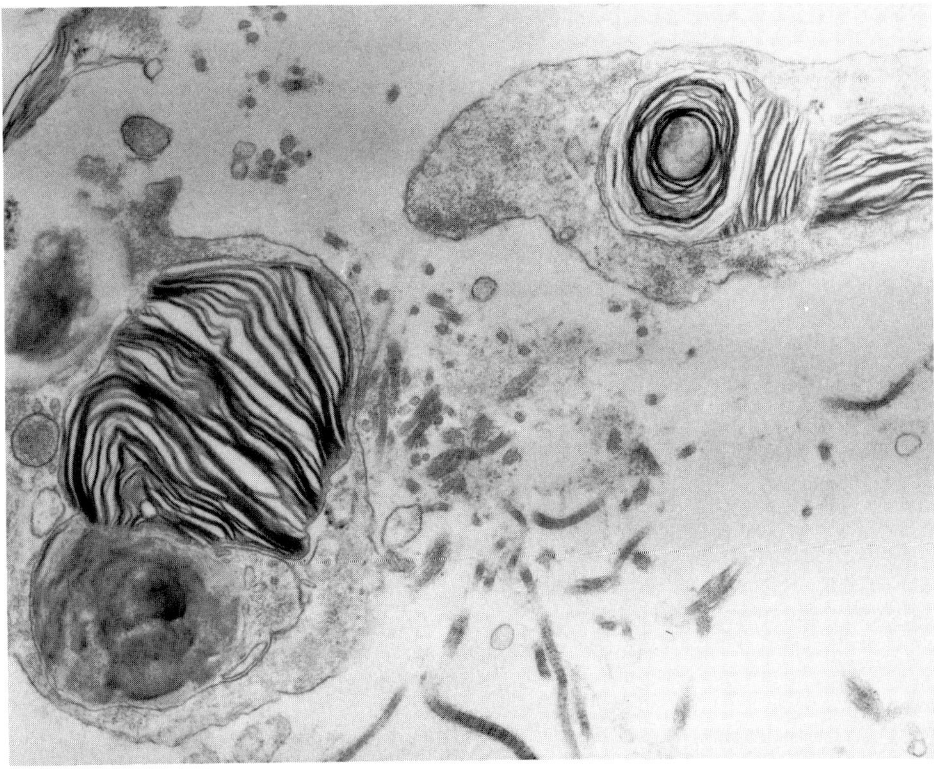

Figure 8–17. The interstitial cells also contain myelin figures. The configuration of the inclusions varies from concentric layers to parallel arrays of electron-dense lamellae. (×10,000.)

there are alternating layers of dense and light material with a periodicity ranging from 3.9 to 9.8 nm. This configuration is considered characteristic of glycolipids.

The glomeruli are conspicuously involved, and all cells may contain large inclusions that may seriously distort the architecture of the glomerulus. Endothelial and mesangial cells contain fewer inclusions than do epithelial cells. The extracellular matrix is initially normal; however, as the disease progresses, the mesangial matrix increases in amount and the peripheral basement membranes become wrinkled and thickened.

Tubular cells also contain inclusions, in rough proportion to that appreciated by light microscopy. The distal tubules are more severely affected than proximal tubules.

The interstitium may also contain cells filled with inclusions. The peritubular capillaries and the arterial tree contain inclusions in the endothelial cells. The medial cells are less often involved.

Prognosis

Renal failure occurs in the fifth decade in most kindreds. The patients have been maintained by both dialysis and transplantation. Patients may have an increased incidence of serious infections, but this is not well established.

SELECTED READINGS

1. Brady TO, Gal AE, Bradley RM, et al: Enzymatic defect in Fabry's disease: Ceramidetrihexosidase deficiency. N Engl J Med 276:1163, 1965.
2. Desnick RJ, Sweeley CC: Fabry's disease: Alpha-galactosidase A deficiency. *In* Stanbury JB, Wyngaarden JB, Frederickson DS, et al (eds): The Metabolic Basis of Inherited Disease, 5th ed. New York, McGraw-Hill, 1983, pp 906–944.
3. Gubler MC, Lenoir G, Grunfeld JP, et al: Early renal changes in hemizygous and heterozygous patients with Fabry's disease. Kidney Int 13:223, 1978.

LECITHIN-CHOLESTEROL ACYLTRANSFERASE DEFICIENCY DISEASE

Deficiency of lecithin-cholesterol acyltransferase (LCAT) is a rare genetic disorder resulting in the accumulation of free cholesterol in many tissues. In the kidneys, these deposits are associated with progressive organ failure. The renal lesions are relatively characteristic, but the diagnosis is made on other grounds.

Pathogenesis

This deficiency was first described in Norway. It affects both sexes equally and has an autosomal recessive inheritance pattern. The relationship between the biochemical defect and the development of the renal lesions is unknown.

Patient Presentation

The characteristic features include corneal opacities, anemia, increased plasma levels of lipids and cholesterol, and undetectable levels of esterified cholesterol and LCAT. Proteinuria is a common early finding, signaling the presence of significant glomerular injury. The nephrotic syndrome may occur, but the most common finding is a progressive decline in renal function that becomes evident during the second decade of life. Hypertension occurs as a complicating factor in the renal disease and promotes the rapid loss of renal function.

Histology

Light Microscopy

The glomeruli are the principal site of the lesions in the initial phases of the disease. They have a honeycomb appearance because of the fact that the lipid accumulations are dissolved during the preparation of the tissue for sectioning (Fig. 8–18). Lipids are found in the cytoplasm of the endothelial and mesangial cells and in the glomerular basement membranes and the mesangial matrix. Silver stains reveal a mottling of the glomerular basement membranes and mesangial spaces. The vascular lumina contain large, eosinophilic coagula of material containing lipids. Later in the disease, progressive sclerosis occurs, leading to a pattern indistinguishable from the lesion of focal glomerulosclerosis. The glomeruli eventually become totally obsolescent as the sclerosis proceeds. Modest

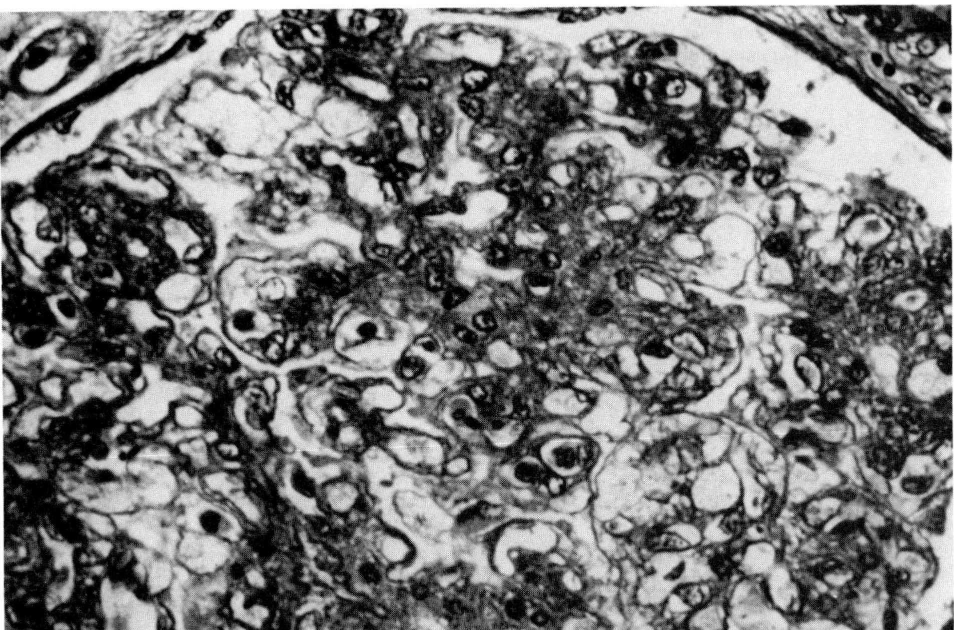

Figure 8–18. The glomerular endothelial and mesangial cells are extensively vacuolated. (PASM, ×400.) (Courtesy of Drs. R. Sibley and J. Churg.)

mesangial proliferation has been reported. The lipids are only faintly oil red O positive.

The distinction between LCAT deficiency and Fabry's disease at the light microscopic level can be based on the location of the lipid-laden lysosomes. In Fabry's disease, the visceral epithelial cells are prominently affected, whereas in LCAT deficiency, the endothelial and mesangial cells are most involved. The interstitium and the tubules also contain lipid, although the lesions are not so marked as those in the glomeruli and occur at a later time in the course of the disease.

The other condition that has similar histologic findings by light microscopy is Alagille's syndrome (a condition associated with congenital biliary atresia).

The arteries and arterioles show an atherosclerotic process that is much more advanced than would be expected for the age of the affected population.

Immunofluorescence Microscopy

The areas of focal glomerulosclerosis contain coarse, segmental deposits of IgG and C3. This pattern is consistent with that seen in other patients with focal glomerulosclerosis. Granular mesangial deposits of apolipoprotein B in the mesangium and along the glomerular basement membranes have been seen in these patients. Again, this is not a unique finding, because it has been described in membranous glomerulonephritis.

Electron Microscopy

The glomerular basement membrane and mesangial matrix contain large lacunae filled with electron-dense, often lamellated, material (Fig. 8–19). Similar material is found in the lysosomes of endothelial and mesangial cells. It is also found in the subepithelial and subendothelial spaces. The mesangial matrix is increased in amount and contains many profiles of hyalin.

Foam cells may fill the glomerular vascular lumen. Like the endothelial and mesangial cells, the lysosomes of these cells contain electron-dense material that may have a lamellated material with a serpentine, cross-striated substructure. Comparable lesions are seen in patients with congenital biliary atresia (Alagille's disease).

The mesangial matrix and peripheral glomerular basement membranes increase in width and substance as the disease progresses.

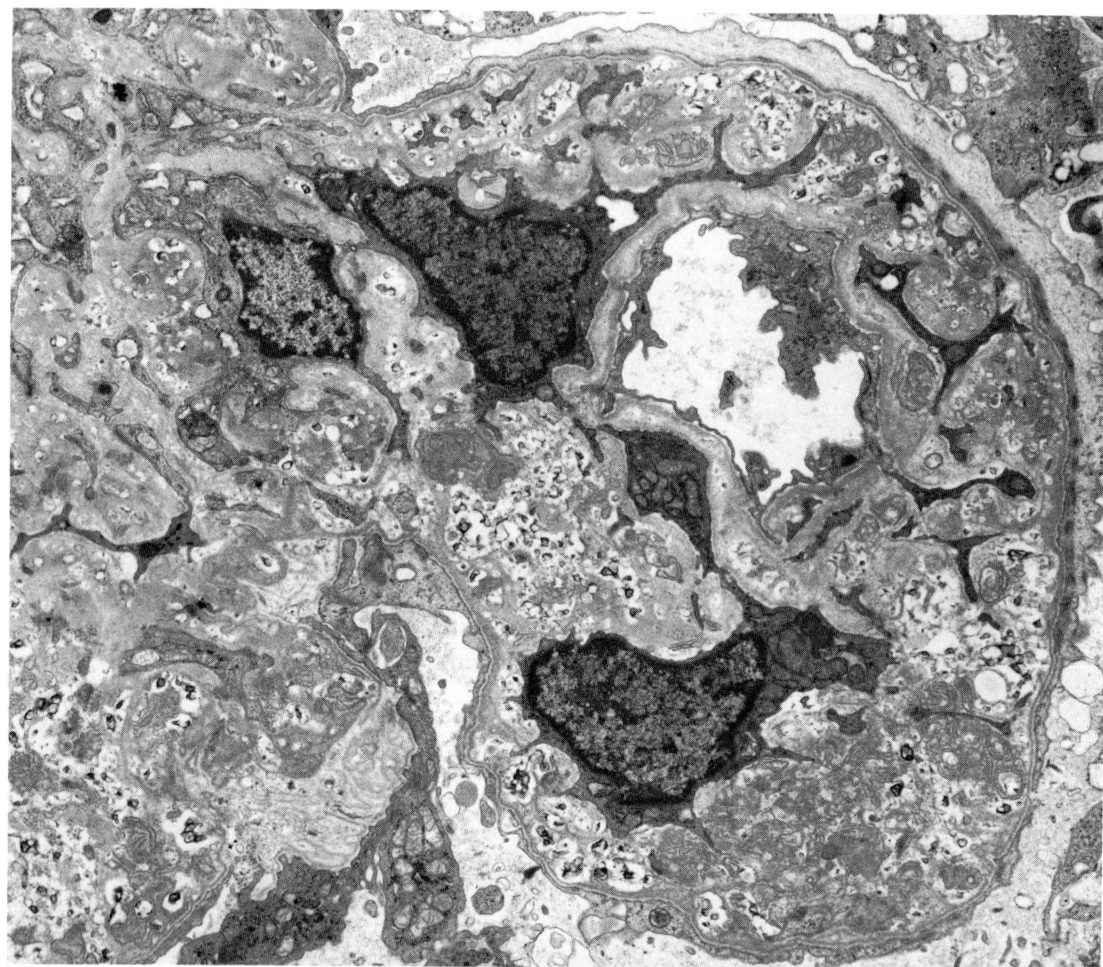

Figure 8–19. The extensive sclerosis involving the mesangium and the peripheral glomerular basement membranes is evident. The multiple vacuoles within the mesangial cells contain electron-dense lipid-laden material. (×5300.) (Courtesy of Drs. R. Sibley and J. Churg.)

Prognosis

The course of the renal disease is one of slow, inexorable deterioration in function to end stage. Unfortunately for these patients, the renal disease rapidly recurs in renal transplants.

SELECTED READINGS

1. Chevet D, Ramee MP, Thomas R, et al: Hereditary lecithin cholesterol acyltransferase deficiency: Report of a new family with two afflicted sisters. Kidney Int 10:185, 1976.
2. GJone E, Norum KR: Familial serum cholesterol ester deficiency. Clinical study of a patient with a new syndrome. Acta Med Scand 183:107, 1968.
3. Magil A, Chase W, Frohlich J: Unusual renal biopsy findings in a patient with familial lecithin-cholesterol acyltransferase deficiency. Hum Pathol 13:283, 1982.
4. Norum KR, GJone E: Familial plasma lecithin-cholesterol acyltransferase deficiency: Biochemical study of a new inborn error of metabolism. Scand J Clin Lab Invest 20:231, 1967.
5. Utermann G, Menzel HJ, Dieker P, et al: Lecithin-cholesterol-acyltransferase deficiency: Autosomal recessive transmission in a large kindred. Clin Genet 19:448, 1981.

Chapter

9

RENAL DISEASES ASSOCIATED WITH LYMPHOPLASMACYTIC DISORDERS

MULTIPLE MYELOMA

Multiple myeloma is characterized by the proliferation of a malignant clone of plasma cells that produces a monoclonal immunoglobulin and/or light chain (the so-called M component). There is a slight male predominance, and the incidence is 3:100,000 persons in the 50- to 70-year age-group.

One of the most prominent features of this disease is the frequent occurrence of renal failure. This complication appears in almost 50% of the patients and is a frequent cause of mortality. The renal lesion is thought to be due to the renal toxicity of the free light chains, leading to damage or dysfunction of tubular epithelial cells.

Other diseases due to the M component, light-chain deposition disease and AL amyloid, will be considered separately, although they may occur in individuals with multiple myeloma.

Pathogenesis

Although patients with renal disease due to myeloma always excrete light chains, some patients with multiple myeloma who do not have renal disease excrete equally large or greater amounts of light chains. These data and information obtained in experimental animals injected with light-chain preparations suggest that light chains are not the only factor leading to the renal toxicity. Nonetheless, both clinical and laboratory data indicate that free monotypic light chains possess renal tubular cell cytotoxicity. One factor may relate to their size and composition. These properties, combined with their high concentration, may enhance their propensity to precipitate in the hypertonic, acidic milieu of the distal tubules. The resultant casts (Bence Jones casts) may obstruct the lumen, magnifying the cytotoxicity. There is evidence that Tamm-Horsfall protein favors cast formation.

The renal disease in multiple myeloma may be multifactorial (Table 9–1), and cast nephropathy is not the only cause of renal failure.

Patient Presentation

Weakness, fatigue, infection, and bone pain are the most common presenting features. These all are suggestive of a malignant process replacing the normal bone marrow. Many patients have proteinuria at the onset. Those who have overt renal failure most

Table 9–1. Factors Contributing to Renal Failure in Myeloma

Hypercalcemia
Hyperuricemia
Pyelonephritis
Dehydration
Contrast media

often are found to have large amounts of circulating light chains, rather than intact immunoglobulins.

Histology

Light Microscopy

In contrast to the tubules, which have florid lesions, the glomeruli are usually completely normal. Glomerular lesions ranging from mild mesangial sclerosis to crescentic glomerulonephritis have been infrequently reported. These reports antedated the recognition of light-chain systemic disease as a disease entity.

The tubular lesion, light-chain cast nephropathy, consists of dilated and atrophied tubules whose lumina are filled with large and distinctive Bence Jones casts (Fig. 9–1). The casts are typical of myeloma and are characterized by an uneven size, a refractile and multilaminated appearance, and the presence of a surrounding cellular reaction that may consist of multinucleated cells (Fig. 9–2). The cellular response is composed of both tubular cells and infiltrating mononuclear cells. The casts often appear hard and may show fracture lines. They are markedly eosinophilic, polychromatophilic, and periodic acid-Schiff (PAS) but not silver positive. They may also stain with thioflavine S and T. The periphery of the casts may be of a darker color than the center. The casts rarely exhibit the histochemical characteristics of amyloid, and when present, the "amyloid casts" are not associated with systemic amyloidosis.

Tubular epithelial cell changes are marked in the regions of the casts, the most common lesions being atrophy and/or degeneration. However, acute tubular lesions may also be found in the absence of myeloma casts. Elsewhere, the tubular cells contain lysosomes filled with proteins and other substances. The presence of crystals in the proximal tubular epithelial cells is considered characteristic of the existence of Fanconi's syndrome. The crystals are dark, elongated, PAS-positive, intracytoplasmic structures.

Interstitial changes parallel the tubular lesions in severity. Interstitial fibrosis is the predominant change in areas of tubular atrophy (Fig. 9–3). Infiltrates of malignant plasma cells are found in approximately 10% of patients. Calcium deposits, related to hypercalcemia, are generally found along tu-

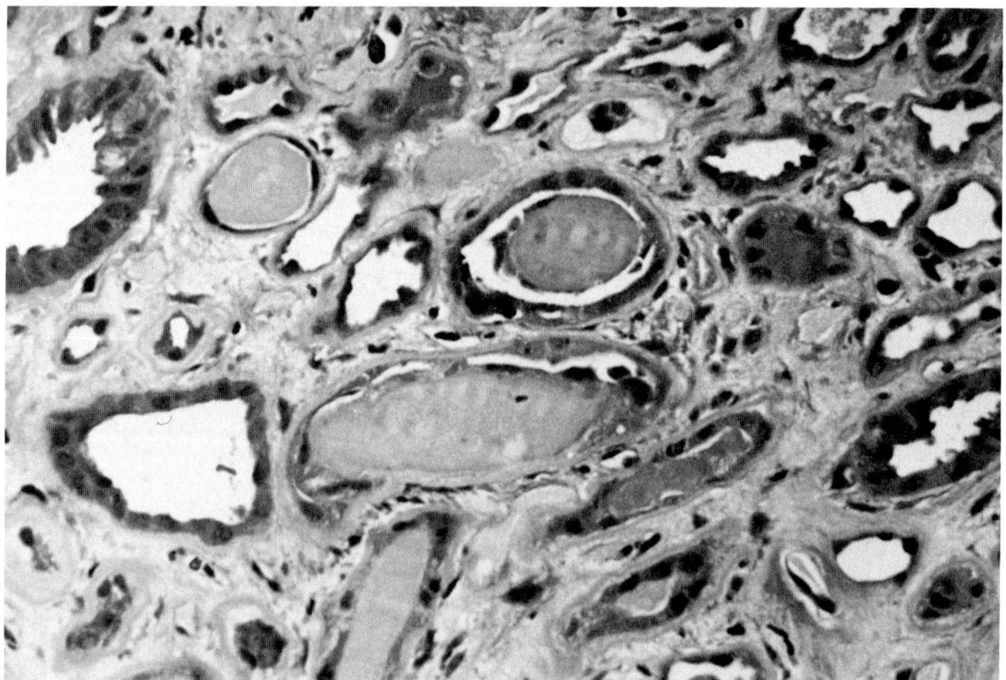

Figure 9–1. Most tubules contain casts similar to that noted in the periphery of this photomicrograph. The casts have a "hard" appearance—that is, the margins are sharp and the casts contain multiple lamellae. The interstitium is expanded and contains scattered inflammatory cells. (H&E, ×300.)

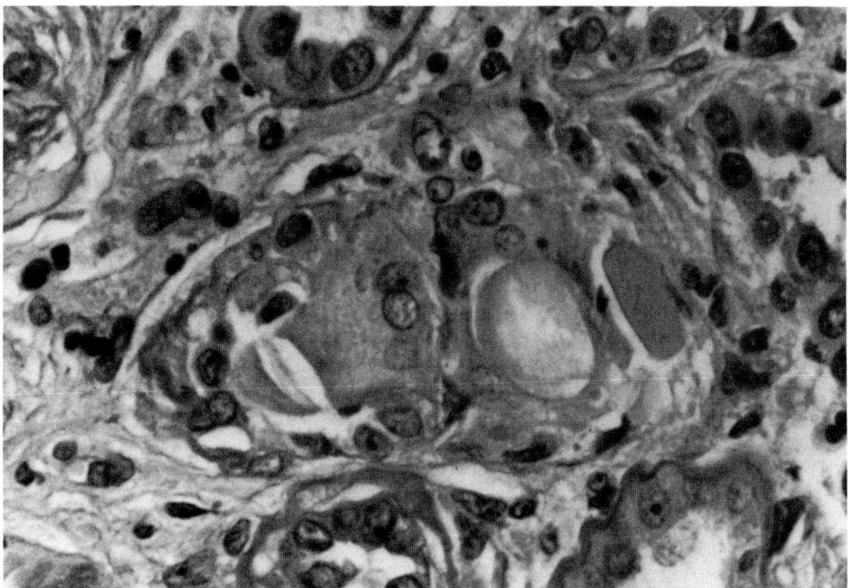

Figure 9–2. The characteristic tubular change is the presence of multinucleated epithelial cells surrounding the hard, waxy casts. (H&E, ×400.)

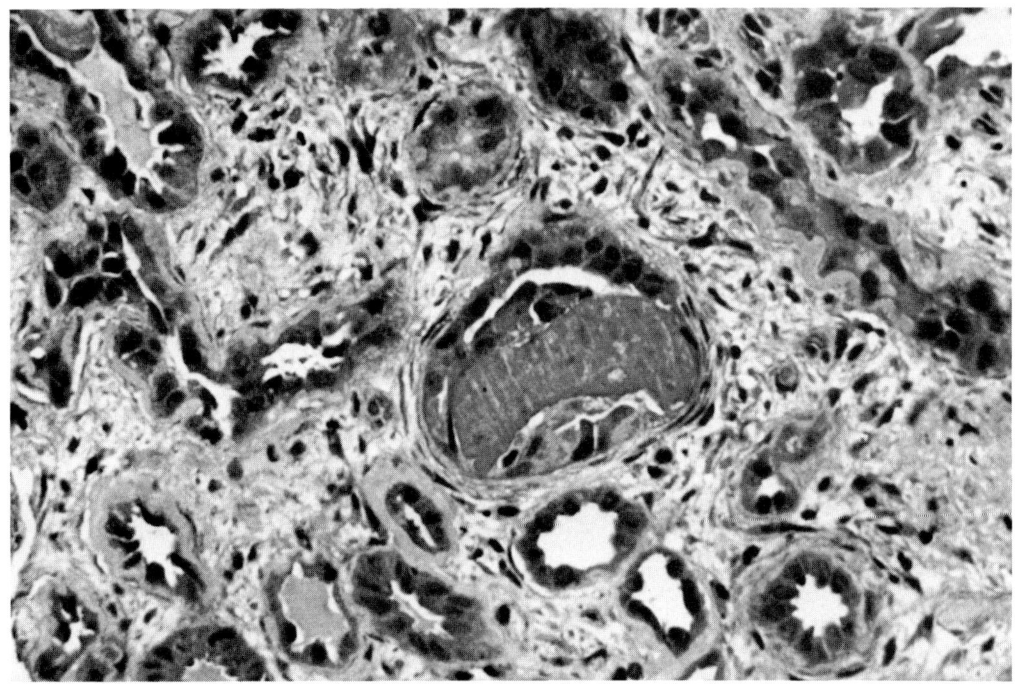

Figure 9–3. The interstitium may contain multiple foci of inflammatory cells, particularly adjacent to tubules containing casts. (H&E, ×300.)

bular basement membranes, but they may also be seen within casts and areas of interstitial fibrosis by von Kossa's stains.

Acute inflammation, representing acute pyelonephritis, may be present.

There are no vessel lesions apart from those expected within this age-group of patients.

Immunofluorescence Microscopy

The glomeruli are negative, unless the patient has either amyloidosis or light-chain systemic disease.

The casts contain immunoglobulin components, Tamm-Horsfall protein, albumin, and occasionally fibrinogen (Fig. 9–4). The staining pattern is unusual in that the central regions may be translucent, and the periphery is brightly stained. Casts containing only the monoclonal M component are thought to be recently formed, whereas those with multiple other serum components are thought to be older, and the heterogeneity is assumed to arise from trapping materials during a period of time.

The tubular basement membranes and the tubular cell cytoplasm are generally free of immunoglobulins.

Electron Microscopy

There are few reports of the electron microscopic appearance of glomeruli in these biopsies, presumably because of the paucity of findings.

There is considerable heterogeneity in the appearance of the casts. Some contain fibrillar material, resembling Tamm-Horsfall protein, and others contain homogeneous, dense material. Others contain fibrils in parallel arrays, but they lack the periodicity characteristic of amyloid.

Crystals of various sizes are a frequent finding. They may have a fibrillar or lattice-like substructure, and the surrounding multinucleated giant cells may contain similar structures. The multinucleated giant cells resemble macrophages. The tubular cells may also contain crystals.

Prognosis

Renal disease is a frequent complication, occurring in 30% of patients at presentation and in almost 50% at some time in the course of the disease. Although acute renal failure may be present (seen in 10% of patients at presentation), the usual course is a slowly progressive decline in renal function. Amyloidosis is found at autopsy in 10% of all patients with multiple myeloma, but it may be encountered in as many as 40% of patients with IgD myeloma.

The presence of renal failure portends a poor prognosis. It was thought to be irreversible, but the development of new thera-

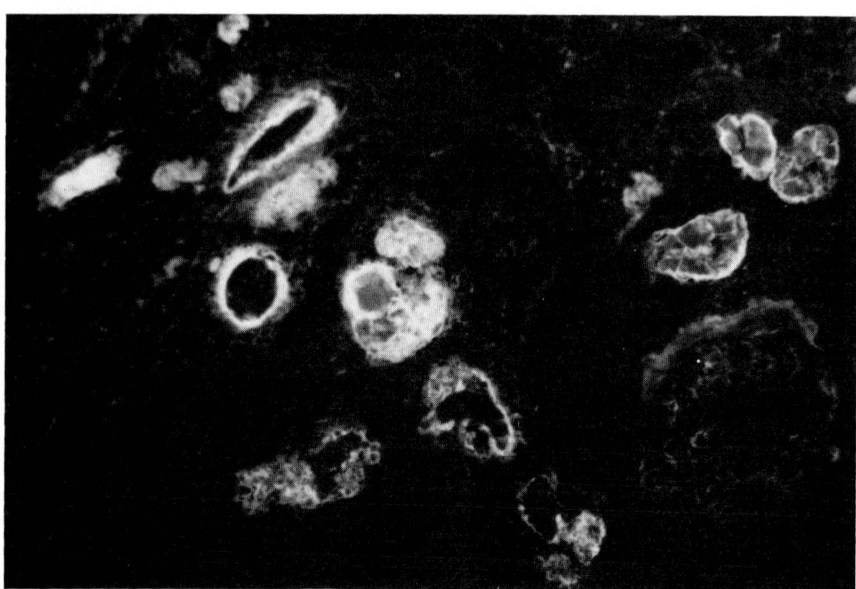

Figure 9–4. Immunofluorescence micrograph demonstrating IgA in myeloma casts. (×150.)

peutic strategies has altered this pessimistic viewpoint.

SELECTED READINGS

1. Cohen AH, Border WA: Myeloma kidney: An immunomorphogenetic study of renal biopsies. Lab Invest 42:248, 1980.
2. Factor SM, Winn RM, Biempica L: The histiocytic origin of the multinucleated giant cells in myeloma kidney. Hum Pathol 9:114, 1978.
3. Levi DF, Williams RC, Lindstrom FD: Immunofluorescent studies of the myeloma kidney with special reference to light chain disease. Am J Med 44:922, 1968.
4. MacKay K, Striker L, d'Amico G, et al: Dysproteinemias and paraproteinemias. *In* Tisher C, Brenner B (eds): Renal Pathology. JB Lippincott, Philadelphia, 1989.
5. Meyrier A, Simon P, Mignon F, et al: Rapidly progressive ("crescentic") glomerulonephritis and monoclonal gammopathies. Nephron 38:156, 1984.
6. Pirani CL, Silva F, D'Agati V, et al: Renal lesions in plasma cell dyscrasias: Ultrastructural observations. Am J Kidney Dis 10:208, 1987.

LIGHT-CHAIN SYSTEMIC DISEASE

Among the renal consequences of the presence of the M component (abnormal immunoglobulins) is the development of light-chain systemic disease. This disease has only recently (1976) been recognized as a clinical entity. Light-chain systemic disease shares features with AL amyloidosis in that it is associated with an extracellular accumulation of immunoglobulin light chains. However, the deposits in light-chain systemic disease have a granular ultrastructure, rather than the fibrillar/beta-pleated sheet structure, which is characteristic of amyloid. Therefore, the deposits in light-chain systemic disease do not have the staining patterns typical of amyloid.

The majority of patients with light-chain systemic disease have a malignant lymphoplasmacytic proliferative lesion, usually myeloma. However, one-third of the patients do not have this association.

Although the light-chain deposits may be widespread, the kidney is the most frequently involved organ, and renal involvement may dominate the clinical condition. The morphologic features of light-chain systemic disease may be recognized by light microscopy; however, the diagnosis can only be made with certainty by immunofluorescence microscopy using antisera to kappa and lambda chains.

It seems likely that this disease is the cause of a previously perplexing observation of a nodular sclerosing glomerular disease, resembling diabetic nephropathy, in patients who did not have diabetes mellitus. These reports antedated the commercial availability of antisera to light chains and did not include a long-term follow-up of the patients.

Pathogenesis

The inappropriate release of large quantities of immunoglobulin light chains, either as single entities or as a part of intact immunoglobulin molecules, leads to the development of light-chain systemic disease. It is likely that all patients with light-chain systemic disease have circulating light chains, although the plasma levels might be low or undetectable (possibly as a result of rapid tissue deposition, low levels of synthesis, or accelerated rates of degradation).

Attempts to study the pathogenesis of this disease have focused on two avenues, the cause of the deposition and the structure of the deposits. Some studies of the light chains have demonstrated a structural abnormality. This observation may explain, in part, both the tendency of these molecules to localize to basement membranes and the absence of the formation of beta-pleated sheets. The molecular or configurational alterations in light chains that favor deposition in basement membranes remain completely unknown.

The composition of the deposits in AL amyloid and light-chain systemic disease differ; those in the former contain mostly lambda light chains, whereas kappa chains predominate in light-chain systemic disease.

Although the emphasis has been on the differences between amyloidosis and light-chain systemic disease, both diseases may be found in the same patient, although this is certainly rare. It is not known whether the presence of both diseases in these patients reflects differences in processing the light chains at different body sites or whether they have two diseases.

Patient Presentation

The patients are typically males over the age of 55 years (male:female ratio is 4:1). Non-selective proteinuria, often in the nephrotic range, and renal failure are frequent at presentation. A patient who has multiple myeloma and has the nephrotic syndrome should be suspected of having either light-chain systemic disease or amyloidosis.

Although the renal disease dominates the presentation, deposits in the liver, heart, and brain may produce symptoms and signs.

The diagnosis rests on the histology at the immunofluorescence microscopic level, especially in patients who do not have overt myeloma.

Histology

Light Microscopy

The glomeruli are large, and the vascular spaces are markedly diminished in size. The characteristic glomerular lesions, mesangial nodules, are present in more than one-half of patients (Fig. 9–5). The nodules are eosinophilic and PAS positive, and do not stain with silver impregnation techniques (Fig. 9–6). Almost all glomeruli contain nodules and, in contrast to those in diabetes mellitus, do not vary in size between and within glomeruli. The peripheral vascular lumina are always decreased in size. The glomerular basement membranes appear to be "stiff" and slightly thickened. The basement membranes of Bowman's capsule may be thickened and infiltrated with material similar in composition to the mesangial nodules.

That there are differences between the glomerular nodules, basement membranes, and arterioles in diabetes mellitus and light-chain systemic disease is summarized in Table 9–2.

The nodules are present in approximately 60% of the patients. In the other 40%, the glomerular changes vary from essentially no lesions to mild mesangial sclerosis and hypercellularity (Fig. 9–7) and/or glomerular basement membrane changes (rigidity, eosinophilia). The lesions must be differentiated from type II membranoproliferative glomerulonephritis. In the latter, the peripheral glomerular basement membrane ribbonlike deposits are brightly refractile and the mesangial proliferation is more pronounced. This differentiation must be carried to the immunofluorescence microscopic level for an accurate interpretation.

One patient with crescentic glomerulonephritis has been reported.

Deposits of a refractile, PAS-positive material in a ribbonlike distribution along the outer aspects of the tubular basement membranes are a uniform finding (Fig. 9–8). The amount of deposits may vary, but they are predominately found in the basement membranes of the distal medullary loop and collecting tubules. The deposits thicken the basement membranes, resulting in the presence of homogeneous, wrinkle-free outlines that may be as thick as those in diabetic patients.

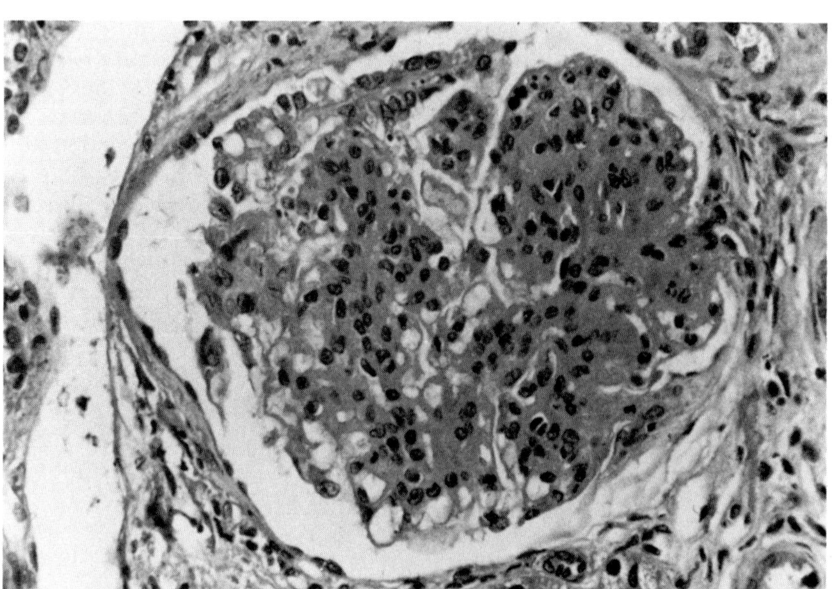

Figure 9–5. There are diffuse, homogeneous mesangial nodules containing an increased number of mesangial cells. This is the characteristic lesion. (Masson's trichrome, ×250.)

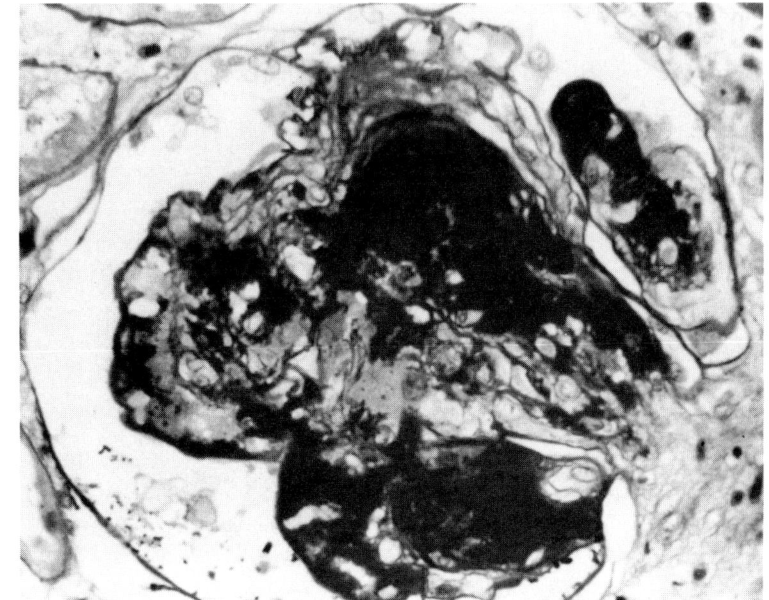

Figure 9–6. The large nodules are PAS positive. They displace the glomerular lumen to the periphery. In contrast to the glomerular basement membranes in diabetes mellitus, those in LCSD are not markedly thickened. (PAS, ×400.)

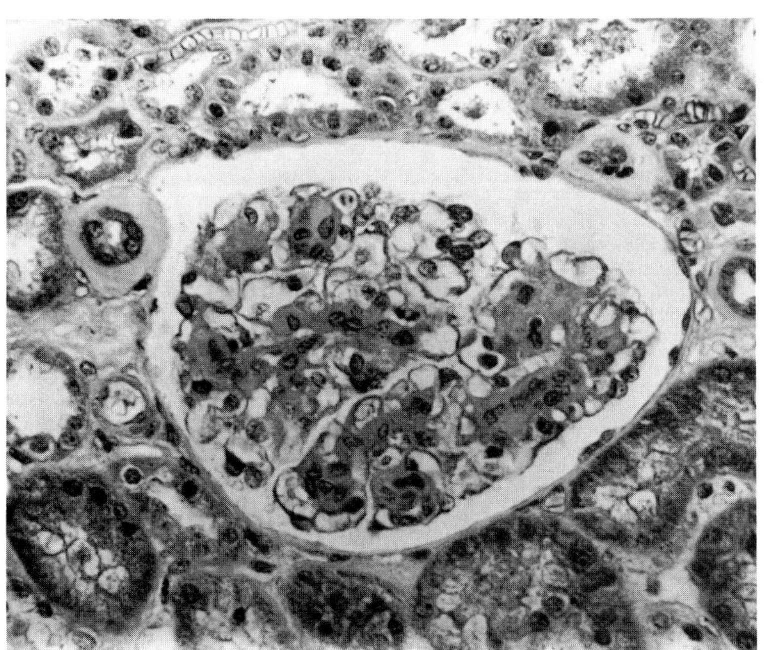

Figure 9–7. In some cases, the mesangial proliferation and sclerosis are less conspicuous and nodules are absent. (Masson's trichrome, ×250.)

Table 9–2. Comparison of the Lesions in Diabetes Mellitus and Light-Chain Systemic Disease

	Diabetes	**Light-chain Systemic Disease**
Nodules		
Argyrophilia	Strongly positive	Negative
Size	Variable	Uniform
Number	Variable	Uniform
Glomerular basement membranes	Thickened, aneurysms	Mild thickening
Arterioles		
Efferent arteriolar sclerosis	Present	Absent
Capsular drops	Present	Absent

The epithelial cells are flattened and often atrophied. We found occasional Bence Jones casts in 8 of 17 patients. The casts were not numerous and the surrounding cellular reaction was scanty in these patients in contrast to those in multiple myeloma.

There are no specific interstitial lesions, although interstitial deposits similar to those found in basement membranes have been described.

The basement membranes in the vascular walls contain the same type of deposits as described previously.

Immunofluorescence Microscopy

This diagnosis cannot be made without using antibodies to immunoglobulin light chains. Kappa chains are found in most patients, but lambda chains as the principal light chains have also been reported in a few cases.

The light chains may be found either along the peripheral glomerular basement membranes or in the nodules (Fig. 9–9). Granular C3 deposits have also been found in the mesangium of such patients. Patients who do not have mesangial nodules may have no glomerular deposits.

In contrast, peritubular deposits are always present, and the diagnosis is most often made by the finding of brightly staining deposits in this region (Fig. 9–10). The distal parts of the nephron are most frequently involved, but the proximal tubular basement membranes may also be affected. The peritubular deposits stain more intensely than do those in the glomeruli. They are distributed in a smooth, linear pattern even if they appear to be sparse and irregular by PAS stains. In rare instances, monotypic heavy chains may be detected. The disease in these patients has

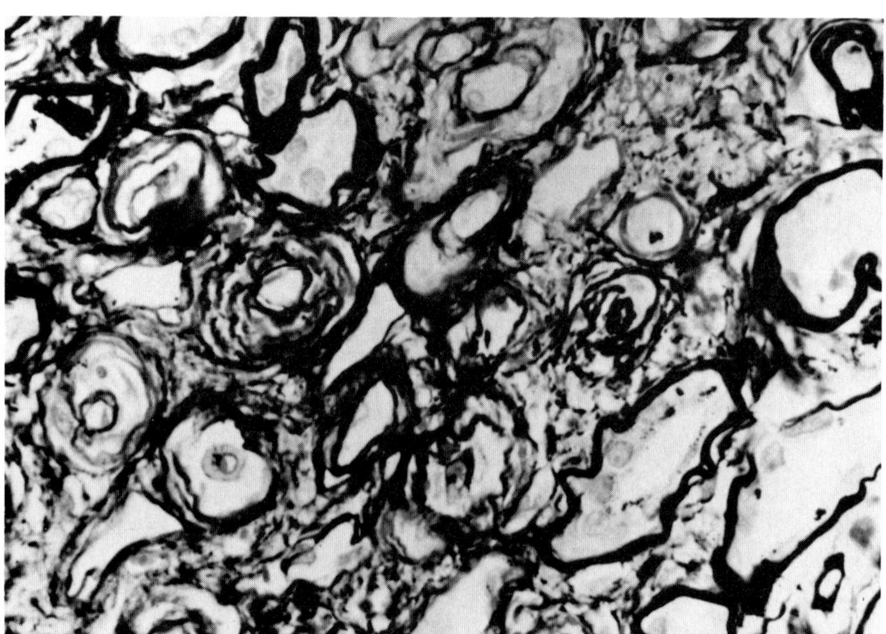

Figure 9–8. Thickened, multilaminated basement membranes in the medulla. (PAS, ×400.)

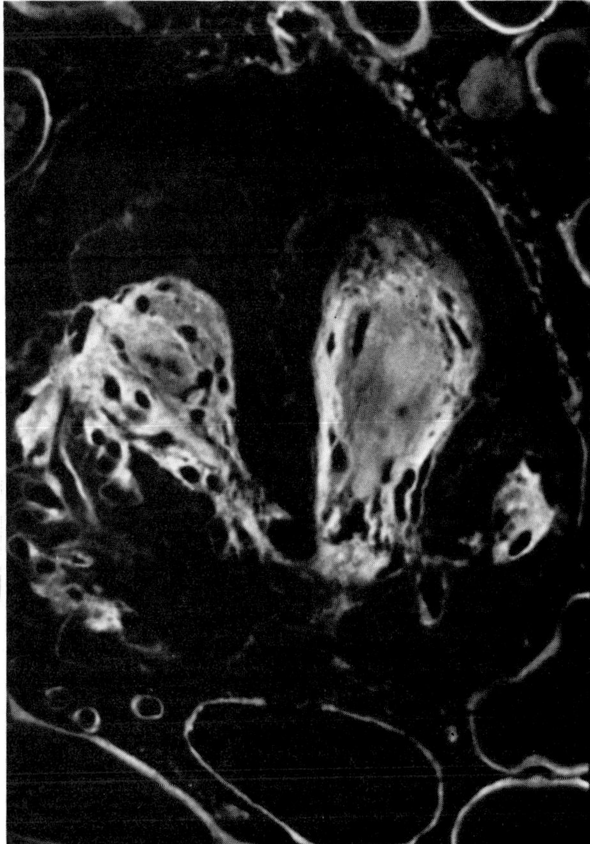

Figure 9–9. Immunofluorescence micrograph, anti-kappa light chain. The glomerular nodules and basement membranes are diffusely positive. (×400.)

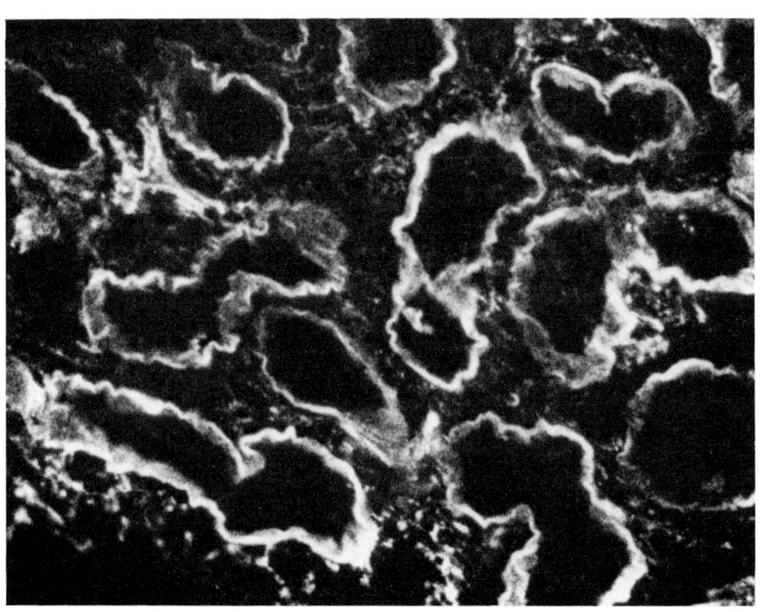

Figure 9–10. Immunofluorescence micrograph, anti-kappa light chain. There are diffuse, linear tubular basement membrane deposits. (×250.)

been called monoclonal immunoglobulin deposition disease.

Deposits may be present along capillary and arteriolar basement membranes.

Electron Microscopy

The glomerular lesions consist of deposits of a non-fibrillar, electron-dense material in both the mesangial nodules and along the glomerular basement membranes. The deposits are finely granular and generally lie in the lamina rara interna, separated from the endothelial cells by electron-lucent, fluffy material. They rarely are seen within the lamina densa, although the exact limits between the two elements may be difficult to discern. No substructure is seen in most biopsy samples, although fibrils of varying types have occasionally been reported. The cellular changes in the glomerulus consist of effacement of some pedicels, patchy mesangial encroachment on the vascular spaces, and an increase in the number of cells in the mesangium.

Like the immunofluorescence microscopic findings, the electron microscopic changes in the tubular compartment are diagnostic. Finely granular deposits are present along the interface of the tubular basement membranes and the interstitium of almost all tubules (Fig. 9–11). They may be quite large, but a substructure is not present. The adjacent tubular cells contain many lysosomes and sometimes crystalline inclusions.

Prognosis

Although it has been speculated that some patients who have mild mesangial changes may subsequently develop more diffuse lesions and even nodular glomerulosclerosis, this transition has only been documented in rare patients. The rarity of light-chain systemic disease makes it difficult to determine its normal pattern of evolution. Some patients have a fulminant course with multiorgan involvement, whereas others may de-

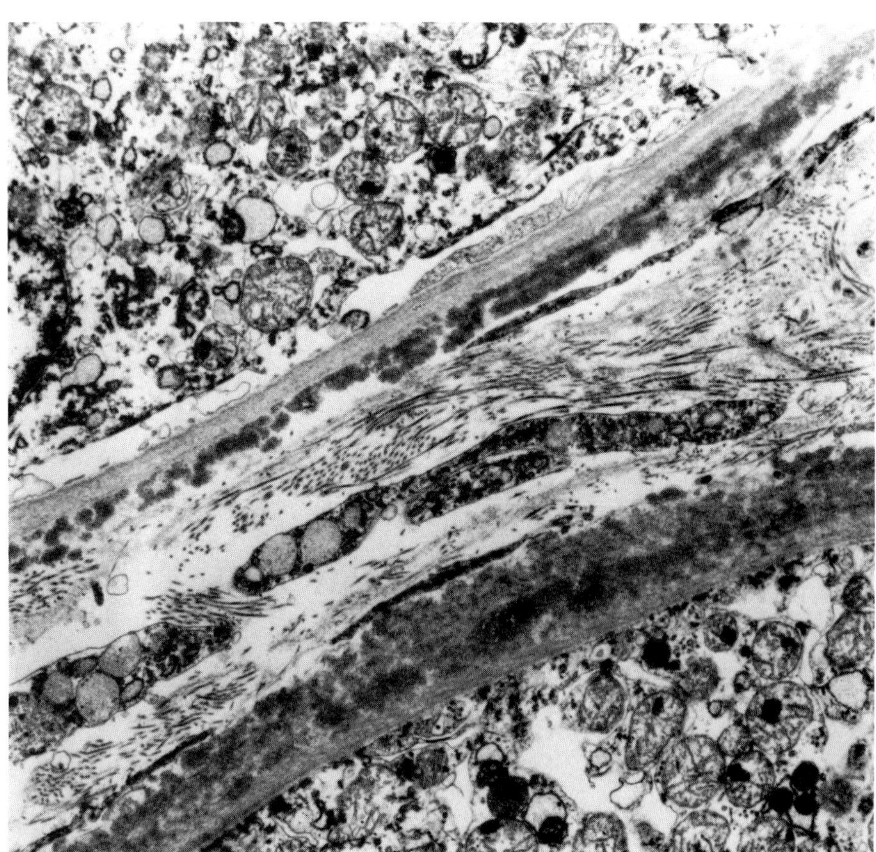

Figure 9–11. Finely granular deposits at the interface of the tubular basement membranes and the interstitium. (×10,000.)

velop renal failure and remain quite well managed on dialytic therapy without other sequelae. The survival appears to parallel that of patients with multiple myeloma with renal failure. Some patients with light-chain systemic disease do not manifest signs of multiple myeloma for months or even years.

Chemotherapy is indicated in patients in whom multiple myeloma is diagnosed. It is less well established whether the indications are the same in the absence of overt myeloma, although some patients are reported to have shown a decrease or stabilization of the amount of deposits after therapy.

SELECTED READINGS

1. Gallo GR, Feiner HD, Katz LA, et al: Nodular glomerulopathy associated with nonamyloidotic kappa light chain deposits and excess immunoglobulin light chain synthesis. Am J Pathol 99:621, 1980.
2. Ganeval D, Mignon F, Preud'homme JL, et al: Visceral deposition of monoclonal light chains and immunoglobulins: A study of renal and immunopathologic abnormalities. *In* Grunfeld JP, Maxwell MH (eds): Advances in Nephrology. Year Book Medical Publishers, Chicago, 1982, pp 25–63.
3. Hofmann-Guilaine C, Nochy D, Jacquot C, et al: Association light chain deposition disease (LCDD) and amyloidosis. One case. Pathol Res Pract 180:214, 1985.
4. Preud'homme JL, Morel-Maroger L, Brouet JC, et al: Synthesis of abnormal immunoglobulins in lymphoplasmacytic disorders with visceral light chain deposition. Am J Med 69:703, 1980.
5. Randall RE, Williamson WC Jr, Mullinax F, et al: Manifestations of systemic light chain deposition. Am J Med 60:293, 1976.
6. Silva FG, Meyrier A, Morel-Maroger L, et al: Proliferative glomerulonephropathy in multiple myeloma. J Pathol 130:229, 1980.

AMYLOIDOSIS

The term *amyloidosis* refers to accumulations of amorphous, homogeneous-appearing extracellular deposits with a fibrillar structure at the ultrastructural level and a characteristic beta-pleated sheet structure by x-ray diffraction. The beta-pleated sheet structure lends the characteristic tinctorial and optical properties evident by Congo red staining. More importantly, this configuration leads to the resistance of this material to proteolytic digestion. As a consequence, amyloid accumulates and progressively impairs the function of the kidneys. The amyloid substances are derived from various precursors, and it has been well established that the accumulation of amyloid fibrils may complicate the course of various diseases. The current classification system for amyloidosis is based on the protein composition of amyloid fibrils in different disease states (Table 9–3).

Other precursors of the amyloid fibrils have been described. These include beta$_2$-microglobulin, hormones, and albumin, but they have not been described in the kidneys.

Pathogenesis

Each of the several varieties of amyloidosis has a separate origin, biochemical composition of the fibrils, and pathogenesis. Despite this heterogeneity, the histologic and electron microscopic patterns are indistinguishable. The two species of amyloid (i.e., AA and AL) that affect the kidney may thus reflect many different diseases.

AL Amyloidosis

AL amyloid components are synthesized from the variable portion of light chains, usually lambda chains. Patients who have AL amyloidosis either have a myeloma or synthesize monoclonal light chains and may be considered as having a plasma cell dyscrasia.

AL amyloidosis complicates the course of approximately 10% of cases of multiple myeloma. It is most frequent in patients with IgD

Table 9–3. Classification of Amyloid Fibrils

Clinical Classification	Fibril Type	Precursor
Myeloma associated	AL	Immunoglobulin light chain (mostly lambda)
Primary amyloidosis	AL	Immunoglobulin light chain (mostly lambda)
Secondary amyloidosis	AA	Serum amyloid A
Familial amyloidosis		
Familial Mediterranean fever	AA	Serum amyloid A
Ostertag	?	Unknown

myeloma, followed by those with light-chain myeloma. The other patients with AL amyloidosis are considered to have primary amyloidosis; nonetheless, they have a population of cells responsible for the production of monoclonal light chains. These data suggest that there may be a continuum between primary amyloidosis and myeloma.

AA Amyloidosis

Although the morphologic and ultrastructural characteristics are similar to those in patients with AL amyloidosis, the biochemical composition of the fibrils in AA amyloidosis is completely different. The origin of the deposits in AA amyloidosis is a large serum precursor, serum amyloid A protein. The serum levels of this protein are increased in chronic infectious and inflammatory diseases, in certain neoplasias, and in familial Mediterranean fever. Serum amyloid A protein is a high-density lipoprotein synthesized by the liver and belongs to the family of proteins collectively designated as acute phase reactants. The exact relationship between the elevated levels of serum amyloid A protein and the development of amyloidosis is not known, because only a small number of patients with the previously listed diseases develop amyloidosis. The amino acid structure of serum amyloid A protein varies among individuals, a fact that may partially explain the variability among patients with respect to the propensity to develop amyloidosis. It has also been suggested that individuals who develop amyloidosis have an impaired ability to degrade serum amyloid protein.

All amyloid deposits, without regard to the nature of the precursor protein, contain a glycoprotein that has been given the designation of the P component. This component represents as much as 10 to 15% of the total fibril weight. The P component is identical to a serum protein called serum amyloid P component. The biologic function of the P component is unknown, but it has also been identified in normal glomerular basement membranes.

Patient Presentation

Although the nature of the fibrils and the inciting causes of AA and AL amyloidosis are quite different among patients, the renal findings are comparable. Massive proteinuria, often associated with the nephrotic syndrome, is the most common presentation in these patients. Hematuria is most often absent, and hypertension is only found in advanced cases. Enlargement of the kidneys is a characteristic finding and reflects infiltration of the renal parenchyma by the amyloid deposits. Renal function, often normal at onset, rapidly deteriorates to end-stage renal failure in the majority of the patients. Glycosuria and other signs of tubular dysfunction are often found.

AA amyloidosis often affects younger patients. In developing countries, chronic infections such as tuberculosis and leprosy are the major underlying disease. Elsewhere, the most commonly associated diseases include rheumatoid arthritis, chronic inflammatory diseases, and cancer. Adenocarcinoma of the kidney is the most common carcinoma associated with the development of AA amyloidosis. Drug abuse, especially when associated with subcutaneous injections, is also commonly associated with the development of AA amyloid. Finally, patients with familial amyloidosis and most of those with familial Mediterranean fever have deposits consisting of AA amyloid fibrils. AA amyloid is rarely found as an isolated event.

By contrast, AL amyloid occurs as part of a plasma cell dyscrasia or as a primary process. Ninety per cent of patients with AL amyloid have an M component in the plasma or the urine. There is a clear male predominance, and the median age at diagnosis is 65 years. AL amyloidosis is characterized by peripheral neuropathy, congestive heart failure, and hypertension. The median survival is very poor, being approximately 1 year.

Newer therapeutic avenues including the use of colchicine in AA amyloid and melphalan in the AL type may delay the deterioration of renal function. Thus it is useful to determine the composition of the renal deposits.

Histology

Light Microscopy

Amyloidosis is characterized by the extracellular deposition of an amorphous, weakly eosinophilic material (Figs. 9–12 and 9–13). The deposits may be present in glomeruli, tubular basement membranes, interstitium, or blood vessels. Large deposits are easily

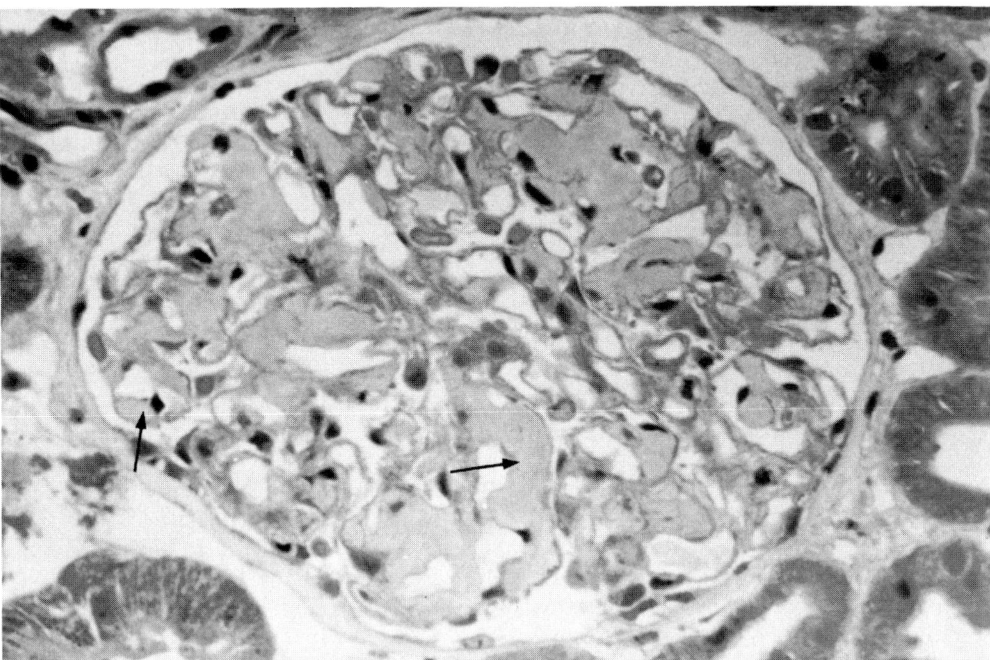

Figure 9–12. A glomerulus that contains irregular, nodular masses of homogeneous, poorly staining material displacing the normal structures (arrows). This material is largely restricted to the mesangium, but a small amount was found along the peripheral glomerular basement membranes. (H&E, ×300.)

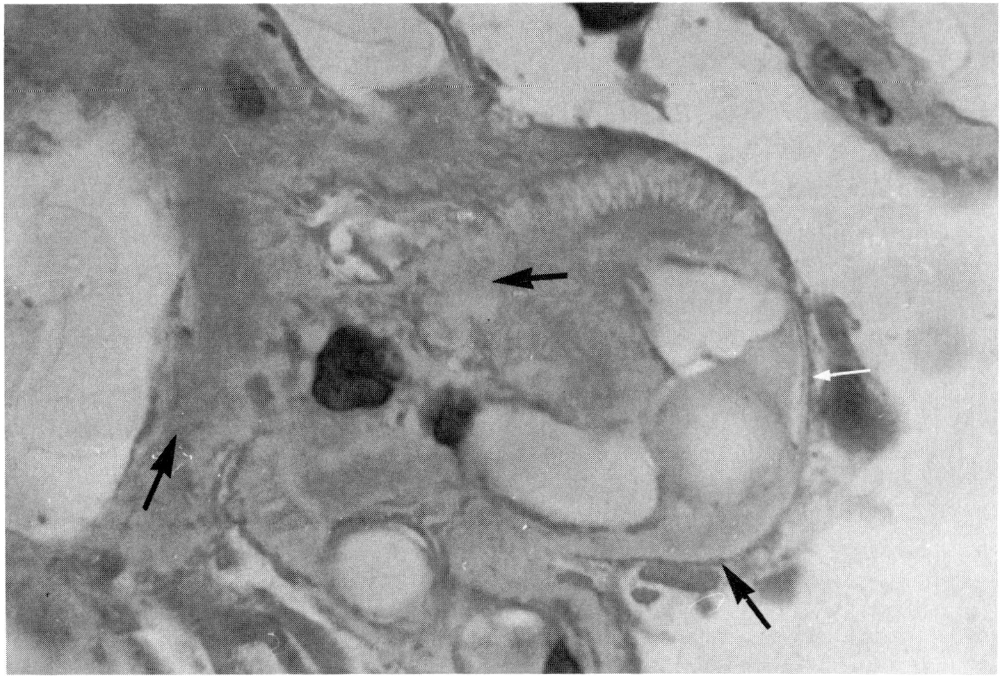

Figure 9–13. At higher magnification, the basement membranes are pale staining (light arrow), in contrast to a more dense material on its endothelial aspects and in the mesangium (heavy arrows). This dark material is amyloid. (H&E, ×1200.)

recognizable, but small deposits, especially when localized to the mesangial areas, may easily be overlooked. Special attention should be paid to biopsies of nephrotic patients who are older than 50 years and who have minimal lesions or a mild increase in the mesangial extracellular matrix material. In these cases, thick sections (8 μm at a minimum) should be stained with Congo red or crystal violet. The metachromasia following crystal violet staining is most easily detectable on cryostat sections from frozen tissue.

The glomerular mesangium is invaded by the extracellular material that presents a smooth, homogeneous appearance. This histologic feature is often referred to as hyalin. Apart from the acidophilia, amyloid is very weakly stained pale pink by PAS and is not stained by silver impregnation (Fig. 9–14). As a rule, no glomerular cell proliferation is associated with the presence of amyloid deposits. There is a decrease in the number of nuclei. Congo red staining reveals orange to rose deposits that show a characteristic apple-green birefringence when examined with polarizing light. This staining pattern is considered the most reliable diagnostic criterion for the presence of amyloid fibrils at the light microscopic level. The deposits stain with thioflavine T by fluorescence microscopy, but this feature is not specific for amyloid fibrils. Although the amyloid deposits are initially localized to the mesangial spaces, as they increase in amount the peripheral glomerular basement membrane becomes progressively invaded. As an end result, there is a gradual loss in the patency of the glomerular vascular loops. In some cases, the mesangial deposits form nodular masses, but unlike those seen in diabetes, the nodules are acellular.

The differentiation of an advanced amyloidotic lesion from that of light-chain systemic deposit disease may be difficult, but the pale, glassy appearance of amyloid deposits and their typical Congo red fluorescence pattern allow their differentiation.

At early stages, the amyloid deposits are restricted to the vascular pole and exist in a segmental and focal distribution. As the peripheral vascular loops become involved, the deposits are first observed in the paramesangial and subendothelial regions. As the amount of deposit increases further, subepithelial deposits are observed, and these are often associated with conspicuous subepithelial glomerular basement membrane abnormalities consisting of irregular spikelike pro-

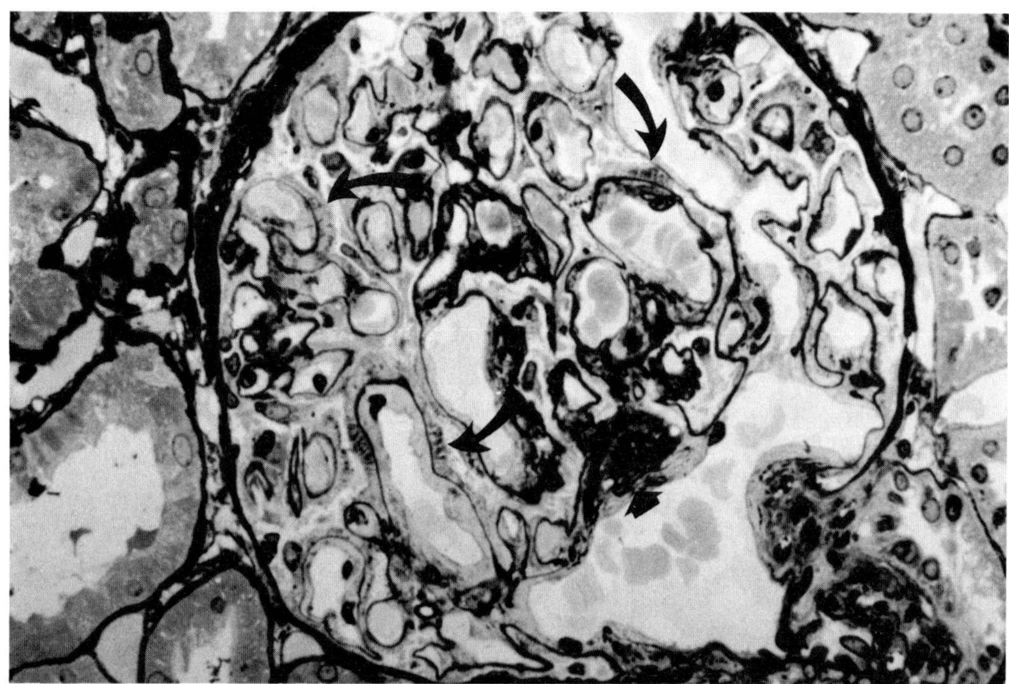

Figure 9–14. Amyloid is not stained with PASM, either in the subendothelium or the expanded mesangial areas. (PASM, ×300.)

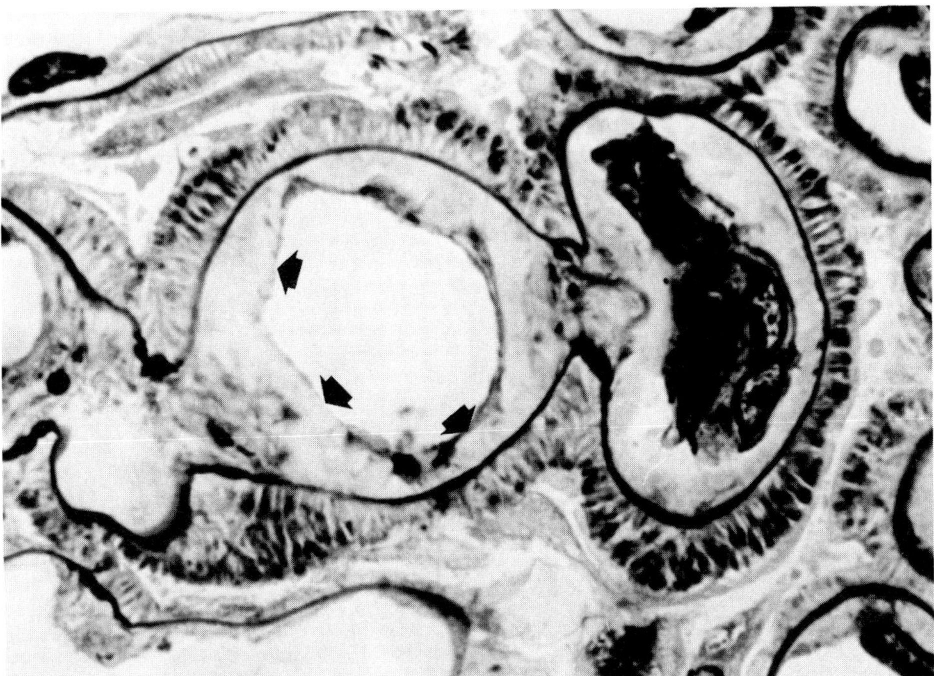

Figure 9–15. The subendothelial amyloid deposits (dark arrows) lie between the glomerular basement membrane and a thin layer of endothelial cytoplasm. The subepithelial amyloid deposits are interspersed with spikelike projections of basement membrane. (PASM, ×1200.)

jections (Fig. 9–15). These spikes are large and usually irregular in distribution. Thus they should not be confused with the subepithelial spikes present in membranous glomerulonephritis. Although an uncommon finding, multinucleated cells may be found surrounding the periphery of the amyloid deposits. The giant cells are assumed to be derived from macrophages. Cellular crescents occur in some advanced cases, but in the vast majority of cases the glomeruli are striking by their acellularity. Even when completely invaded by amyloid deposits and completely obsolescent, the glomeruli remain large. In late cases, the deposits may lose some of the histochemical properties of amyloid.

Tubular basement membranes often contain amyloid deposits recognizable as ribbonlike, bright refractile deposits. These are preferentially localized to the basement membranes of distal tubules. Epithelial cells often show atrophy and/or hyalin droplets. Bence Jones casts have been described in patients with amyloidosis, but they are very rare in our experience. However, large proteinaceous casts are extremely common and often numerous. Amyloid plaques may be found in the interstitial tissue, especially in the medulla.

The interstitium often contains a disseminated lymphocytic and plasmocytic infiltrate in patients with advanced disease.

Amyloid deposits may be found in each of the layers of the arterial and arteriolar walls (Figs. 9–16 and 9–17). As in other structures, the deposits are acellular and irregularly invade and displace the native extracellular matrix. In patients with minimal or no proteinuria, the arterioles may be the only element of the renal parenchyma containing amyloid deposits.

The differentiation between AL and AA amyloid at the light microscopic level may also be possible using the differential sensitivity of the fibrils to trypsin digestion. When slides are prestained with Congo red, they are subjected to trypsin digestion. Only AA amyloid deposits are degraded, when assessed for the loss of apple-green birefringence.

Immunofluorescence Microscopy

It has been suggested that amyloid deposits nonspecifically trap serum component in-

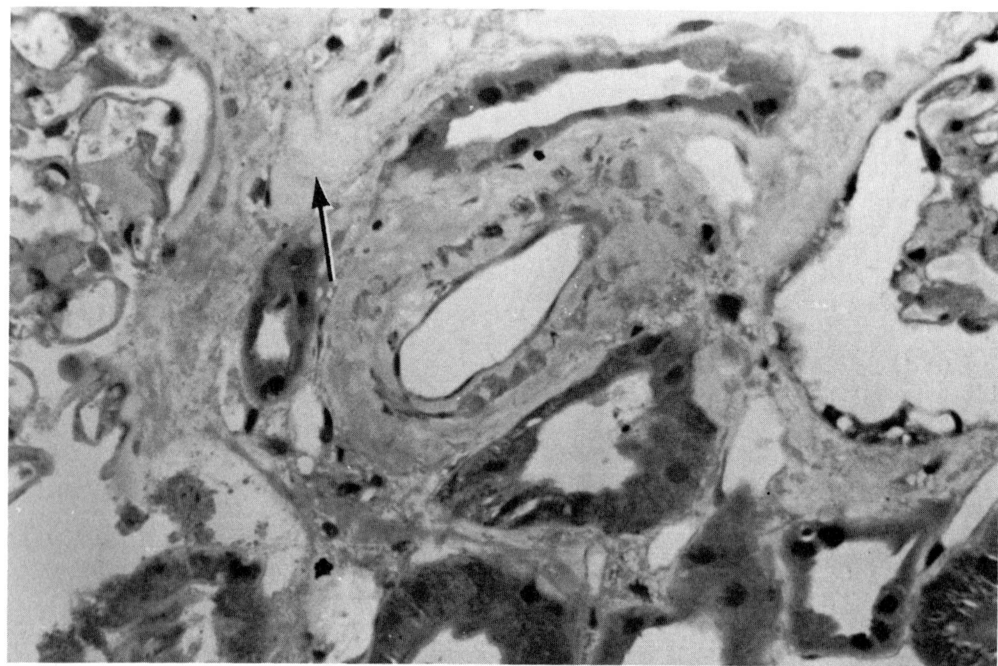

Figure 9–16. Homogeneous, eosinophilic amyloid deposits lie within the interstitium (arrow) and in the wall of an artery. The arterial smooth muscle cells are displaced and distorted by the deposits. (H&E, ×600.)

cluding immunoglobulins, complement, and fibrinogen. Although this may be true, it should not lead to confusion, because commercially available antibodies to AA allow the differentiation of amyloid and immunoglobulin deposits (Fig. 9–18).

Conversely, in AL amyloid the deposits react only with the antibody directed against the light chain (usually lambda chains) composing the fibrils (Fig. 9–19). Therefore, immunofluorescence microscopy may be used to categorize the type of amyloid in the de-

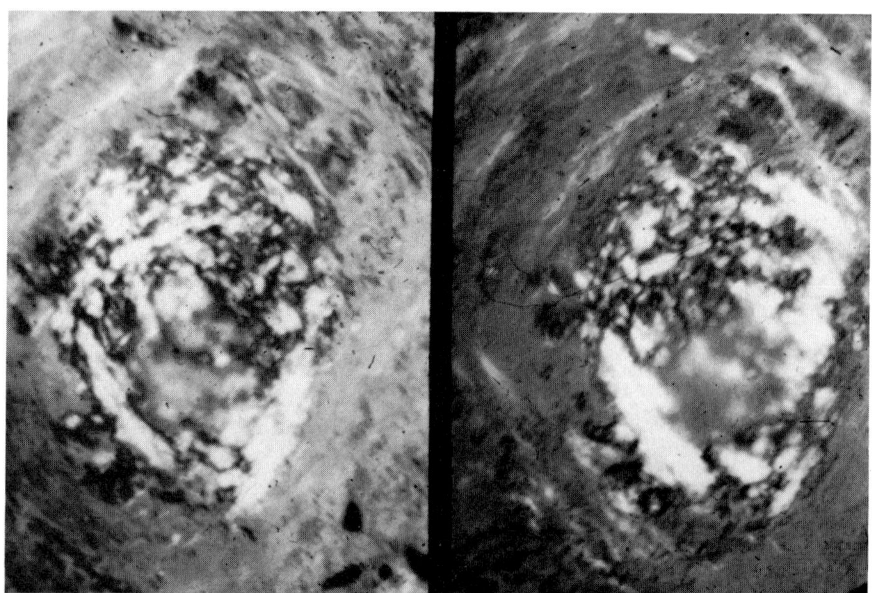

Figure 9–17. The amyloid deposits in this artery, stained with Congo red, show the characteristic apple-green birefringence with polarized light. (×300.)

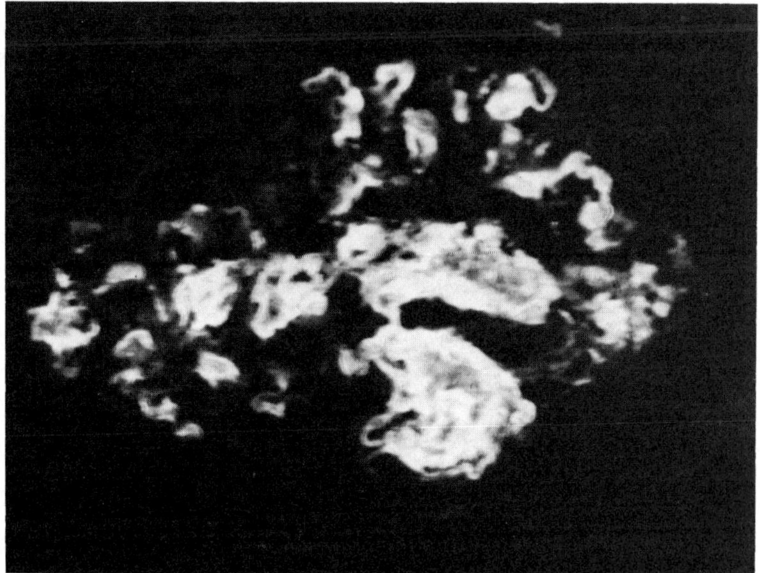

Figure 9–18. Immunofluorescence micrograph, anti-AA amyloid. The glomeruli contain large deposits. (×250.)

posits. In addition, immunoperoxidase methods yield good results on paraffin-fixed material.

Electron Microscopy

The use of electron microscopy is critical to confirm the presence of amyloid fibrils, especially when the deposits are small. The ultrastructural features allow one to make the diagnosis of amyloidosis, but they do not allow differentiation between the different types of fibril composition. Their identical morphologic appearance provides the best justification for their aggregation under the generic descriptor of amyloidosis. Amyloid deposits consist of fibrils with a regular nonbranching topography (Fig. 9–20). They vary in width from 80 to 100 nm and in length from 330 nm to several micrometers. They exist in disorderly arrays, appearing like straws in a haystack. Individual fibrils may show a beaded substructure with a 50-nm periodicity. The deposits exist as compact aggregates when they are adjacent to the cell profiles but appear more loosely arranged when they are at a distance. The fibrils are extracellular and initially invade the mesan-

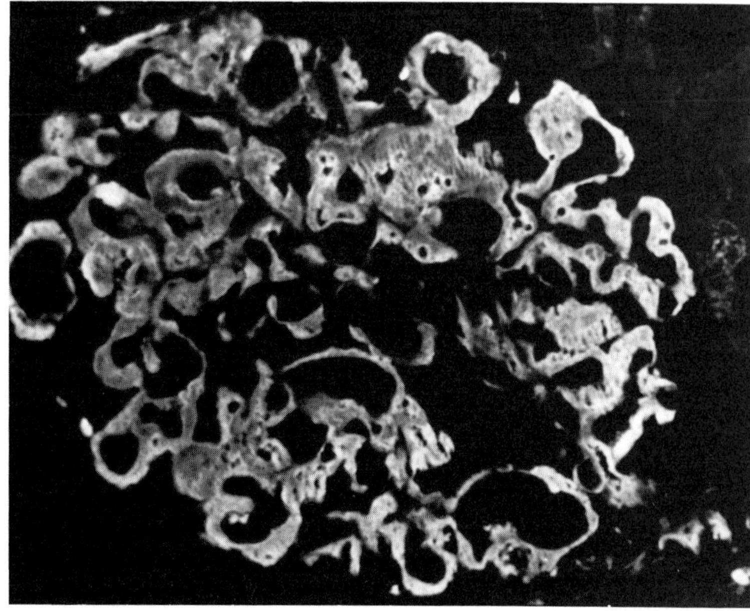

Figure 9–19. Immunofluorescence micrograph, anti-lambda light chain. The subendothelial and mesangial deposits are strongly positive. (×400.)

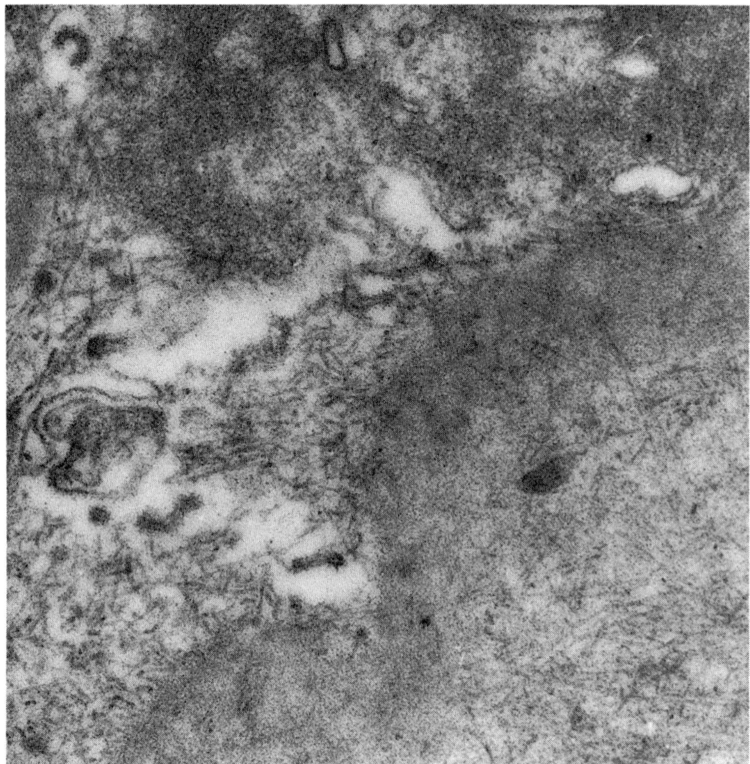

Figure 9–20. The electron microscopic appearance of amyloid fibrils is one of a tangled array of straight, non-branched fibrils that are randomly arrayed. (×10,000.)

gial matrix. The cell limits, which are often imprecise, may give the impression that the fibrils are present in the cytoplasm of mesangial cells. It seems likely that the cells in the mesangium, which have been said to contain fibrils in certain rare occasions, are bone-marrow derived macrophages. In the early stages, the extracellular matrix adjacent to the deposits remains normal, but with time it becomes distorted and increased in amount. The fibrils may extend through the basement membrane, and the basement membrane itself may undergo marked alteration. The endothelial cells loose their fenestrae in the areas adjacent to the deposits. When podocytes are in contact with the deposits, the pedicels may show spreading. In addition, a new layer of basement membrane may appear between the epithelial cells and the fibrils, appearing to encircle them.

Deposits in the other renal basement membranes share the same ultrastructural features as those in the glomeruli.

Prognosis

Patients who do not have treatable underlying causes of amyloidosis have a poor prognosis. Patients with AL amyloid, especially those with an overt myeloma, have a much more rapidly progressive course than those with AA amyloid. Patients with AA amyloid on the basis of an underlying chronic inflammatory or infectious process may show arrest or regression of the deposits if the underlying process is resolved.

New forms of therapy show promise for the resolution of deposits, but the evidence is too fragmentary to make generalizations at this point. One patient has been recently reported who had amyloid deposits secondary to chronic drug abuse, and in whom proteinuria markedly diminished when drug abuse was stopped. The amount of renal deposits did not appear to diminish, however.

Finally, amyloid deposits have been shown to recur in renal transplants, if the underlying condition is not resolved before placement of the graft.

SELECTED READINGS

1. Crowley S, Feinfeld DA, Janis R: Resolution of nephrotic syndrome and lack of progression of heroin-associated renal amyloidosis. Am J Kidney Dis 13:333, 1989.
2. Dickman SH, Churg J, Kahn T: Morphologic and clinical correlates in renal amyloidosis. Hum Pathol 12:160, 1981.

3. Gallo GR, Feiner HD, Chuba JV, et al: Characterization of tissue amyloid by immunofluorescence microscopy. Clin Immunol Immunopathol 39:479, 1986.
4. Glenner GG: Amyloid deposits and amyloidosis. The beta-fibrilloses. N Engl J Med 302:1283, 1980.
5. Isobe T, Osserman EF: Patterns of amyloidosis and their association with plasma-cell dyscrasia, monoclonal immunoglobulins and Bence-Jones proteins. N Engl J Med 290:473, 1974.
6. Nolting SF, Campbell WG: Subepithelial argyrophilic spicular structures in renal amyloidosis: an aid in diagnosis. Hum Pathol 12:724, 1981.
7. Wright JR, Calkins E, Humphrey RL: Potassium permanganate reaction in amyloidosis. Lab Invest 36:274, 1977.

MIXED CRYOGLOBULINEMIA

Glomerular lesions have been a recognized occurrence in mixed cryoglobulinemia for more than 20 years. It is still debated whether or not this disease is a plasma cell dyscrasia. *Cryoglobulin* is the generic term given to immunoglobulins that precipitate on cooling and resolubilize on warming. The cryoglobulins most often associated with renal disease contain at least two different immunoglobulins and are called mixed cryoglobulins.

A syndrome consisting of purpura, weakness, arthralgias, and (frequently) glomerular disease was first described in the mid-1960s. This multisystem involvement is characteristic of the acute disease.

Cryoglobulins may be present in a number of diseases, but the term *mixed essential cryoglobulinemia* is restricted to those patients with the characteristic clinical symptoms and cryoglobulins of the IgM anti-IgG type. There is disagreement about the number of patients who develop renal disease, between 20 and 55%, often several years after the onset.

The disease is common, several hundred cases being reported. There are wide, unexplained variations in the incidence of the disease among different geographic regions. It occurs only in adults, and there is a slight female predominance. Many of the reported cases are in northern Italy.

Pathogenesis

The glomerular lesions are thought to be due to the localization of the immunoglobulin aggregates to the glomeruli. The complexes fix complement and serve as chemoattractants for macrophages. The released products from these processes have been implicated in the proliferation of resident glomerular cells. This simplistic explanation does not account for the fact that only one-third of the patients with cryoglobulinemia develop a renal lesion, that the glomerular lesions are so diverse, and that there are wide regional and geographic variations.

It is clear that the presence of IgM rheumatoid factor is important in the development of the renal lesion. It is a monoclonal response against polyclonal IgG. It is not known whether the IgG is directed against a single antigen or whether it is a collection of immunoglobulins. Some researchers have suggested that the IgG is directed against hepatitis antigens, but this remains speculation.

The mechanism of the cryoprecipitation is also unknown, but the cryoglobulin concentration in the circulation does not appear to be directly related to the presence, absence, or intensity of the underlying glomerular lesion.

It has been suggested that the IgM is an anti-idiotypic anti-IgG antibody. The single most well-established fact is that when the cryoglobulins are composed of a single type of immunoglobulin, they are not usually associated with a glomerular lesion.

Patient Presentation

The signs and symptoms vary widely. The acute nephritic syndrome is present in 20 to 30% of patients and is characterized by hematuria, heavy proteinuria, hypertension, and the sudden onset of renal failure. Renal involvement may not be obvious. Oliguric acute renal failure may occur in 5%.

The majority of patients with mixed cryoglobulinemia have a more indolent and protracted renal course, presenting with proteinuria, hypertension, and hematuria. The renal disease most often appears several years after the onset of the extrarenal systemic signs and symptoms. Most patients have depressed serum complement component levels.

Histology

Light Microscopy

The glomerular lesions in patients with cryoglobulinemia are diverse, and several patterns have been recognized:

Diffuse proliferative and exudative glomerulonephritis

Membranoproliferative glomerulonephritis
Focal and segmental glomerulonephritis

Any of these histologic patterns may be associated with an acute small vessel vasculitis. Although rare, this association contributes to the diagnosis of the lesion.

Exudative Glomerulonephritis

This is the characteristic lesion of the glomerulonephritis of cryoglobulinemia. The glomeruli are large, with diffuse, marked intraglomerular hypercellularity (Fig. 9–21). The intravascular cells are mainly macrophages, which can be recognized by a nonspecific esterase stain. Their clear cytoplasm is also useful to differentiate them from resident glomerular cells. Neutrophils are present in small numbers. The vascular loops are distended, but the glomerular basement membranes are not thickened.

The lumina are almost obliterated by the infiltrating macrophages, proliferating resident glomerular cells, and deposition of an eosinophilic, amorphous proteinaceous mass that is often called a "thrombus." This material represents local precipitates of cryoglobulins in the vascular spaces (Fig. 9–22). There may be multiple profiles of this material within a single glomerulus, particularly if there is an associated nephritic syndrome. The presence of this material in combination with a proliferative and exudative glomerulonephritis is very suggestive of mixed cryoglobulinemia. These thrombi are not always plentiful and may be absent if the biopsy is performed at a time when the disease is relatively quiescent.

Membranoproliferative Glomerulonephritis

This is the lesion most frequently found in patients with chronic renal involvement. There is diffuse mesangial cell proliferation and infiltration with macrophages. Neutrophils are uncommon. The peripheral glomerular basement membranes are extensively duplicated, and there is diffuse mesangial sclerosis. In contrast to the acute glomerulonephritis described earlier, there are few luminal thrombi at this stage. Crescents may be seen, but they are not present in a large number of glomeruli.

A lobular pattern may be seen after treatment in patients with long-standing disease. In these instances, the macrophage infiltrate is inconspicuous and the mesangial nodules are large and strongly PAS positive.

Focal and Segmental Proliferative Glomerulonephritis

The mesangial proliferation is focal, and there often is a mixture of cellular and fibroepithelial crescents.

The tubules and interstitium do not have

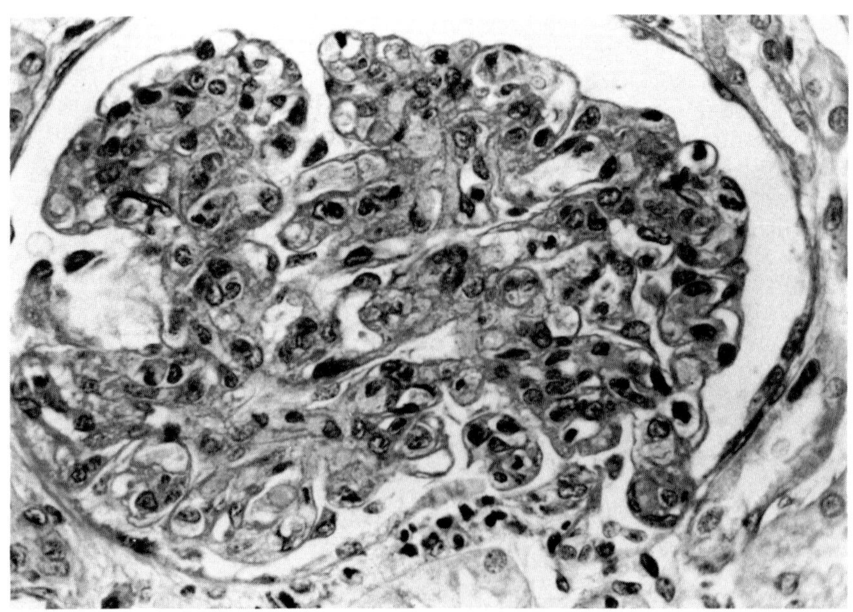

Figure 9–21. There is marked, diffuse intraglomerular hypercellularity. (Masson's trichrome, ×400.)

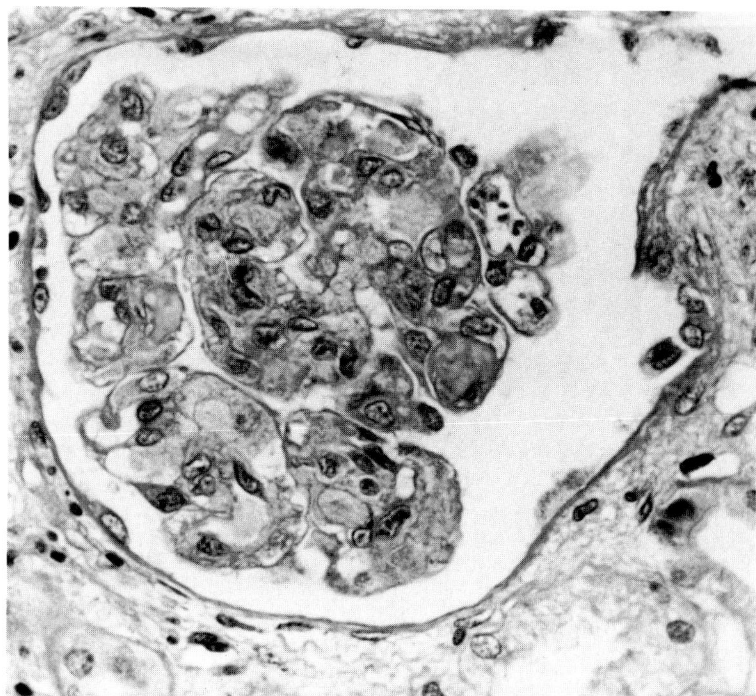

Figure 9–22. Multiple rounded, pale-staining "hyalin thrombi" are found within the glomerular lumen. (Masson's trichrome, ×250.)

specific abnormalities; rather they reflect those in the glomerular compartment.

No matter what type of glomerular lesion exists, a small vessel vasculitis is quite common. This is one of the few conditions in which a small vessel vasculitis coexists with a proliferative and exudative glomerulonephritis. The lesions affect either the interlobular or the afferent arterioles. They vary from an acute necrotizing arteritis involving the whole arterial wall, including the intima and media, to various degrees of perivascular inflammatory infiltrate (Fig. 9–23). Occlusion of the small arterioles by material similar to that found within glomeruli may also occur. In our experience, the most common vascular lesion is an abundant, periadventitial infiltrate. The interlobular arteries are frequently affected. The lesions are often quite

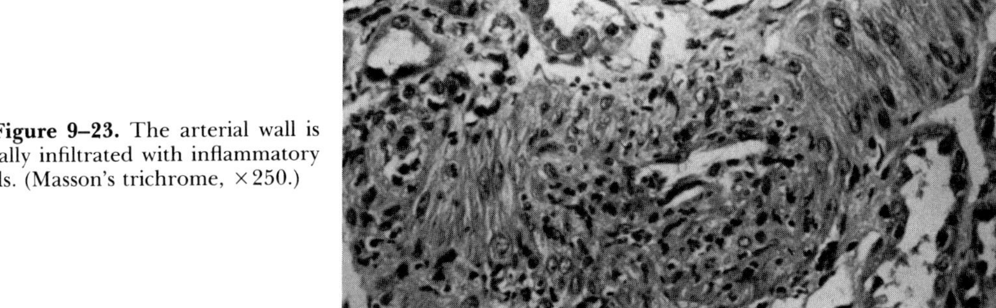

Figure 9–23. The arterial wall is locally infiltrated with inflammatory cells. (Masson's trichrome, ×250.)

focal, so multiple sections should be obtained in search for these lesions.

Immunofluorescence Microscopy

The glomerular deposits have the same composition as the circulating cryoglobulins. Thus deposits of IgG and IgM are present in many locations of the glomeruli. The large intravascular thrombi contain IgG and IgM as well as complement components (Fig. 9–24). These large intraluminal aggregates may be the only deposits found in patients with acute cryoglobulinemic glomerulonephritis, but diffuse granular deposits may also be present.

IgG, IgM, C1q, C4, and C3 are found in a peripheral glomerular basement membrane distribution in patients with membranoproliferative glomerulonephritis.

The deposits in patients with the focal lesions by light microscopy have the same types of immunoglobulins as in acute glomerulonephritis. However, in contrast to the focality of the lesions by light microscopy, there are diffuse, granular mesangial deposits by immunofluorescence microscopy.

As might be expected, in patients with IgA cryoglobulinemia, the glomerular deposits contain IgA.

Electron Microscopy

The similarity between the substructure of the glomerular aggregates in the luminal thrombi and that of circulating cryoglobulin precipitates has been noted by many investigators. Thus, the diagnosis of cryoglobulinemia can be made by the finding of deposits with this characteristic fibrillar substructure containing annular or cylindric structures with spokes. The curved cylinders are 250 nm in width and are arranged in pairs. They may show parallel striations. The fibrillar material is often surrounded by amorphous osmiophilic extracellular material. The deposits that represent the cryoglobulin precipitates in the glomeruli are the most characteristic finding in this glomerulonephritis.

A large number of macrophages are seen within the glomerulus, particularly in the vicinity of the fibrillar material (Fig. 9–25).

Prognosis

The lesions in the patients with acute glomerulonephritis are said to resolve without sequelae. Although probably true, this conclusion is based on the study of only a few patients. In some patients, the deposits disappear but the mesangial proliferation persists and mesangial sclerosis develops. Persistence of the glomerular disease is usually associated with the findings of either focal and segmental or membranoproliferative glomerulonephritis.

Recurrent episodes of acute nephritis have been documented. The exact course and

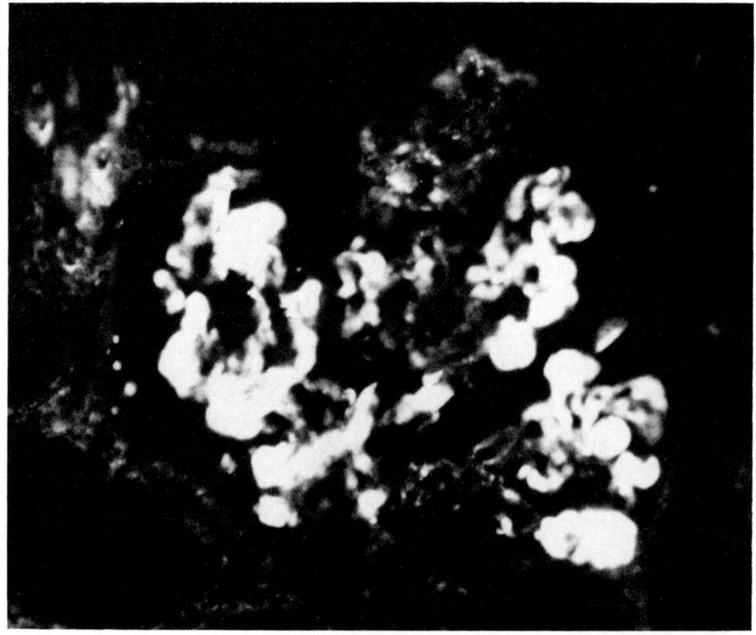

Figure 9–24. Immunofluorescence micrograph, anti-IgM. The hyalin thrombi are brightly positive. (×400.)

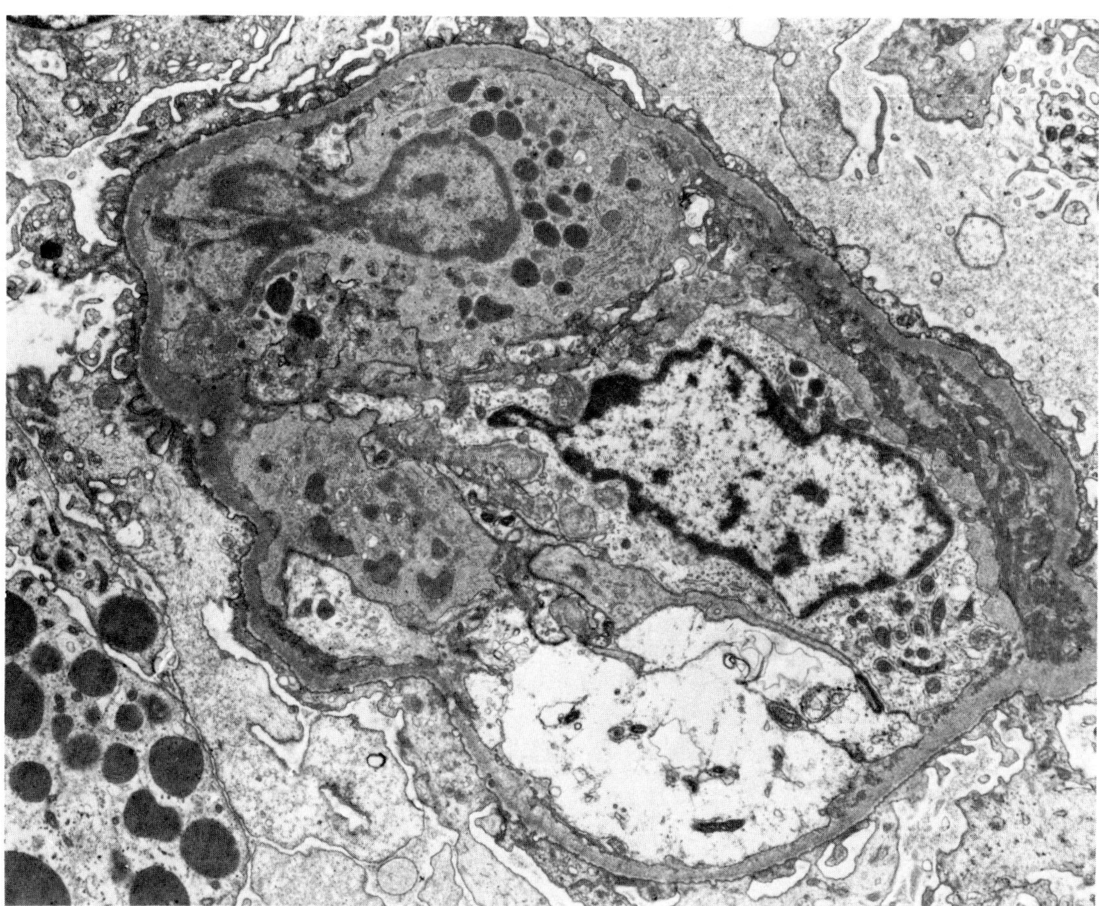

Figure 9–25. The glomerular basement membranes are focally duplicated, and there are subendothelial deposits. These changes, along with the infiltrate of monocytes, lead to occlusion of the glomerular loops. (×4230.) (Courtesy of Dr. G. d'Amico and the Department of Pathology, San Carlo Hospital, Milan, Italy.)

renal prognosis are not clear from either the literature or the personal experience of those who have seen many such patients. It is most likely true that no more than 10 to 20% of the patients with mixed cryoglobulinemia develop end-stage renal disease.

Many immunosuppressive regimens have been promulgated, but the small number of patients, coupled with the wide variety of renal manifestations, has not allowed the development of meaningful broad generalizations about therapy.

SELECTED READINGS

1. D'Amico G, Ferrario F, Colasanti G, et al: Glomerulonephritis in essential mixed cryoglobulinemia. Proceedings Eur Dial Transplant Assoc Eur Ren Assoc 21:527, 1984.
2. Feiner H, Gallo G: Ultrastructure in glomerulonephritis associated with cryoglobulinemia. Am J Pathol 88:145, 1977.
3. Ferrario F, Castiglione A, Colasanti G, et al: The detection of monocytes in human glomerulonephritis. Kidney Int 28:513, 1985.
4. Meltzer M, Franklin EC, Elias K, et al: Cryoglobulinemia. Clinical and laboratory study. Am J Med 40:837, 1966.
5. Morel-Maroger L, Verroust P: Glomerular lesions in dysproteinemias. Kidney Int 5:249, 1974.
6. Sinico RA, Winearls CG, Sabadini E, et al: Identification of glomerular immune deposits in cryoglobulinemic glomerulonephritis. Kidney Int 34:109, 1988.
7. Verroust P, Mery JP, Morel-Maroger L, et al: Glomerular lesions in monoclonal gammopathies and mixed essential cryoglobulinemias. Adv Nephrol 1:161, 1971.

MONOCLONAL GAMMOPATHY

Monoclonal gammopathy, the presence of a peak of an electrophoretically homogeneous immunoglobulin, may occur in individuals without myeloma or Waldenström's macroglobulinemia. Other terms have been used to define this benign condition: *benign, atypical, idiopathic paraproteinemia*. This anomaly appears to be associated with glomerular disease with an increased frequency.

Pathogenesis and Patient Presentation

The pathogenesis of the glomerular lesions in this syndrome is unknown.

Monoclonal gammopathy most commonly affects adults after the age of 50 years. A monoclonal cryoglobulin has been reported in several patients.

Histology

Light Microscopy

In most of the cases there is some degree of endocapillary glomerular proliferation. The proliferation may be diffuse or focal and segmental. Infiltration of the glomeruli by macrophages has been reported in patients with the acute nephritic syndrome.

Patients who also have cryoglobulinemia may show glomerular lesions resembling those with mixed cryoglobulinemia—namely, intraluminal deposits, macrophages in the glomerular loops, and occasionally membranoproliferative glomerulonephritis. Membranous glomerulonephritis and minimal change disease have also been described.

Immunofluorescence Microscopy

No clear-cut pattern has emerged from the various case reports of this syndrome. A relationship between the circulating pathologic immunoglobulin and the glomerular deposits can only be confirmed when they have the same composition. This has been the case in a few patients who had an IgG monoclonal gammopathy and cryoprecipitates in the glomeruli containing IgG. One is tempted to attribute those cases to mixed cryoglobulinemia, in which these components are found both in the circulation and in the glomeruli.

Electron Microscopy

The absence of large series and the lack of documented cases make it difficult to describe the renal lesions accurately. Intracellular crystals and fibrillar deposits have been reported in a few patients with diffuse proliferative glomerular lesions. The fibrils form parallel bundles, are most frequently found in patients with cryoglobulinemia, have a width of 20 to 40 nm, and lack the periodicity of amyloid fibrils.

Prognosis

Too few cases have been reported to establish a prognosis for this condition.

GLOMERULAR LESIONS IN MALIGNANCIES

Glomerular Lesions in Carcinoma

Membranous Glomerulonephritis

The most common renal lesion noted in patients with carcinoma is membranous glomerulonephritis. It accounts for more than one-half of the glomerular lesions in carcinoma. Most authors point out the strong relationship between membranous glomerulonephritis and carcinoma, although this link is the subject of some controversy.

The association between the nephrotic syndrome and cancer was first recognized in 1966 in a 10-year follow-up study of 101 patients in the United States. It was observed that in adults presenting with the nephrotic syndrome, neoplasia was discovered within a period of 14 months in 10.9%. Membranous glomerulonephritis was the renal lesion in nine of these ten patients. A similar incidence was found in another study of 44 British adults with membranous glomerulonephritis; 4 were found to have carcinomas. We reported that in a series of patients with membranous glomerulonephritis in France, 7 of 86 had a carcinoma. Finally, in a report on 3476 patients with proteinuria in the United Kingdom, 42 had an underlying carcinoma, and the principal histologic lesion in this group was membranous glomerulonephritis. Thus, there appears to be a privileged relationship between membranous glomerulonephritis and carcinoma in adults.

Pathogenesis

The pathogenesis is not clear. Attempts to isolate substances from the circulation are too sparse to draw general conclusions. The cancers most commonly associated with membranous glomerulonephritis are pulmonary, with bronchogenic being the predominant lesion. Other sites include the colorectal area, kidney, breast, and stomach.

Histology

The features are the same as those described in Chapter 4.

Prognosis

The prognosis is essentially determined by the underlying tumor.

Membranoproliferative Glomerulonephritis

Membranoproliferative glomerulonephritis has been most often reported in association with gastrointestinal carcinomas. However, it has also been reported that in a series of 40 patients with hypernephromas, 35% had mesangial deposits of immunoglobulins and complement. In a series of 57 patients with renal cell carcinoma, we also found mesangial changes ranging from moderate to severe sclerosis. A few specimens showed glomerular epithelial cell proliferation with or without synechiae or crescents.

Amyloidosis

The renal amyloid deposits in patients with carcinomas have been shown to be of the AA type, in those few cases studied by modern techniques, and it seems reasonable to assume that many of the others are similar. The incidence of amyloidosis in one series of 4033 autopsies of patients with cancer was 0.4%. Only 7 of 16 affected patients had an associated carcinoma, but membranous glomerulonephritis was the most frequent renal lesion. In this and other series, the most frequent tumors associated with renal amyloidosis are hypernephromas.

Glomerular Lesions in Lymphoma

Hodgkin's Disease

Amyloidosis was the most common renal lesion before 1963, but it has largely disappeared as a complication. The most frequent is minimal lesion. This change may antedate the diagnosis of Hodgkin's disease. Its appearance correlates with the initial onset and recurrences, and it disappears with remissions.

Renal lesions of other types are much less frequently associated with Hodgkin's disease. They include focal sclerosis, membranous glomerulonephritis, membranoproliferative glomerulonephritis, proliferative glomerulonephritis, and crescentic glomerulonephritis with circulating anti-glomerular basement membrane antibodies.

Non-Hodgkin's Lymphoma

The renal lesions are of quite diverse types, in contrast to those associated with Hodgkin's disease. In these cases, it has been difficult to

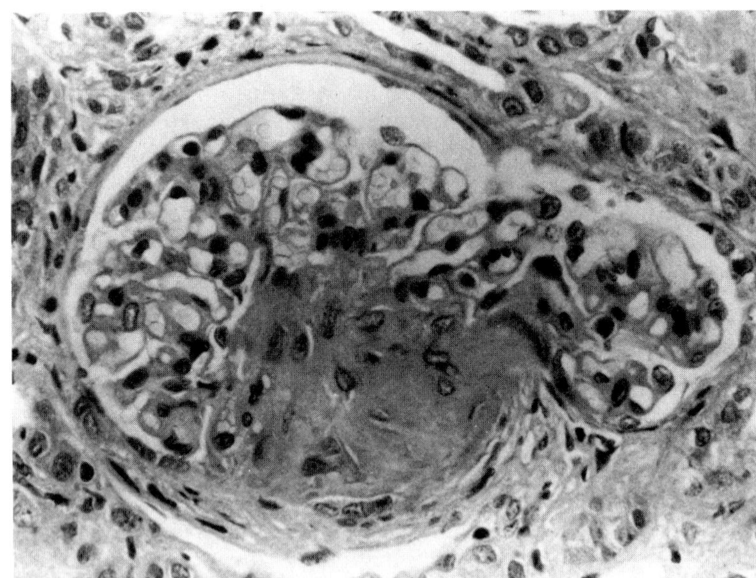

Figure 9–26. Focal sclerosis affecting one-half of the glomerulus. There is also interstitial fibrosis and an infiltrate of mononuclear cells. (Masson's trichrome, ×250.)

directly implicate the hematologic malignancy in the pathogenesis of the renal lesion.

Glomerular Lesions in Leukemias

Chronic Lymphocytic Leukemia

Glomerular lesions, although uncommon in most types of leukemia, are as frequently found in chronic lymphocytic leukemia as in lymphoid malignancies (Fig. 9–26). The most commonly reported histologic type is membranoproliferative glomerulonephritis. Monoclonal gammopathy has been found in several patients, and cryoglobulinemia was reportedly present in another series. Our experience is similar and would suggest that in patients with chronic lymphocytic leukemia with a proliferative glomerular lesion, slightly more than one-half have an associated monoclonal gammopathy.

SELECTED READINGS

1. Dabbs D, Striker L, Mignon F, et al: Glomerular lesions in lymphomas and leukemia. Am J Med 80:63, 1986.
2. Davison AM: The United Kingdom Medical Research Council's glomerulonephritis registry. Contrib Nephrol 48:24, 1985.
3. Eagen JW, Lewis EJ: Glomerulopathies of neoplasia. Kidney Int 11:297, 1977.
4. Gilboa N, Durante D, Guggenheim S, et al: Immune deposit nephritis and single-component cryoglobulinemia associated with chronic lymphocytic leukemia. Nephron 24:223, 1979.
5. Lee JC, Yamaushi H, Hopper J: The association of cancer and the nephrotic syndrome. Ann Intern Med 64:41, 1966.
6. Silva FG, Pirani CL, Mesa-Tejada R, et al: The kidney in plasma cell dyscrasias: A review and a clinicopathologic study of 50 patients. *In* Fenoglio C, Wolff M (eds): Progress in Surgical Pathology. New York, Masson, 1984, pp 131–176.

IMMUNOTACTOIDS AND FIBRILS IN THE GLOMERULI

The name *immunotactoid glomerulonephritis* was coined to designate a glomerular disease with fibrillar non-amyloid glomerular deposits that could only be detected by electron microscopy.

Patient Presentation

Hypertension and chronic microscopic hematuria and proteinuria are common presenting findings. The patients described so far have not had plasma cell dyscrasias. Nonamyloid fibrils have also been described in patients with other types of glomerular diseases, such as cryoglobulinemia and IgG monoclonal benign gammopathy.

Histology

Light Microscopy

The amount of mesangial matrix is increased, with various degrees of mesangial cell proliferation.

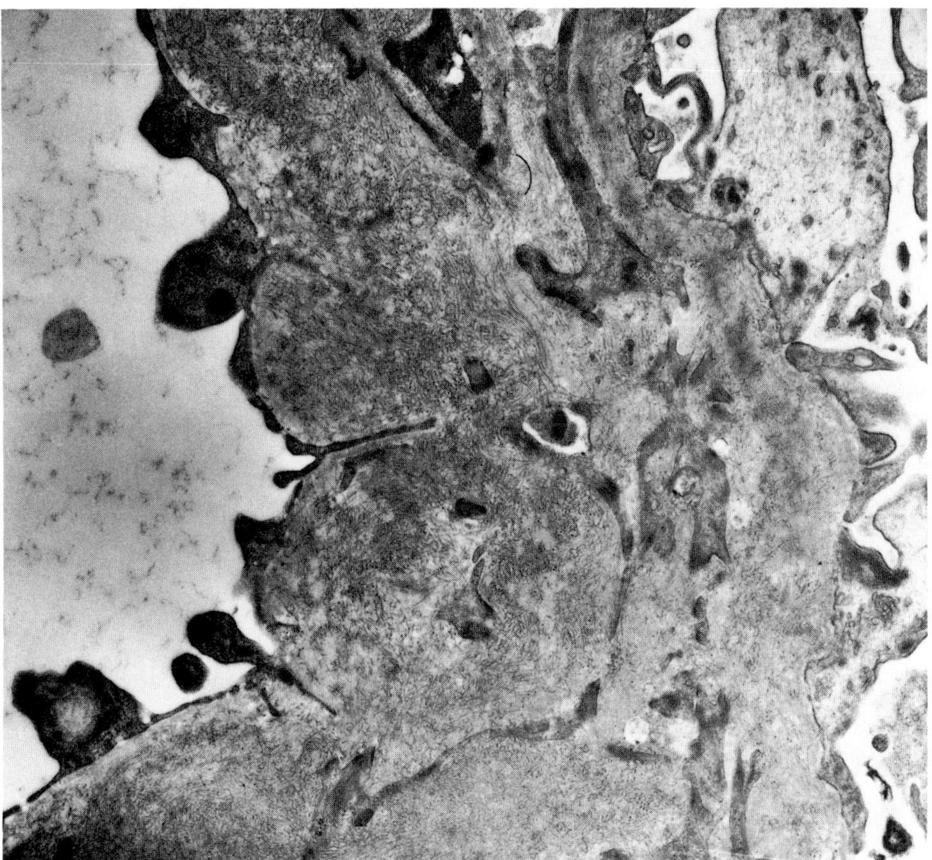

Figure 9–27. Bundles of non-branched fibrils are present in both the mesangial and subendothelial regions. (×14,000.)

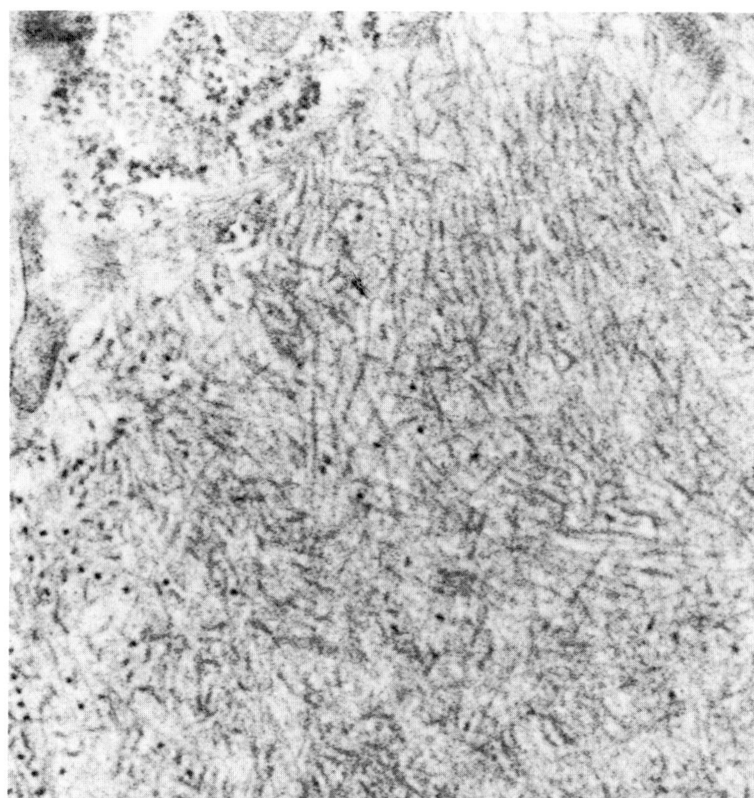

Figure 9–28. At higher power, the fibrils are irregularly arranged, and no substructure is visible. (×35,000.)

Immunofluorescence Microscopy

Irregular granular deposits of IgG, IgM, and C3 are seen in the mesangial and subendothelial areas.

Electron Microscopy

Bundles of fibrils without a recognizable periodicity have been described in the mesangial and subendothelial areas (Fig. 9–27). The individual size of the microfibrils approximates 20 μm (Fig. 9–28). They are usually distributed in the same regions as the deposits seen by immunofluorescence microscopy. It has been suggested that they represent altered immunoglobulins, but this point has not been fully elucidated.

Prognosis

The significance of fibrils is unknown, and whether or not this histologic finding justifies a separate disease category, that is, immunotactoid nephropathy, needs further discussion.

SELECTED READINGS

1. Alpers CE, Rennke HG, Hopper J Jr, et al: Fibrillary glomerulonephritis: An entity with unusual immunofluorescence features. Kidney Int 31:781, 1987.
2. Duffy JL, Khurana E, Susin M, et al: Fibrillary renal deposits and nephritis. Am J Pathol 113:279, 1983.
3. Hsu HC, Churg J: Glomerular microfibrils in renal disease: A comparative electron microscopic study. Kidney Int 16:497, 1979.

Chapter

10

GLOMERULAR DISEASES ASSOCIATED WITH PREGNANCY

TOXEMIA OF PREGNANCY

Pregnancy may be associated with a number of diseases. It may for instance exacerbate renal diseases that existed before the pregnancy. The only syndrome that is specific for pregnancy is preeclampsia, or toxemia of pregnancy. Although the frequency of the disease is decreasing, preeclampsia still represents a common problem during the third trimester of pregnancy. This condition was clearly delineated in the 1960s with the help of detailed pathologic studies, but the use of biopsies in this setting is much more restricted now.

Many diseases that antedate a pregnancy, in particular those with a hypertensive component, may be exacerbated during the late part of pregnancy. A pathologist thus may have to recognize an underlying glomerular disorder from those abnormalities characteristic of toxemia of pregnancy.

Pathogenesis

Toxemia of pregnancy is associated with intravascular coagulation, and as in thrombotic microangiopathies, the glomerular endothelium is the principal site affected. The pathogenesis, although not completely elucidated, is presumably related to a combination of factors. Pregnancy predisposes to intravascular coagulation and to the effect of endotoxins, as shown in a number of experimental conditions. In the third trimester of pregnancy, ischemia of the uterus and placenta may trigger the release of thromboplastic substances. Finally, there may be a genetic propensity to develop preeclampsia in response to immunologic reactivity against the fetal antigens. A vasospasm of the arterioles may be the initiating factor leading to the endothelial damage sometimes referred to as endotheliosis, progressing to local thrombosis in the glomeruli.

Patient Presentation

The disease typically affects primiparas and occurs during the third term of pregnancy. Hypertension, proteinuria, and

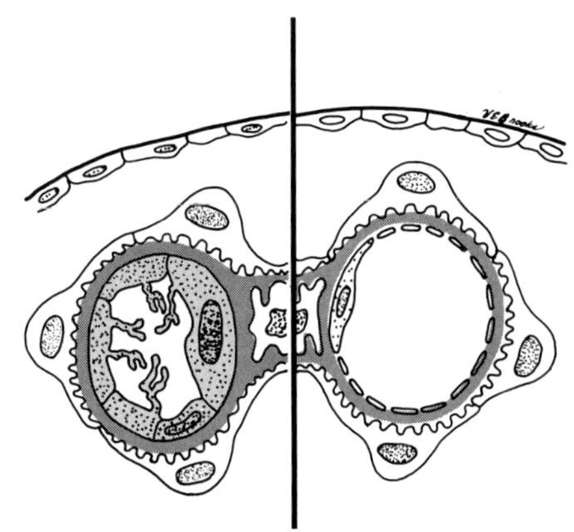

Figure 10–1. Diagram of endothelial cell swelling.

edema are characteristic. Another feature is retinal arteriolar spasm, which correlates with the severity of the glomerular lesions. Other clinical findings include a decline in glomerular filtration rate and hyperuricemia. Proteinuria is moderate, and the nephrotic syndrome, although possible, is a rare event.

Histology

Light Microscopy

The glomerular changes are diffuse and regular, consisting of enlargement and loss of the vascular spaces by an expanded mesangium and endothelial cell swelling (Figs. 10–1 and 10–2). Hypercellularity is not a feature of this disease, although the glomeruli may appear to have an increased number of cells because of the cytoplasmic swelling. The glomerular basement membranes appear thickened (Fig. 10–3) on hematoxylin and eosin (H&E) stains, but silver stains reveal normal contours (Fig. 10–4). The subendothelium is widened and filled with a flocculent material (Fig. 10–5).

Aside from endothelial swelling, the blood vessels do not show lesions.

The tubules and interstitium are generally unremarkable, unless tubular necrosis is present. Hyalin droplets may be present in tubular epithelium, and casts may be seen in the lumina if the patient has significant proteinuria.

Immunofluorescence Microscopy

There is considerable discussion about the amount and type of deposits in this syndrome. Suffice it to say that there is little evidence to implicate an immunologic component in this process at the present time. Deposits of IgG and IgM have been found along the glomerular basement membranes in approximately 10% of biopsies and are most frequently present in the severe forms of the disease. Fibrin may also be found in the glomeruli. As was the case with immunoglobulin deposits, fibrin is most commonly found in biopsies on patients with severe lesions.

Electron Microscopy

The major changes occur on the luminal aspects of the glomerular basement mem-

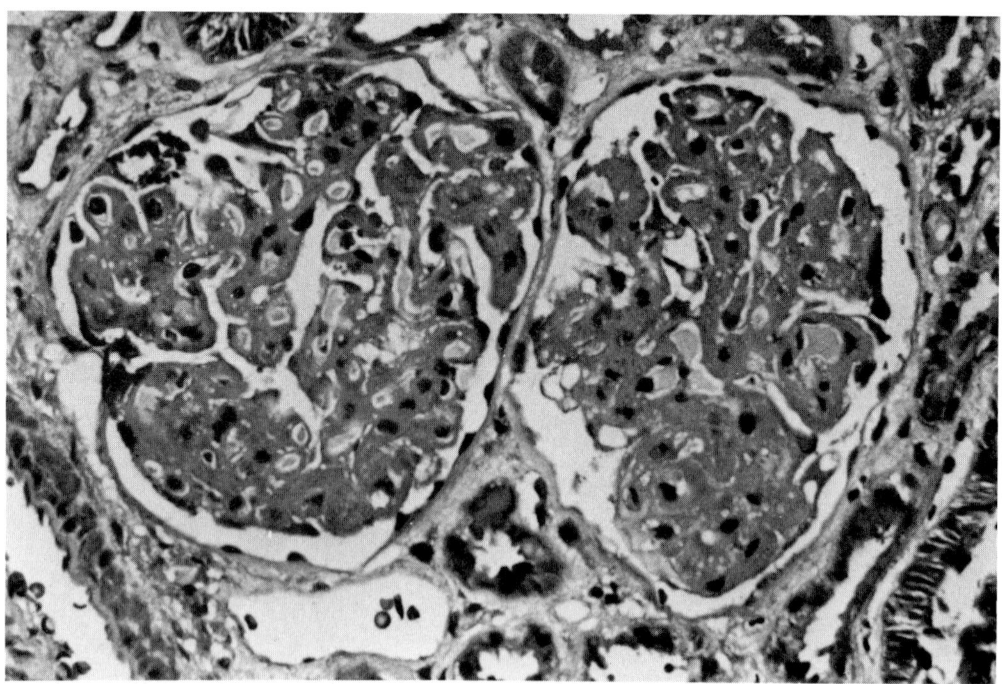

Figure 10–2. The glomerular basement membranes in all glomeruli have a thickened, refractile profile. The vascular spaces are markedly compressed. The number of intraglomerular cells is not increased. The interstitium is edematous. (H&E, ×300.)

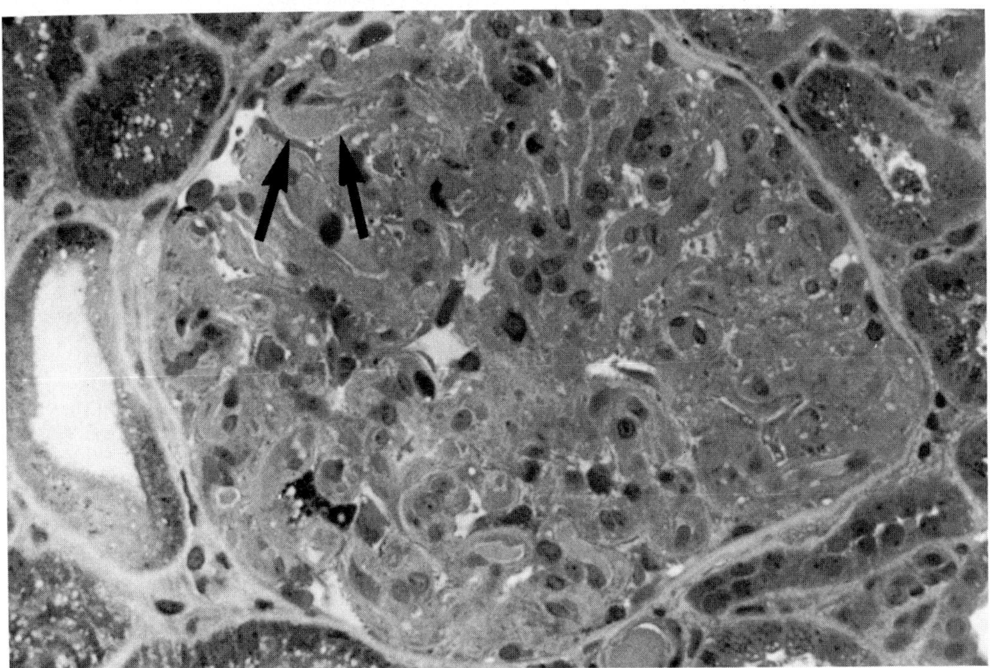

Figure 10–3. At higher power, the details of the glomerular basement membranes (pale refractile lines) are outlined by the subendothelial deposits (arrows). The vascular spaces are almost completely occluded. (H&E, ×500.)

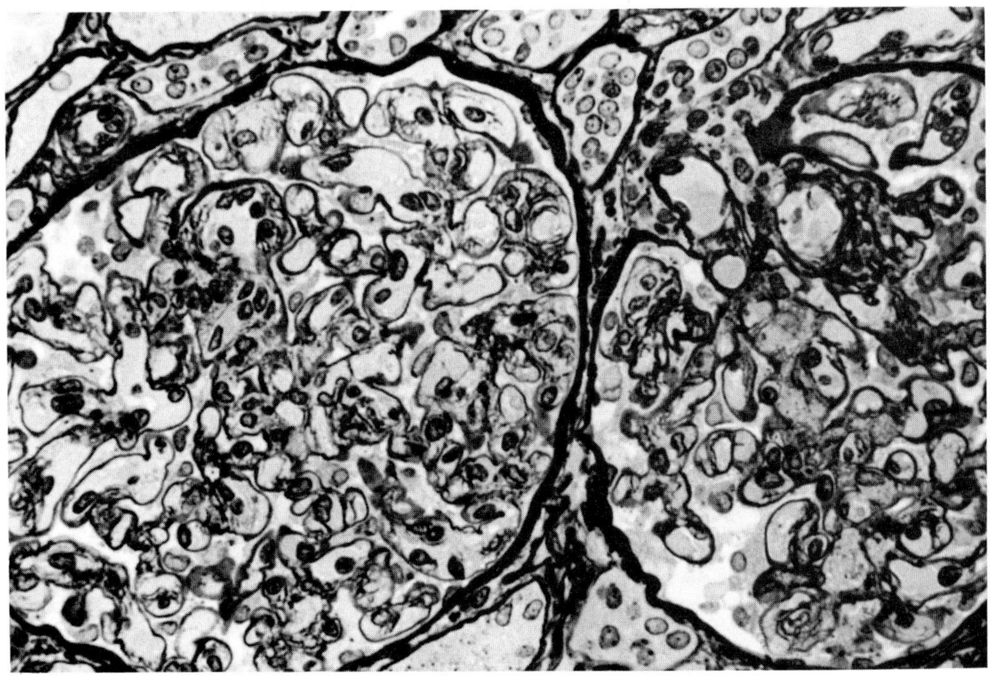

Figure 10–4. The basement membranes and mesangial matrix are not increased in amount. (PASM, ×300.)

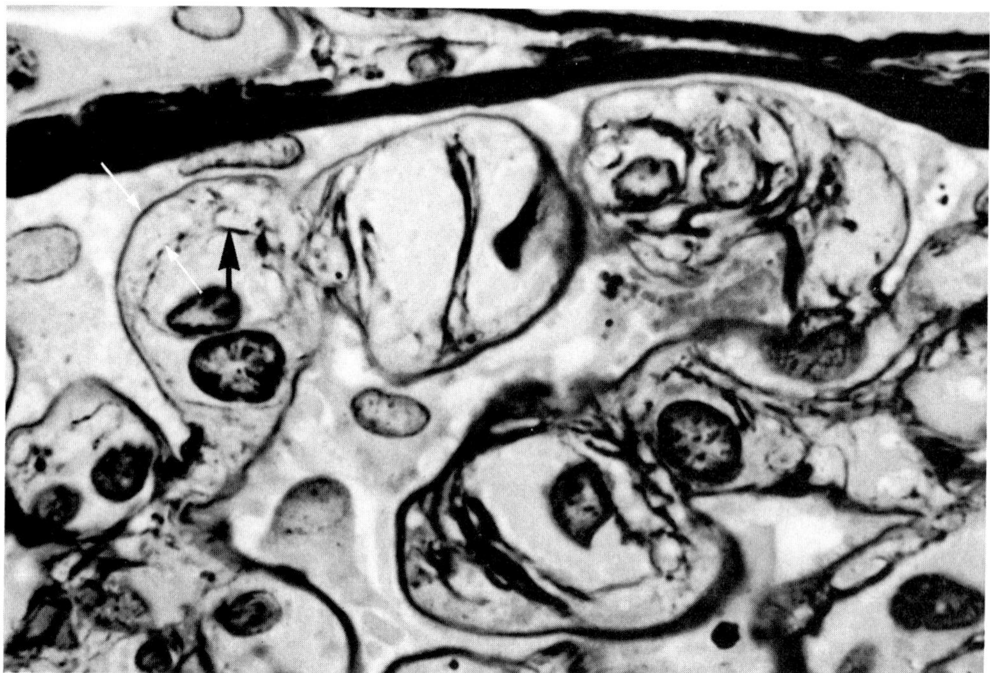

Figure 10–5. At higher power, the widened subendothelial spaces are clearly visible. The luminal aspect of the endothelial cell cytoplasm (dark arrow) is widely separated from the glomerular basement membrane by deposits (light arrows). (PASM, ×1200.)

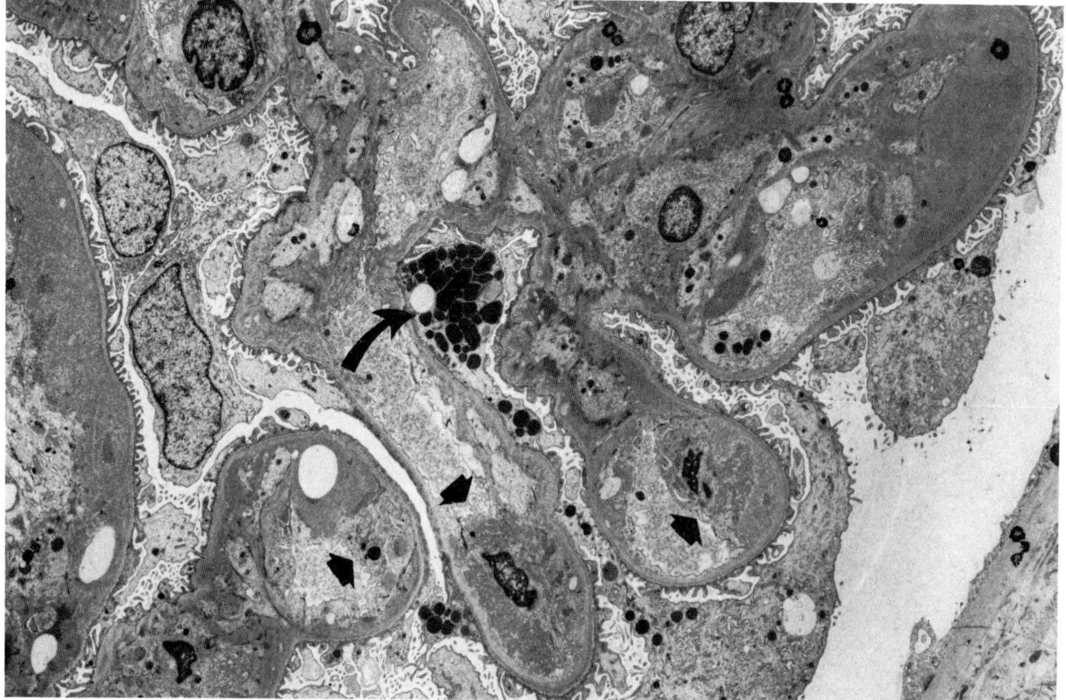

Figure 10–6. The endothelial cell cytoplasm is prominent (arrowheads). There are large subendothelial deposits in most glomerular loops. The epithelial cell cytoplasm is filled with dense lysosomes (curved arrow). (×2000.)

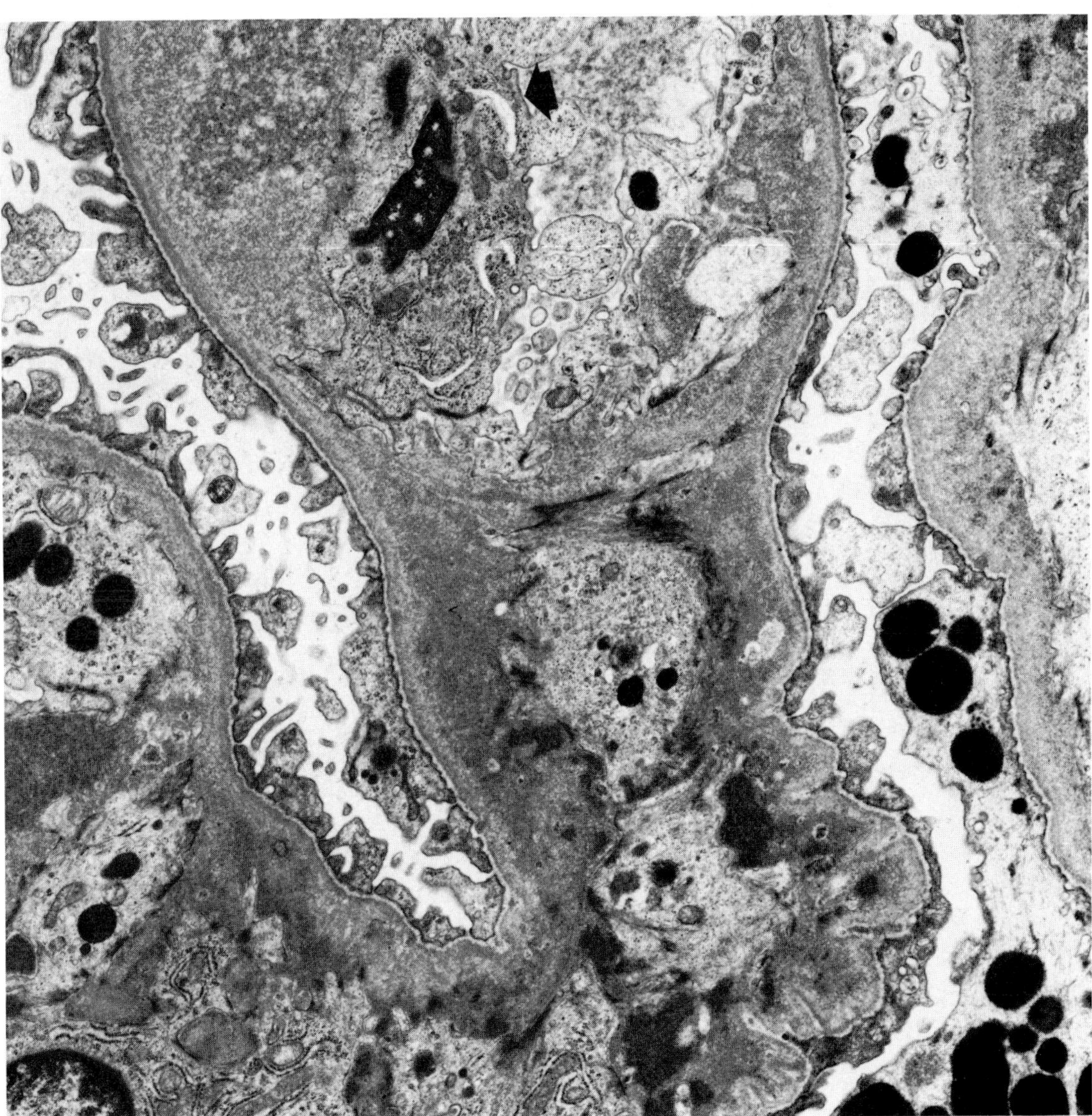

Figure 10–7. At higher magnification, the endothelial cell cytoplasmic prominence is apparent (arrowhead), and the large subendothelial deposits are easily appreciated. Large lysosomes are present in both endothelial and mesangial cells. (×4000.)

branes. The endothelial cells are swollen and vacuolated (Fig. 10–6). The lamina rara interna is markedly expanded and contains flocculent material and electron-dense strands of material resembling basement membranes (Fig. 10–7). As noted by light microscopy, the mesangial cells also appear swollen, and the mesangial matrix is expanded. Material resembling fibrin may be seen in the vascular spaces.

The epithelial cells may contain an increased number of lysosomes, but they are otherwise unremarkable.

Prognosis

Most investigators agree that the lesions associated with preeclampsia are completely reversible. However, few long-term studies have been performed, and renal biopsies have not been a part of the follow-up evaluation.

SELECTED READINGS

1. Kincaid-Smith P: Participation of intravascular coagulation in the pathogenesis of glomerular and vascular lesions. Kidney Int 7:242, 1975.
2. Pirani CL: Coagulation and renal disease. *In* Bertani T, Remuzzi G (eds.): Glomerular Injury 300 Years after Morgagni. Wichtig Editore, Milano, Italy, 1983, pp 119–138.
3. Pollak VE, Nettles JB: The kidney in toxemia of pregnancy: A clinical and pathological study based on renal biopsies. Medicine 39:469, 1960.
4. Pollak VE, Pirani CL, Kark RM, et al: Reversible glomerular lesions in toxemia of pregnancy. Lancet 2:59, 1956.
5. Spargo B, McCartney CP, Winemiller R: Glomerular capillary endotheliosis in toxemia of pregnancy. Arch Pathol 68:593, 1959.
6. Wagoner RA, Holley KE, Johnson W: Accelerated nephrosclerosis and post-partum acute renal failure. Ann Intern Med 69:237, 1968.

Chapter

11

RENAL TRANSPLANTATION

Approximately 8000 renal transplants are performed each year in the United States. Graft survival is improving as a result of organ sharing and donation programs and improved methods of immunosuppression. The latter include the use of cyclosporine A in combination with azathioprine and steroids.

The loss of transplant function has many causes. The likelihood of a particular etiology depends, in large part, on the interval since transplantation. Both a renal biopsy and a detailed clinical and laboratory work-up are frequently necessary to establish a definitive diagnosis on which to base proper therapy. This chapter contains a description of the conditions that may cause loss of graft function. They are grouped by the interval following graft placement. At the end of this chapter is a short description of techniques to evaluate the status of the graft.

IMMEDIATE (HOURS) OR HYPERACUTE REJECTION

Immediately after vascularization of the transplant an episode of hyperacute rejection may follow. This event is now uncommon. It is due to the presence of preformed antibodies, predominantly of the ABO groups, which are now detected by prescreening assays. The groups at most risk include multiparous women, recipients of multiple transfusions, and individuals who have previously received a renal graft.

Patient Presentation

The diagnosis is usually made by the transplant surgeon because of the sudden development of graft swelling and cyanosis.

Histology

Light Microscopy

In the first few postoperative hours, the glomeruli are relatively unaffected, but massive infiltration of the peritubular capillaries by neutrophils occurs. There may also be large areas of interstitial hemorrhage (Fig. 11–1).

Within a few hours, the glomerular vascular loops appear dilated and filled with fibrin thrombi and red blood cell aggregates (Fig. 11–2). The arterial tree and the interstitial capillaries also contain thrombi. At this stage, the tubular epithelium also shows massive sloughing and necrosis (Fig. 11–3). Complete cortical necrosis rapidly ensues.

Immunofluorescence Microscopy

Linear deposits of IgG and C3 may be seen along the endothelial aspects of the vasculature within the first few hours. The most prominent finding, however, beginning within the first few hours, is the progressive appearance of massive fibrin/fibrinogen deposits in every vascular compartment of the kidney.

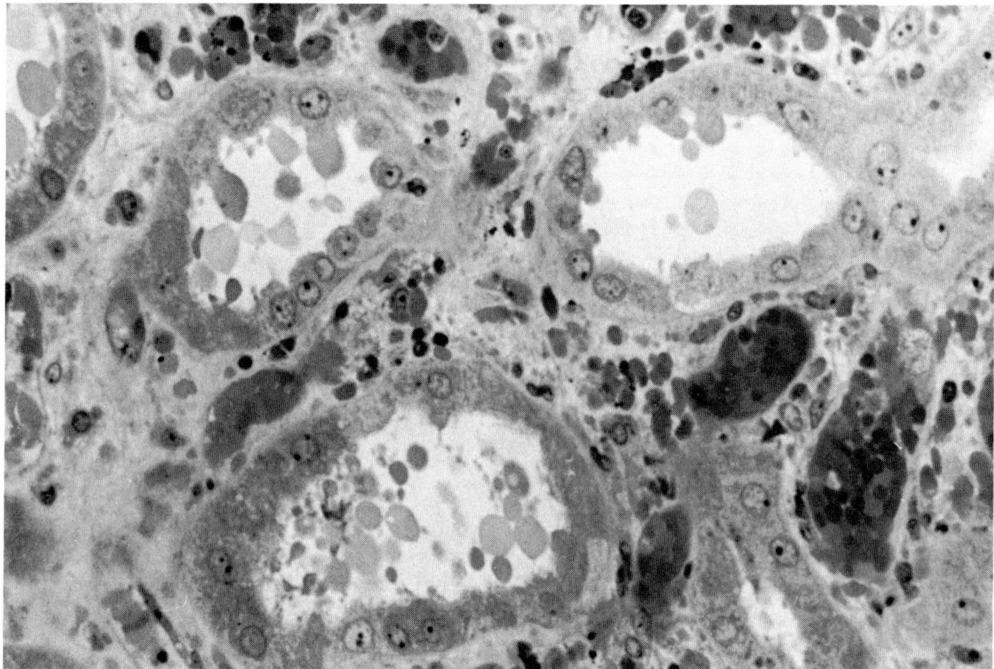

Figure 11–1. Hyperacute rejection. There is an increased number of red blood cells within capillary spaces. There is also diffuse epithelial cell necrosis. (H&E, ×300.)

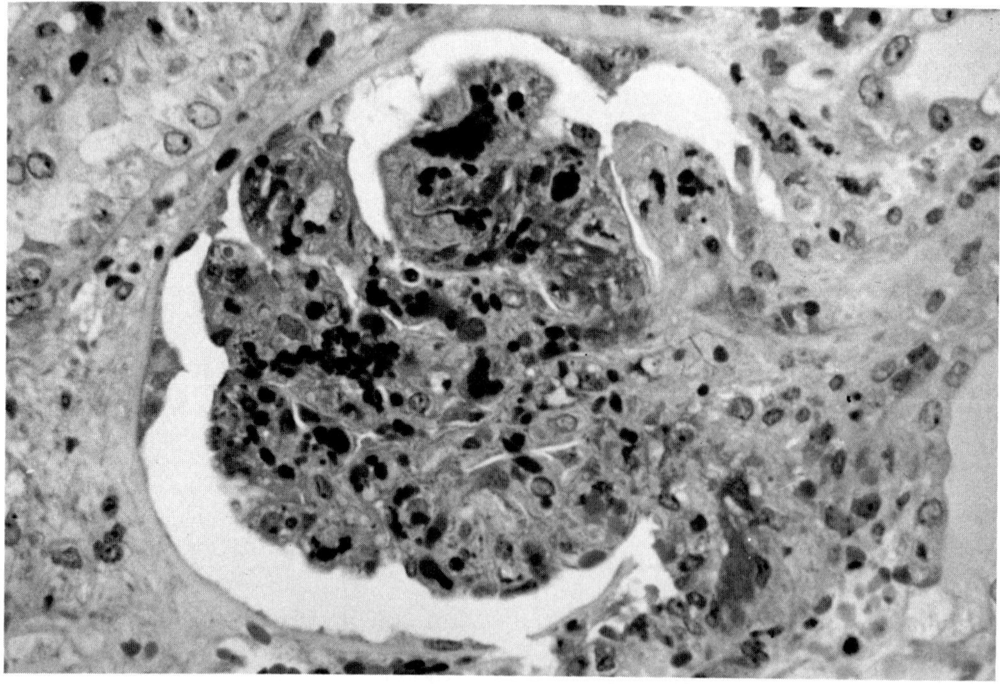

Figure 11–2. Hyperacute rejection. The vascular loops are filled with red blood cells and fibrin thrombi, distorting the architecture. The surrounding tubular epithelium is undergoing necrosis. (H&E, ×300.)

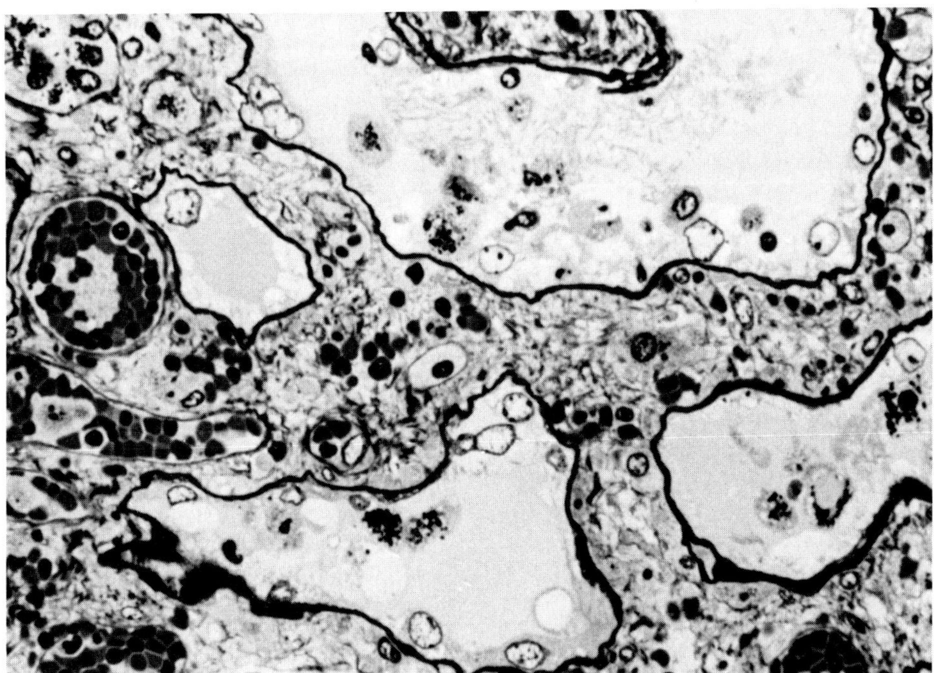

Figure 11–3. Hyperacute rejection. The interstitium is filled with edema and inflammatory cells. The tubules are nearly completely necrotic, and the epithelial cells are sloughing into the lumen. (H&E, ×300.)

Electron Microscopy

The glomeruli are filled with platelet and leukocyte fragments within minutes. Necrosis appears later and involves all cell types.

EARLY (DAYS TO WEEKS) REJECTION

Renal lesions of several different types may be encountered. If there are technical problems related to the operative procedure, a renal biopsy is not performed.

Patient Presentation

During this time, a decrement in renal function may be due to either acute tubular injury (necrosis) or graft rejection. A renal biopsy may be an invaluable tool in the elucidation of the state of the renal graft during this period. It should be noted that a renal transplant may demonstrate lesions that, although not present in a normal kidney, do not necessarily carry a poor prognosis. Examples include interstitial infiltration and edema. The practice of routine allograft biopsy has been crucial in demonstrating the need to exercise extreme caution in the interpretation of graft biopsy specimens.

Acute Tubular Necrosis

Histology

Light Microscopy

Acute tubular necrosis is not unusual during this period, and it seems to have increased in frequency with the advent of cyclosporine A therapy. The histologic features of acute tubular necrosis in the post-transplant patient are not different from those in native kidneys and are described in Chapter 13. However, there may also be evidence of mild transplant rejection, including scattered foci of lymphoid and plasma cells in the interstitium and proliferative changes involving the medium-sized arteries and arterioles. The latter consist of intimal hyperplasia, usually modest, and the finding of an occasional neutrophil or lymphocyte in the vascular wall.

Immunofluorescence Microscopy

Deposits of fibrin along the endothelial aspects of the glomeruli are common, but the lumina remain patent and complete thrombosis is uncommon.

Electron Microscopy

Electron microscopy is not helpful, except to exclude cell necrosis.

Acute Rejection

Introduction and Patient Presentation

The most worrisome of the conditions occurring in the early post-transplant interval is acute rejection. It may be related to the presence of donor leukocytes carried within the graft; these sensitize recipient leukocytes to attack the graft. Acute rejection may appear during the first week, but it may occur at any time. It is most frequent within the first 2 months. Acute rejection is recognized by a decrease in renal function and often by the presence of enlargement and tenderness of the graft. It may be triggered by a change in the immunosuppression regimen.

Histology

Light Microscopy

As noted earlier, a number of interstitial and vascular lesions in biopsies of renal transplants are not harbingers of a bad prognosis. These include mild interstitial edema or fibrosis and scattered infiltrates of lymphocytes in the interstitium. Vascular lesions are also common and may be reflective of native disease in the donor rather than a manifestation of a lesion secondary to its status as a transplanted organ in the recipient.

The glomeruli are usually unremarkable. Glomerular changes are evident on occasion, in the form of so-called transplant glomerulopathy. These changes include simplification of the glomeruli with thickened glomerular basement membranes (Fig. 11–4) and mesangial prominence, which has a basket-weave appearance by silver stain. In certain patients, a fluffy fibrillar subendothelial material is present, resulting in thickening of the glomerular wall. This lesion, which resembles that observed in thrombotic microangiopathy, suggests that chronic endothelial and coagulation abnormalities may underlie transplant glomerulopathy.

Other features that assist in the definition of an acute rejection episode include diffuse interstitial edema and inflammation, as well as infiltration of the tubular epithelium with leukocytes (Fig. 11–5). The character of the interstitial inflammatory infiltrate is variable, but the number of mononuclear cells is often remarkable.

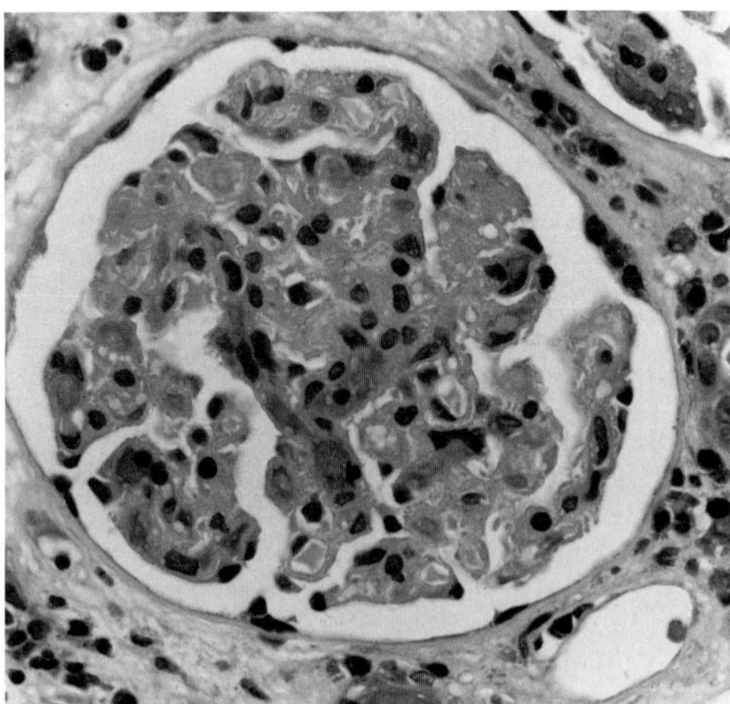

Figure 11–4. Acute rejection. The major glomerular change is endothelial swelling, which results in marked diminution in the size of the vascular spaces. (H&E, ×300.)

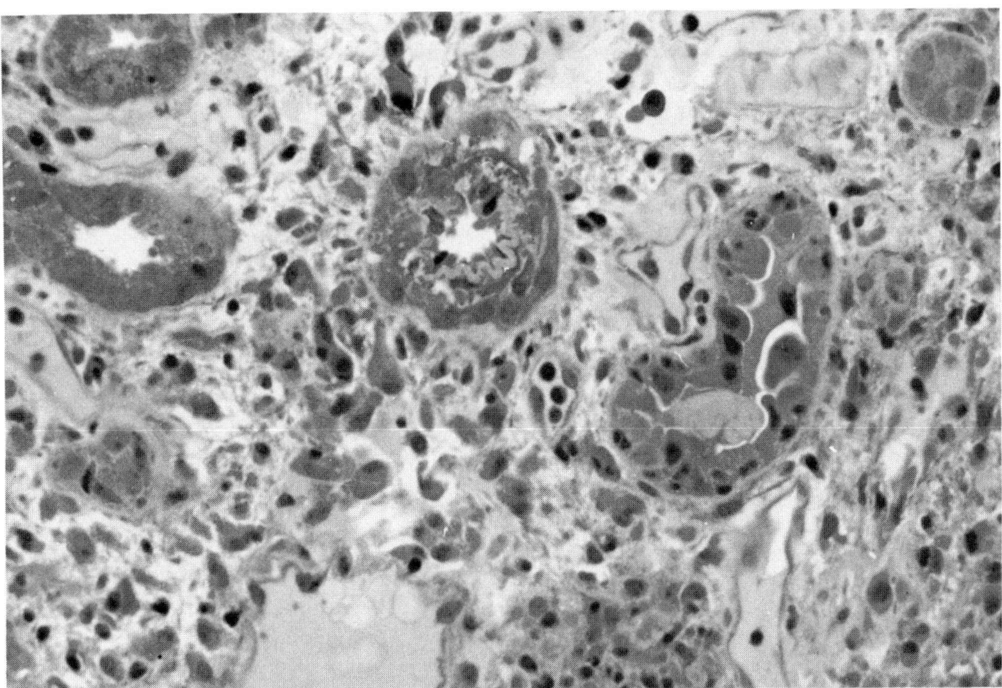

Figure 11–5. Acute rejection. The severity and extent of the inflammatory infiltrate are obvious. The tubular epithelium (right center) is infiltrated by inflammatory cells. (H&E, ×300.)

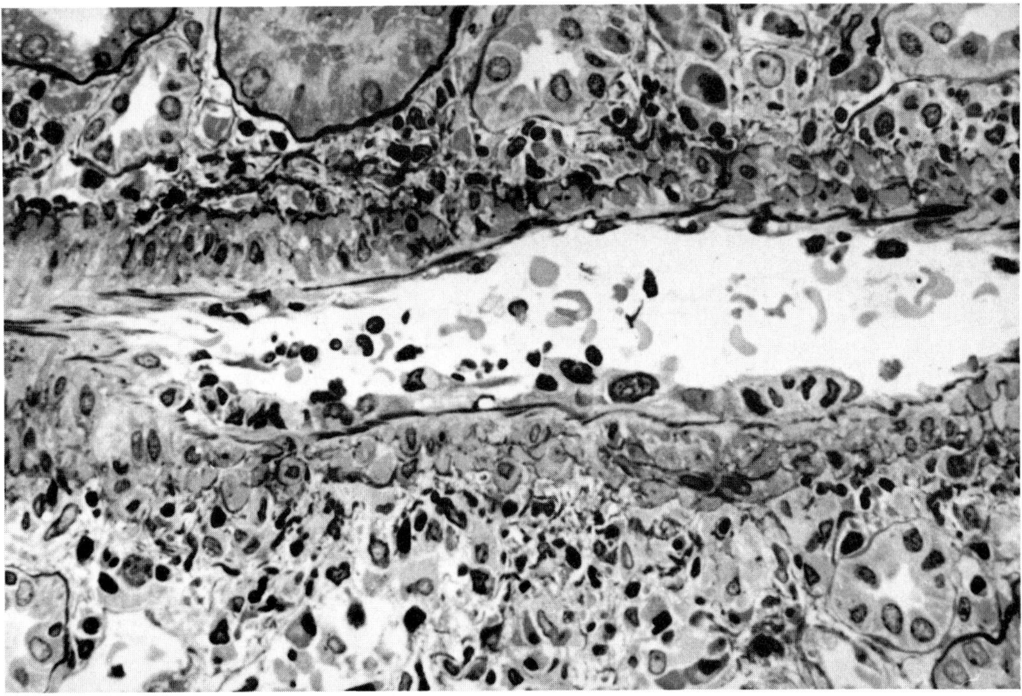

Figure 11–6. Acute rejection. There is marked endothelial injury, manifest by adherent neutrophils, vacuolation and proliferation of endothelial cells, and an inflammatory cell infiltrate in the subendothelial space. (PASM, ×300.)

The intrarenal arteries and arterioles always show lesions. The most characteristic change is the presence of intimal thickening and the appearance of inflammatory cells within and adherent to the endothelium (Fig. 11–6). The media may also contain lipid-laden macrophages as well as an increase in the amount of extracellular matrix. In the most severe lesions, the vessels may be filled with thrombus.

Immunofluorescence Microscopy

Immunofluorescence microscopy does not add substantial information. The glomeruli, as a rule, do not contain immune reactants. The vessels may contain deposits of C3/IgM when there is an associated sclerotic lesion. Fibrin/fibrinogen is occasionally found in blood vessel walls if a severe inflammatory vasculitis is present.

The character of the inflammatory infiltrate varies widely. The use of antibodies to lymphocyte markers with immunoperoxidase staining has failed to show a specific pattern that predicts the presence of rejection. It has been shown that T cells, monocytes, and HLA-Dr-positive populations of lymphocytes are present in the interstitium. Smaller numbers of B cells have been identified. One group has suggested that the presence of Leu-7-positive lymphocytes between cells of the tubular epithelial cells correlates with acute rejection (Fig. 11–7).

Electron Microscopy

The glomerular wall thickening is due to subendothelial widening and the accumulation of flocculent material in that space, as well as thickening of the endothelial cell cytoplasm (Fig. 11–8). These findings are consistent with endothelial cell injury. The mesangium is less dense than normal, with areas of increased lucency admixed with zones of normal density.

Prognosis

When suspected, acute rejection is frequently treated empirically. However, a definitive diagnosis can only be made on renal biopsy. Acute rejection is often reversible, with return of graft function. The long-term prognosis is inversely correlated with the number of rejection episodes and directly with their response to therapy. The presence of transplant glomerulopathy early in the post-transplant period carries a poor prognosis for long-term graft function.

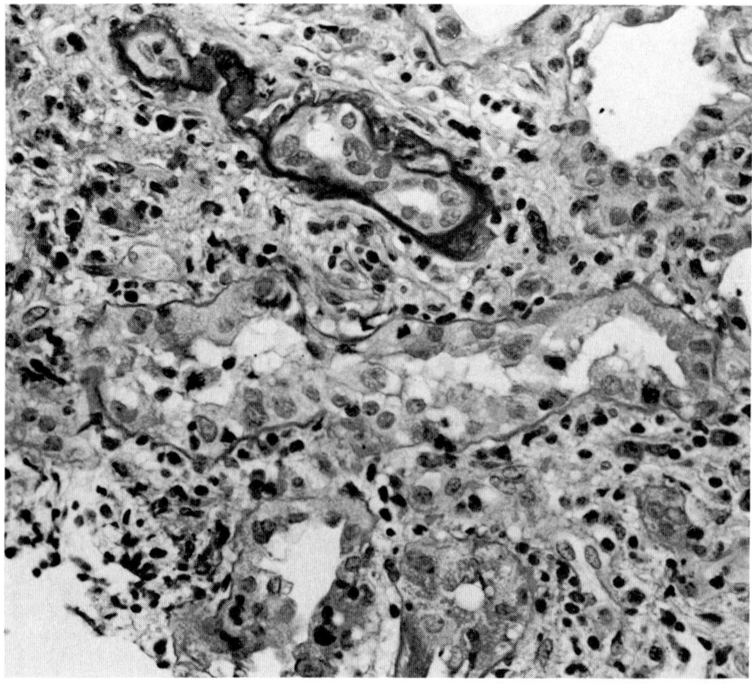

Figure 11–7. Acute rejection. Immunoperoxidase, anti-leu-7. The interstitial infiltrate is composed of many cells that express leu-7 antigen on their surface. (×250.)

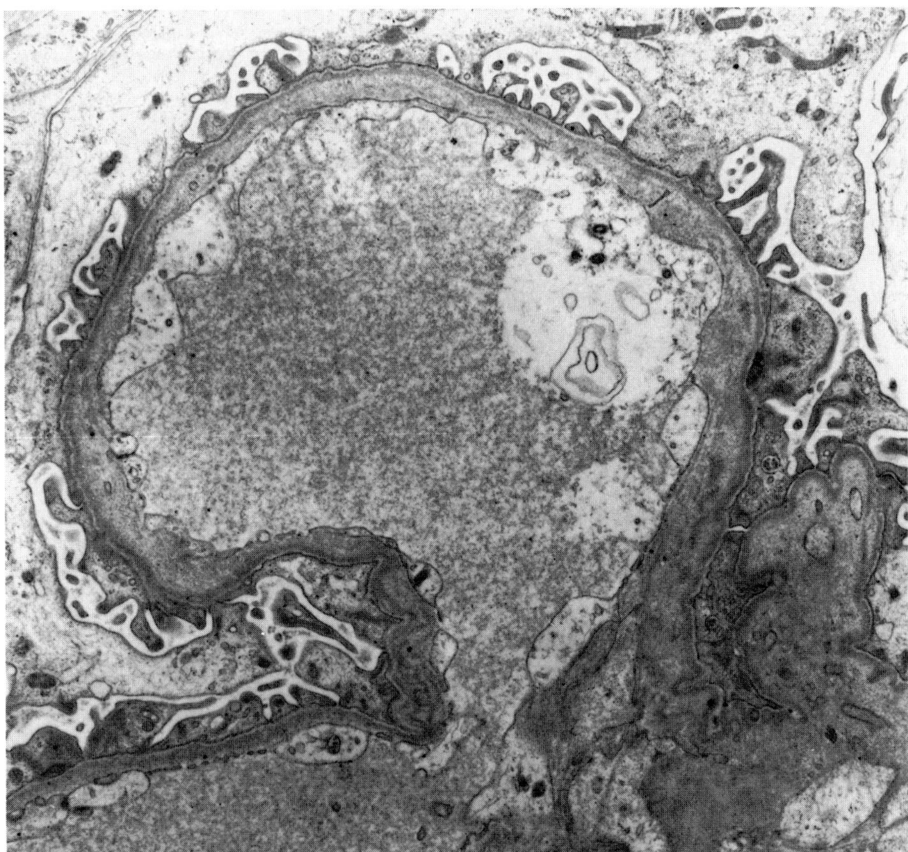

Figure 11–8. Acute rejection. The subendothelial space is diffusely widened and contains a loose, flocculent material. The endothelial cell cytoplasm is swollen. (×4200.)

INTERMEDIATE (MONTHS) REJECTION

In the intermediate period, the cause of graft failure can be traced to one of three processes: acute rejection (discussed earlier), cyclosporine A nephrotoxicity, or infection.

Cyclosporine A Nephrotoxicity

The use of cyclosporine A as an immunosuppressive agent in transplantation has resulted in increased overall cadaver graft survival. However, dose-related nephrotoxicity has limited its usefulness. This toxicity limits the dose of the drug that can be used and restricts its use to the period beginning 7 to 10 days after transplantation rather than in the immediate postoperative period. These restrictions are due to the accentuation of tubular and vascular injury induced by cyclosporine A.

Pathogenesis

The causes and consequences of cyclosporine A nephrotoxicity have been examined in animals. Administration of cyclosporine A to rats produced alterations in renal hemodynamics, including increased renal vascular resistance and decreased glomerular filtration rate. Similar changes have been observed in humans. Chronic administration results in decreased renal blood flow and changes that have been identified as being similar to ischemic alterations.

Histology

Light Microscopy

ACUTE TOXICITY

The early lesions of cyclosporine A toxicity appear to be due to tubular toxicity, leading to acute injury followed by necrosis. However, there may be an element of acute vascular injury as well, because some patients develop lesions that are comparable to those in the hemolytic-uremic syndrome as well as those in recipients of bone marrow transplants.

The tubular lesions consist of isometric vacuolation of the proximal tubular epithelial cells, tubular inclusion bodies, and microcalcification. It is not clear whether these changes represent a toxic response or are reflective of metabolism of the drug by these cells.

Chronic Lesions

The principal glomerular lesion appears to be ischemia. The glomerular basement membranes are wrinkled and contracted, revealing an overall decrease in surface area when examined by detailed morphometric studies. The lesions vary from modest wrinkling affecting occasional glomerular loops to severe sclerosing lesions with massive thickening of the glomerular basement membranes and collapse of the vascular loops. The glomeruli gradually lose their normal cellularity as they undergo ischemic atrophy. The sclerotic glomeruli are small, whereas the remaining patent glomeruli may undergo significant compensatory hypertrophy.

The interstitium always exhibits marked changes, with linear or striped zones of fibrosis and inflammatory infiltrate, which may coalesce to form broad bands of involvement. Tubular atrophy initially is patchy, but it progresses if the drug is not discontinued or the dosage reduced. The result may be marked and diffuse tubular atrophy, which initially preferentially involves the distal tubules and loops of Henle. These segments frequently contain casts and may form large "pseudo-thyroid" areas.

Conspicuous arteriolar and arterial lesions are seen in most cases. They are such a characteristic feature that they have come to be known as cyclosporine A-associated vasculopathy. The arterioles show subintimal and medial hyalinosis, a finding that is not considered to be reversible (Fig. 11–9). Therefore, this vascular lesion is thought to signal the presence of an irreversible course culminating in deteriorating renal function. Extensive eosinophilic deposits appear between the pericytes of the afferent arterioles, contributing to a gradual occlusive process. The deposits are associated with anisonucleosis of the pericytes and progressive atrophy of the media. The arterial lesion consists of fibrointimal thickening and elastic lamina duplication, comparable to that in hypertensive patients. This change is quite reminiscent of hyalin arteriolosclerosis associated with hypertension, although the hyalin deposits tend to have a more peripheral location and are

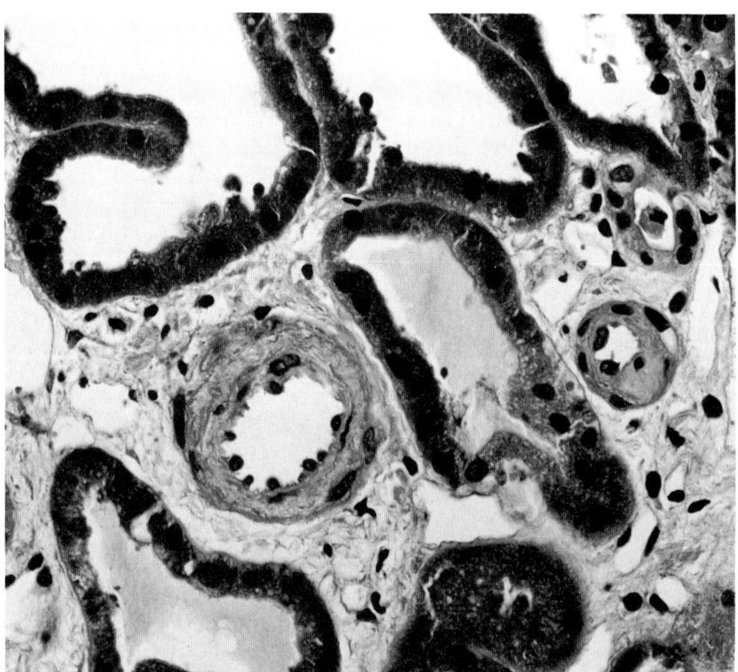

Figure 11–9. Cyclosporine A toxicity. The arterioles and small arteries show subintimal and medial hyalinosis. There is mild interstitial edema and tubular atrophy. (Masson's trichrome, ×250.)

usually circumferential as compared with the eccentric subendothelial nodules seen in hypertension or diabetes. The hyalin is often accompanied by vacuoles within smooth muscle cells and by narrowing of the vascular lumen by either fibrin thrombi or by mucoid intimal thickening. The changes are at times so severe as to resemble those in hemolytic uremic syndrome. These latter lesions may dissipate on cessation of the drug.

Immunofluorescence Microscopy

There are no specific deposits.

Electron Microscopy

In addition to the lesions characteristic of the ischemic process (i.e., wrinkling and thickening of the glomerular basement membranes), there is an accumulation of mesangial matrix in the non-ischemic glomeruli.

Prognosis

The long-term prognosis for patients with cyclosporine A-associated nephropathy is not well established. Some studies suggest that the lesions inevitably progress to end-stage renal failure. This outcome has most often been found in patients treated with high doses of the drug for prolonged periods. It is not clear which, if any, of the lesions revert to normal when the drug is withdrawn. It seems unlikely, however, that significant glomerulosclerosis, tubular atrophy, or vascular hyalinosis would be reversible.

Infectious Complications

Introduction and Patient Presentation

Long-term immunosuppressive therapy increases the risk of infectious complications. Infection in the allograft may result in decreased function. The most common infections to affect the graft are bacterial and viral, although any opportunistic organism that has invaded the donor may affect the transplant. Staphylococcal organisms are the most frequent bacteria to produce renal infections. In this case, abscesses usually occur as a result of hematogenous spread from another site, although ascending infection and pyelonephritis may be encountered. The most typical viruses are cytomegalovirus and herpesvirus. As in bacterial infections, the presence of these viruses in the graft usually represents dissemination from another site, usually the lungs.

Histology

Light Microscopy

The recognition of a viral infection by renal biopsy is difficult and requires a high degree of suspicion. Light microscopy may reveal typical nuclear inclusions. In cytomegalovirus, cytoplasmic inclusions and cytomegaly are seen (Fig. 11–10). These inclusions are typically observed in tubular epithelial cells, in glomerular podocytes, and occasionally in interstitial cells. Immunoperoxidase techniques using antisera against herpes or cytomegalovirus may aid in distinguishing between true inclusions and prominent nucleoli, which may be seen in regenerating tubular cells. Finally, when there are inclusions in cells comprising the inflammatory infiltrate, there is an increased likelihood of an infection as compared to that of simply a carrier state of latent viruses.

CHRONIC REJECTION

With increasing time after placement of the graft, the conditions likely to cause graft dysfunction include chronic cyclosporine nephrotoxicity (discussed earlier), chronic graft rejection, recurrence of the original disease, or de novo glomerulonephritis. The first two are manifest clinically by the insidious loss of renal function. The appearance of glomerular disease, whether recurrent or de novo, may be suspected by the development of proteinuria.

Introduction and Patient Presentation

The earliest morphologic alterations consistent with chronic rejection may become evident as soon as several months after transplantation.

Histology

Light Microscopy

The microscopic changes are first evident in the arteries and consist of striking intimal proliferation resulting in occlusion of arteries

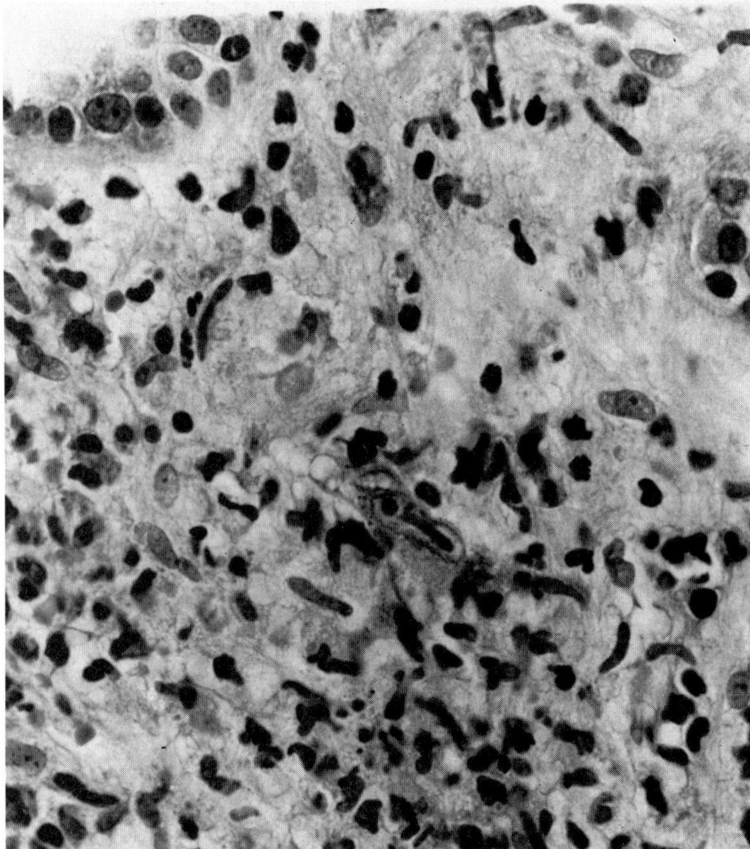

Figure 11–10. Cytomegalovirus inclusions. Large inclusions are found in nuclei and cytoplasm of tubular epithelial cells. (H&E, ×400.)

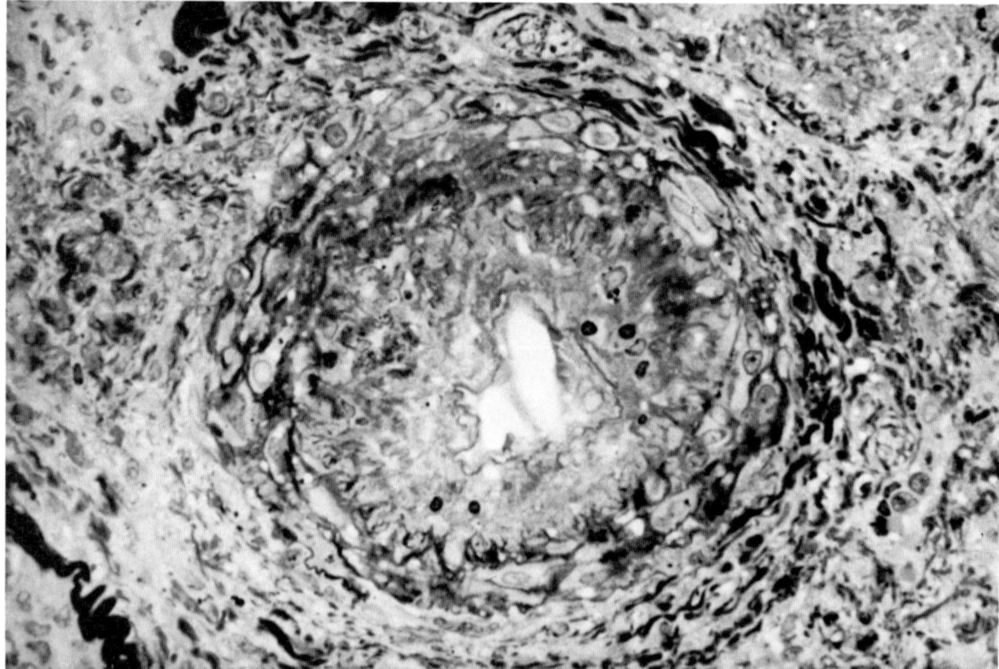

Figure 11–11. Chronic rejection. The arterial lumen is markedly reduced by intimal proliferation, increased extracellular matrix deposition, and duplication of the internal elastic lamellae. The media is also scarred, and the elastic laminae are disorganized. (PASM, ×300.)

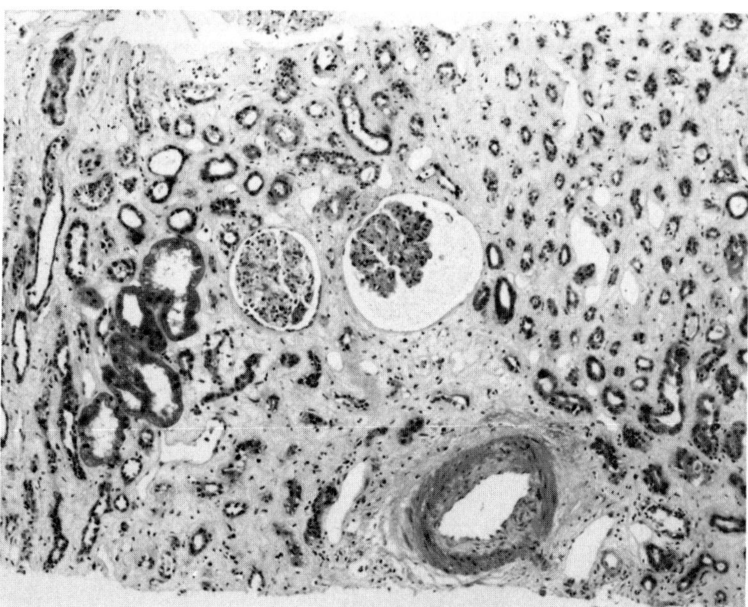

Figure 11–12. Chronic rejection. There is diffuse interstitial fibrosis, tubular atrophy, and glomerular ischemia. The vascular lesions are also widespread. (Masson's trichrome, ×100.)

and arterioles (Fig. 11–11). This is followed by diffuse interstitial fibrosis (Fig. 11–12). The glomerular changes are secondary to the vascular disease and include collapse of vascular loops followed by obsolescence. These vascular changes are diffuse rather than patchy, as is the case with cyclosporine A nephrotoxicity. They also differ in that all sizes of vessels are involved, whereas in cyclosporine A toxicity, the small blood vessels are most severely affected. An acute rejection episode may be superimposed on a kidney that is the site of a chronic rejection process, years after transplantation.

RECURRENCE OF THE ORIGINAL DISEASE

Many types of glomerulonephritis may recur in a transplanted kidney. Their histopathologic appearance and clinical presentations are identical to the original disease. Therefore, the reader is referred to the descriptions of these lesions in previous chapters. In some cases, recurrent disease results in graft loss, but in most instances, it results in neither loss of the graft nor graft dysfunction.

However, there are some diseases in which recurrence regularly results in graft dysfunction and even graft loss. These include the hemolytic-uremic syndrome, focal and segmental glomerulosclerosis with hyalinosis, and diabetic nephropathy. The lesions of the hemolytic-uremic syndrome may recur within months of the graft placement and inevitably lead to graft failure. These lesions must be differentiated from cyclosporine A nephrotoxicity.

It takes longer for focal glomerulosclerosis to recur in the graft. The recurrence rate of the disease is 40%, and graft loss results in 25% of patients. Those who have experienced a recurrence of this lesion in one graft are at very high risk for recurrence in a subsequent graft.

Diabetic nephropathy has been reported to recur within 5 to 10 years after graft placement. This interval may be shorter than the time required for the development of glomerulosclerosis in the native kidneys of diabetic patients.

Some types of histologic glomerular lesions may develop in the graft but result in only mild evidence of renal disease. This group includes membranoproliferative glomerulonephritis (types I and II) and IgA nephropathy. Type I membranoproliferative glomerulonephritis recurs in 35% of patients but results in graft loss in only 10% of those affected. On the other hand, type II membranoproliferative glomerulonephritis (dense deposit disease) recurs in as many as 88% of patients, with laboratory evidence of recurrence in 24% and graft loss in 10%. IgA nephropathy recurs frequently in the allograft but rarely causes graft loss.

It has generally been considered that recurrence of anti-glomerular basement membrane disease and systemic lupus erythematosus nephritis can be avoided by waiting for a sufficient interval for the original disease to dissipate. There have been few long-term studies to document this point, however.

DE NOVO DISEASE

Any renal disease may arise de novo in a renal transplant. Diabetic nephropathy has been reported 7 years after diabetes mellitus had developed during the post-transplant period.

Membranous glomerulonephritis is the most common de novo glomerular lesion. The reasons for this are not clear. Finally, patients who have hereditary nephritis and who have received transplants develop circulating anti-glomerular basement antibodies, but they do not develop renal disease. The presence of anti-glomerular basement membrane disease in this setting suggests that the abnormalities of the glomerular basement membrane in hereditary nephritis result from missing components that serve as antigens that are recognized as foreign by the graft host and the formation of antibodies to these components. It has been shown that these antibodies are similar, if not identical, to those in Goodpasture's disease.

NEW TECHNIQUES IN THE ANALYSIS OF TRANSPLANT BIOPSIES

Needle biopsy of the graft has been the standard method for determining the presence and type of pathologic process affecting an allograft. Recently developed techniques or new applications of older methods have been used in the assessment of renal tissue in an attempt to further the understanding of the immune mechanisms underlying rejection and the pathogenesis of cyclosporine nephrotoxicity. These include the application of immunoperoxidase techniques to the identification of lymphocyte subpopulations. As noted earlier, the analysis of markers for lymphocyte subpopulations has not yet helped to establish the diagnosis of rejection, but the method has considerable potential as our understanding of the rejection process improves. For instance, it may be possible to recognize different types of rejection, allowing the development of individually tailored anti-rejection therapy. Finally, analysis of newly expressed HLA class II antigens may help distinguish between rejection and cyclosporine A nephrotoxicity, because expression of this marker is an indication of an immunologic response rather than a toxic injury. The immunoperoxidase technique may also be used to identify viral antigens in the biopsy specimen.

Several reports have discussed the use of needle aspirations of the graft in the assessment of potential rejection episodes. The types of inflammatory cells are counted and compared with simultaneous counts from peripheral blood. The proportions of the types of cells are used to distinguish between rejection and nephrotoxicity. In the former case, the aspirate contains a predominance of lymphocytes; in the latter case, the aspirate more closely resembles the population in the circulation. The advantages of this technique are that it is less traumatic and less costly than a needle biopsy and that results are available within hours. The disadvantages are that it does not allow analysis of renal structure, thus several common processes such as recurrence of diseases and certain types of viral infections will not be recognized.

SELECTED READINGS

1. Berger J, Yaneva H, Nabarra B, et al: Recurrence of mesangial deposition of IgA after renal transplantation. Kidney Int 7:232, 1975.
2. Boucher A, Droz D, Adafer E, et al: Characterization of mononuclear cell subsets in renal cellular interstitial infiltrates. Kidney Int 29:1043, 1986.
3. Myers BD, Ross J, Newton L, et al: Cyclosporin-associated chronic nephropathy. N Engl J Med 311:699, 1984.
4. Pirani CL, Hardy MA: Hyperacute renal allograft rejection. *In* Remuzzi G, Rossi EC (eds): Hemostasis and the Kidney. Butterworths, Boston, 1989, pp 281–289.
5. Solez K, McGraw DJ, Beschorner WE, et al: Reflections on the use of renal biopsy as the gold standard in distinguishing transplant rejection from cyclosporine nephrotoxicity. Transplant Proc 17:123, 1985.
6. Thiel G, Mihatsch M, Landmann J, et al: Is cyclosporin-A induced nephrotoxicity in recipients of renal allografts progressive? Transplant Proc 17:169, 1985.
7. Toledo-Pereyra LH: Kidney Transplantation. FA Davis, Philadelphia, 1988.

Chapter

12

RENAL LESIONS IN HYPERTENSION

The definition of hypertension established by the World Health Organization is the presence of blood pressure exceeding 140/90 mm Hg.

Hypertension affects approximately 28% of the people in the United States. However, this is an average figure and does not take into account the large variations between different ages and races. For instance, the incidence of hypertension in blacks is 33%. The differences between blacks and non-blacks become even more striking if one considers the risk of developing end-stage hypertensive renal disease. The frequency with which hypertensive patients develop renal disease is unknown. The answer to this important question requires further investigation. It would seem very likely that only a fraction of those with hypertension will develop end-stage renal disease.

Finally, renal biopsies are not a standard part of the work-up of a hypertensive patient, thus a special study would have to be designed to address the question of the incidence and type of renal lesions that precede the development of end-stage renal disease.

The renal lesions in hypertension can be categorized as shown in Table 12–1.

No cause can be discerned in 95% of this group. These patients are thus said to have essential, or idiopathic, hypertension. This condition is generally associated with a slow, progressive loss of nephrons and is manifest morphologically by benign nephrosclerosis. In 1 to 7% of patients with benign hypertension there is a sudden and unexplained progression to more severe levels of hypertension, the malignant phase. This rapid evolution of hypertension and the renal damage it causes, so-called malignant nephrosclerosis, often produce a clinical picture of acute renal failure. Definable causes of hypertension include atherosclerosis of the renal vessels, fibromuscular dysplasia, various endocrinopathies, and chronic renal disease. The clinical presentation of these conditions, known as secondary hypertension, is variable. An additional form of renal vascular disease often accompanied by acute decline in renal function is atheroembolic renal disease.

A progressive loss of nephrons is thought to occur with aging even when hypertension is absent. This change is marked histologically by the development of small, wrinkled glomeruli that become obsolescent and by zones of tubular atrophy and interstitial fibrosis, which are found in a linear distribution radiating from the corticomedullary junction to the cortex. These changes affect the superficial cortical nephrons most severely, causing the capsule to adhere to the kidney. The interlobular arteries show loss

Table 12–1. Causes of Renal Lesions in Hypertension

Cause	% of Total
Idiopathic	
Benign nephrosclerosis	90
Malignant nephrosclerosis	5
Known cause	5
Renal artery stenosis	
Chronic renal disease	
Fibromuscular dysplasia	
Endocrinopathies	
Atheroembolic embolism	

of smooth muscle cells and fibrous intimal thickening. A direct correlation is present between advancing age and both glomerulosclerosis and degree of intimal thickening of the interlobular arteries. These changes appear to be independent of the blood pressure.

As a consequence of the loss of nephrons, renal function also declines continuously. Renal blood flow decreases at a rate of approximately 10% for each decade beginning at age 40 years. Glomerular filtration rate also diminishes but at a slower pace. Recent studies have questioned whether the progressive decline in renal function, which is found in the population as a whole, accurately reflects that in individual patients. It is now being considered that there are two subsets within the aging population. One has vascular disease and develops more rapid loss of nephrons, and another maintains their renal function until an advanced age. This is now a point of active investigation.

BENIGN NEPHROSCLEROSIS

Benign hypertension, which is associated with the changes known as benign nephrosclerosis in the kidneys, is an insidious disease usually producing no symptoms. Hypertension is defined as blood pressure greater than 140/90 mm Hg. It usually begins before the age of 50 and is more common in women than in men and in blacks than in people of other races. The factor or factors responsible for the initiation of essential hypertension are unknown. Several mechanisms are believed to play a part. These include modifications of the renin-angiotensin system, an increase in blood volume, abnormalities in mineralocorticoids, and some type of dysregulation of the autonomic nervous system.

Patient Presentation

In the early stages of benign nephrosclerosis, there is no apparent reduction in renal function. Examination of the urinary sediment may reveal occasional hyalin and fine granular casts and, rarely, red blood cells. Small amounts of protein may be present in the urine. The earliest detectable abnormality of renal function is a decrease in the renal plasma flow. A reduction in the glomerular filtration rate occurs later. Progression of the renal injury eventually results in a slowly rising serum creatinine level, and this may be the factor that brings the patient to medical attention. As noted in Chapter 1, elevation of the serum creatinine level may not occur until the glomerular filtration rate has fallen to less than 50% of normal and is thus not a good screening tool to evaluate renal damage.

Histology

Light Microscopy

Many glomeruli are normal, especially those at a distance from the capsule. Others show ischemic changes characterized by collapse of peripheral capillary loops, a decrease in overall size, and thickening of the basement membrane of Bowman's capsule. These changes tend to occur in linear sclerotic zones characterized by interstitial fibrosis and tubular atrophy. The glomeruli within the fibrotic areas appear to be clustered together because of the tubular atrophy. Periodic acid-Schiff (PAS) or silver stains demonstrate the "wrinkling" of the glomerular basement membranes and decrease in glomerular size (Figs. 12–1 and 12–2). These changes are most evident near the mesangial regions and progressively involve the rest of the tuft. There is a progressive disappearance of nu-

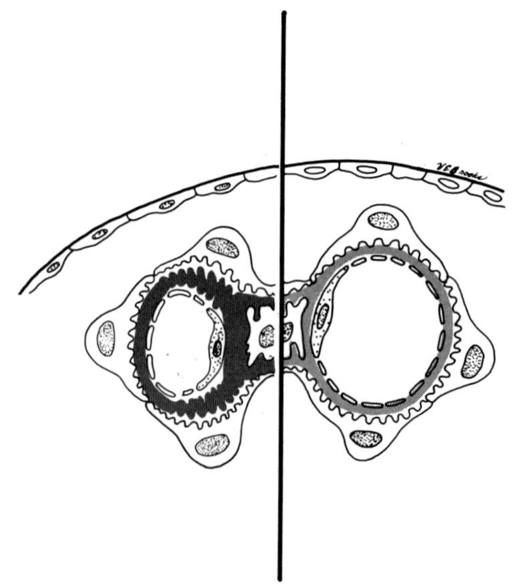

Figure 12–1. Diagram of an ischemic glomerulus. The major change is wrinkling and thickening of the glomerular basement membranes, particularly near the mesangium.

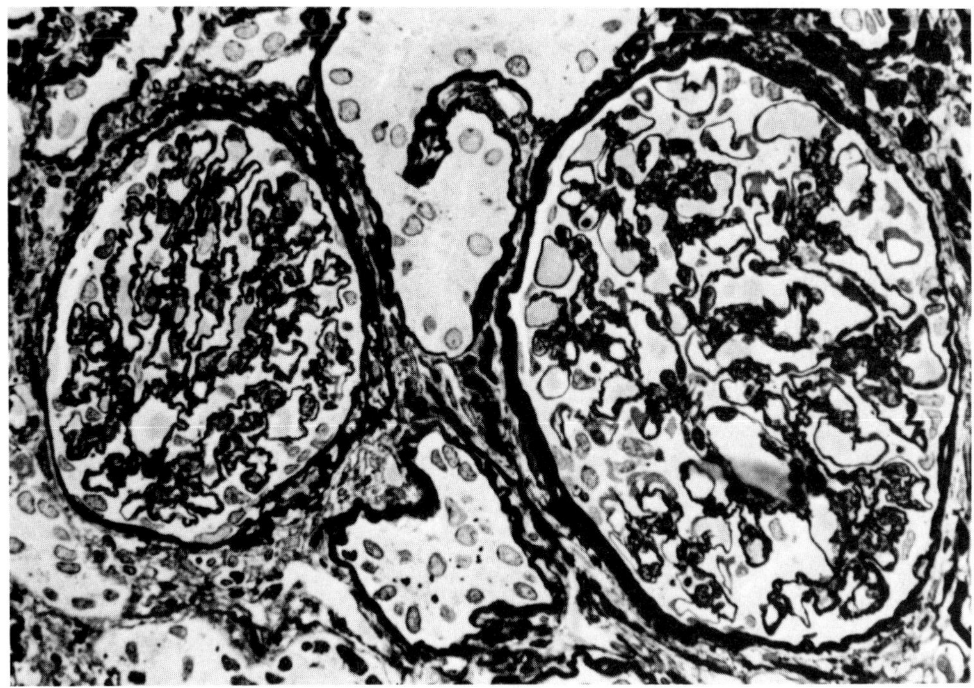

Figure 12–2. The interstitial fibrosis and tubular atrophy with basement thickening attest to the chronicity of the process. The basement membranes of the glomerulus on the right are most wrinkled near the mesangial regions. The wrinkling in the glomerulus on the left extends throughout the entire structure. The basement membrane of Bowman's capsule is thickened in both, but is partially interrupted in the glomerulus on the left. (PASM, ×300.)

clei as the tuft shrinks and becomes obsolescent. Bowman's space fills with extracellular matrix, best seen on trichrome stain. The degree of glomerulosclerosis correlates with the severity of generalized atherosclerosis and with increased intrarenal vascular disease.

Tubular atrophy characterized by flattening of epithelial cells and thickened basement membranes occurs both near affected glomeruli and in areas near normal-appearing glomeruli. These data have been taken as evidence that the tubular epithelia have an increased susceptibility to ischemia.

Interstitial fibrosis is present in a patchy distribution and is frequently accompanied by an inflammatory infiltrate composed of small lymphocytes. The fibrosis surrounds and encompasses atrophic tubules. Hyalin casts are found within the lumen of the atrophied tubules. These areas of atrophied tubules filled with casts superficially resemble thyroid tissue, and the process has been called pseudo-thyroid change. The zones of atrophy vary in size depending on the number of nephrons supplied by the affected vessel and alternate with patches of hypertrophied tubules (Figs. 12–3 and 12–4). This irregularity in the distribution of tubulo-interstitial lesions is characteristic of chronic ischemic lesions.

The vessels present in renal biopsy specimens include the interlobular arteries and afferent and efferent arterioles. The interlobular arteries show intimal thickening with consequent reduction of the lumen (Figs. 12–5 and 12–6). The intimal thickening is frequently accompanied by multilayering (so-called reduplication) of the internal elastic lamina. There are often no changes in the media. The arterioles and small arteries develop hyalin arteriolosclerosis, characterized by the accumulation of a homogeneous, eosinophilic material within the vessel wall often associated with loss of smooth muscle cells (Fig. 12–7). The hyalin contains multiple plasma components, suggesting an abnormality in the permeability of the vascular wall, which may include an element of endothelial injury. Hyalin arteriosclerosis also results in narrowing of the lumen and loss of normal compliance of these resistance vessels. The changes in the arterioles show a positive correlation with generalized atherosclerosis, mean blood pressure, and the occurrence of cardiovascular complications.

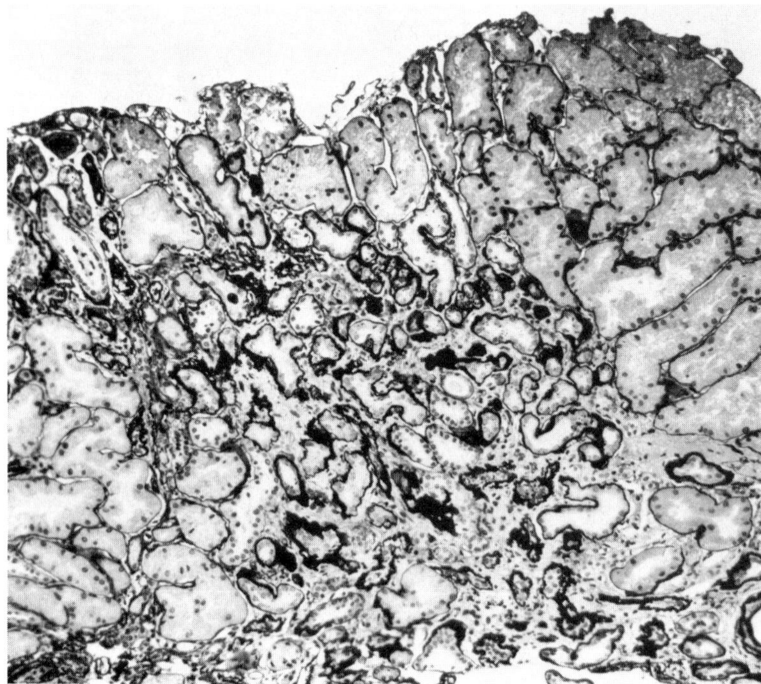

Figure 12–3. Areas of tubular atrophy and interstitial fibrosis (center) alternate with unaffected zones. The tubular basement membranes are thickened around the atrophic tubules. (PASM, ×75.)

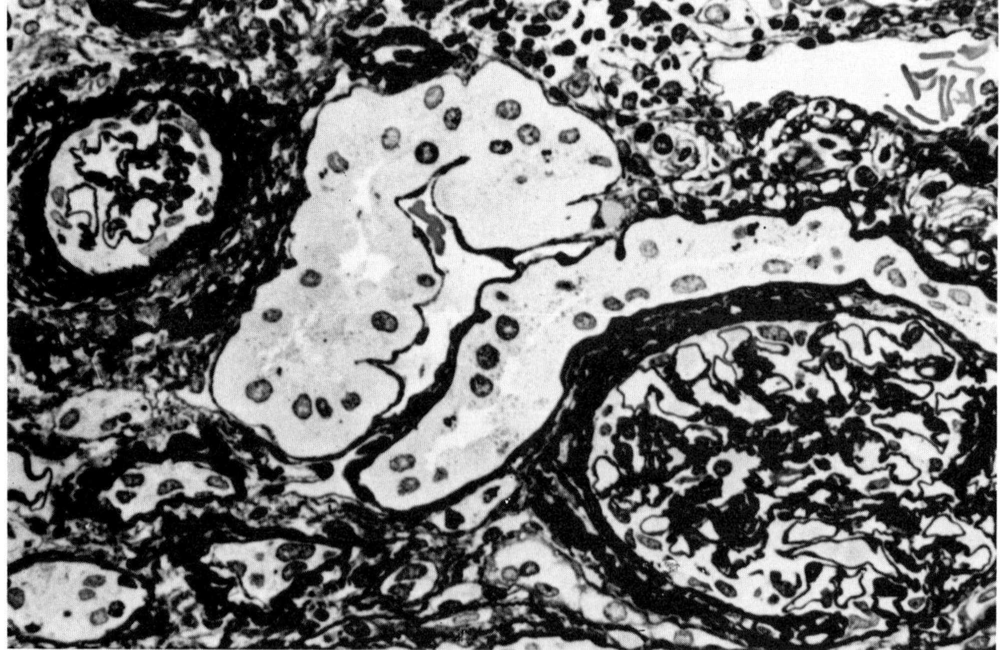

Figure 12–4. The basement membranes of all segments of the nephron are thickened. The interstitium is infiltrated with inflammatory cells, and there is an increase in the amount of interstitial matrix. (PASM, ×300.)

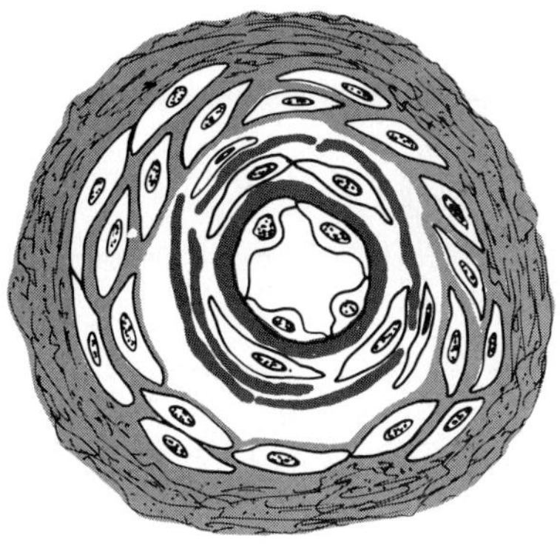

Figure 12–5. Diagram of a small artery with multilayering of the internal elastic lamina and its associated connective tissue.

Immunofluorescence Microscopy

The changes by immunofluorescence microscopy include staining of the hyalin deposits by C3 and very commonly IgM. This pattern is nonspecific and may be seen in aging kidneys as well as in a number of other conditions associated with hyalin deposits and/or sclerosis. There is usually no staining of glomeruli, although scarred glomeruli may contain deposits of C3 and IgM. C1q codistributes with C3, in most instances.

Electron Microscopy

Electron microscopic examination confirms collapse of the capillary loops with extensive wrinkling and thickening of glomerular basement membranes. The wrinkling is most marked near the mesangial regions, often giving the false impression of mesangial sclerosis. However, the mesangial matrix is normal in amount. The glomerulus has a relatively hypocellular appearance.

Hyalin arteriolosclerosis is manifest by the appearance of homogeneous material within the arterial wall, often replacing smooth muscle cells (Figs. 12–8 and 12–9).

Prognosis

Most patients with even mild hypertension are now treated, so it is necessary to examine reports from the 1950s to appreciate the natural history of untreated hypertension. Most patients present before the age of 50 and do not have significant symptoms for approximately 15 years. During the succeeding 5 years, they develop cardiovascular disease, including involvement of the heart, brain, and kidney. However, there is extreme variability between patients.

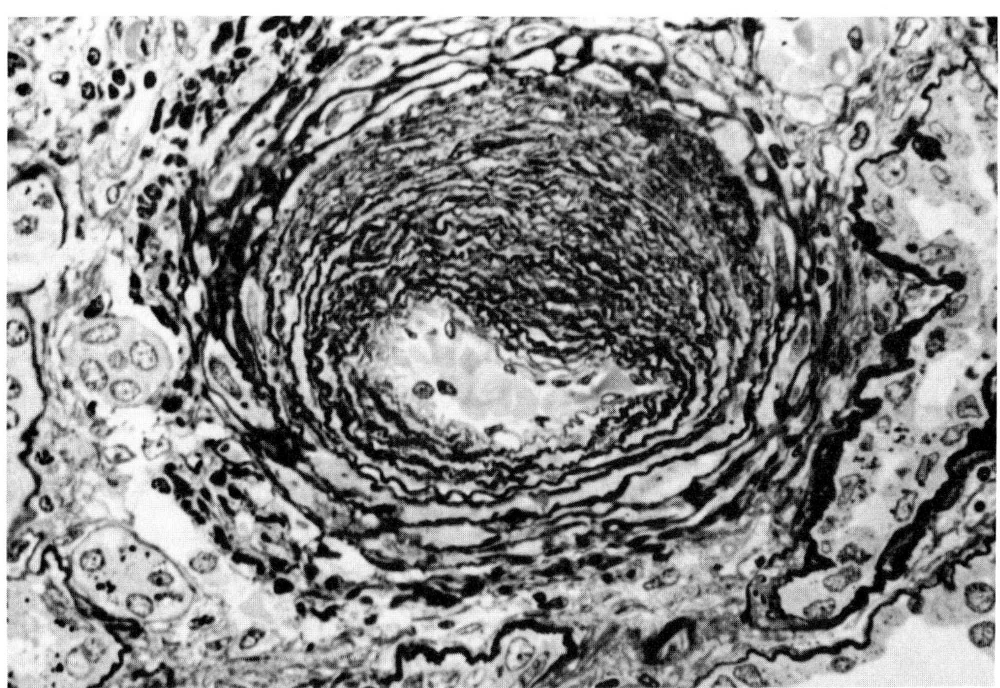

Figure 12–6. The multiple lamellae in the subintima are visible in this silver-stained preparation. (PASM, ×300.)

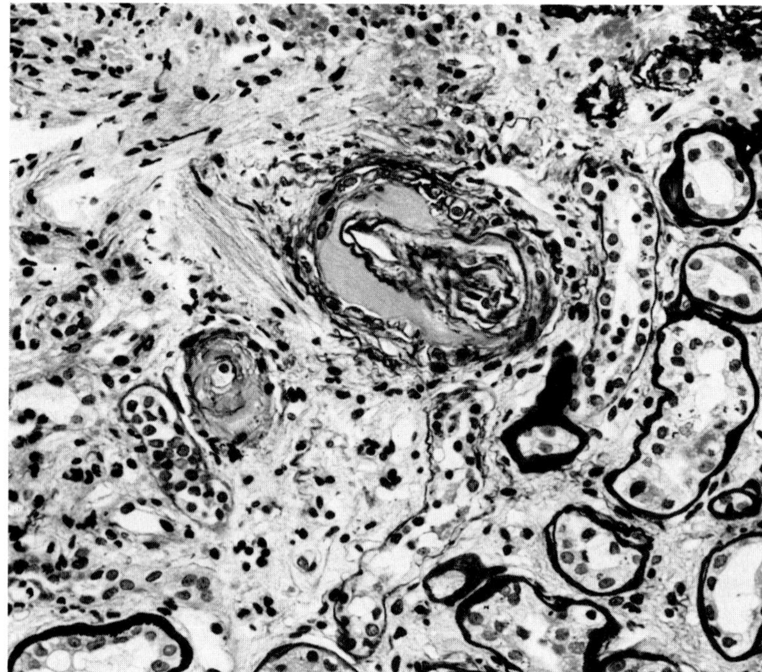

Figure 12–7. Hyalin deposits are present in the subintima of the small artery (right) and throughout the wall of the adjacent arteriole (left). (PASM, ×300.)

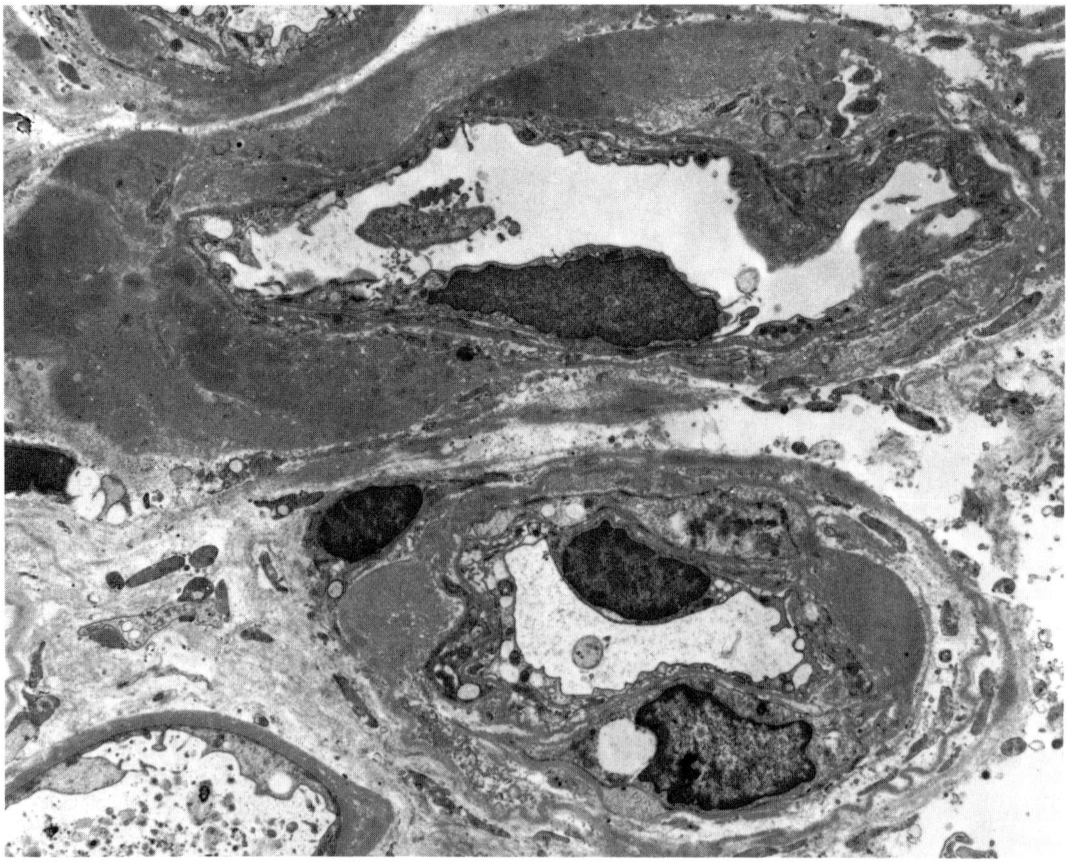

Figure 12–8. The areas between the intima and the surrounding smooth muscle layer contain irregular, large deposits of hyalin. The smooth muscle cells are absent in the regions of the hyalin deposits. (×1000.)

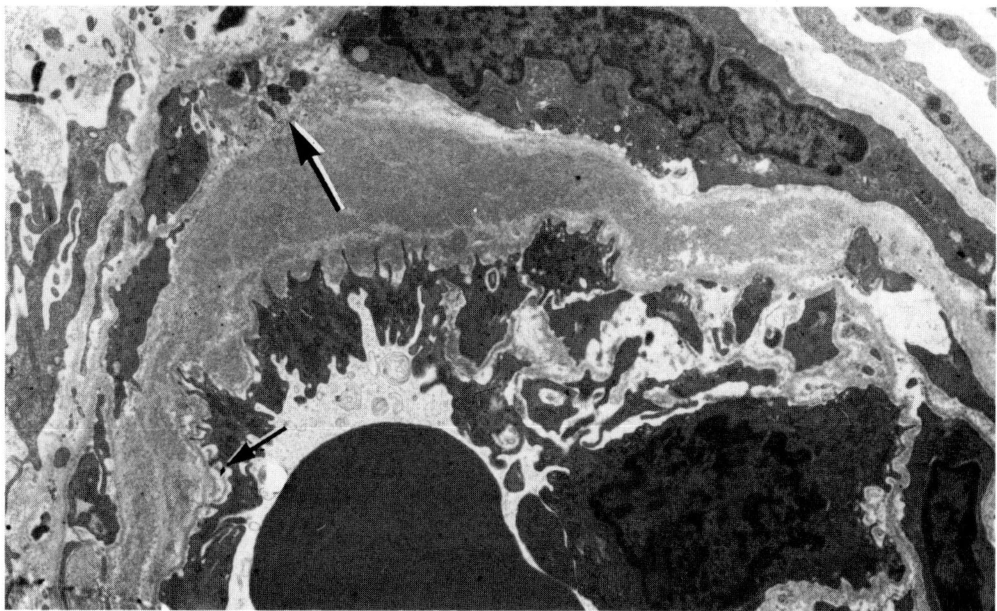

Figure 12–9. The basement membrane of the smooth muscle cells of the media is duplicated near the hyalin deposits (thin arrow). The hyalin has a granular appearance in some areas (heavy arrow), and in others it is more homogeneous. (×2500.)

The Framingham study has shown that both stroke and cardiovascular disease are more common in patients with hypertension. Recent studies indicate that treatment of patients with even very mild elevations of blood pressure results in decreased morbidity and mortality from stroke and cardiovascular diseases. The incidence of renal disease does not appear to have decreased in a like manner, however.

MALIGNANT NEPHROSCLEROSIS

Malignant hypertension most often occurs in patients who have a previous history of benign essential hypertension. This complication occurs in 1 to 7% of patients with essential hypertension. Malignant hypertension is defined as a diastolic blood pressure that is persistently greater than 120 mm Hg and eye changes consisting of papilledema with retinal hemorrhages and exudates. Males are affected more frequently than females, and the highest frequency is in blacks. Malignant nephrosclerosis may also be seen in various other diseases that affect the kidneys, including glomerulonephritis, pyelonephritis, vasculitis, and scleroderma.

Patient Presentation

The presenting symptoms include headache, dizziness, weight loss, and difficulties with vision. The documentation of an extreme elevation of blood pressure, in combination with the typical funduscopic alterations, confirms the diagnosis. Examination of the urine reveals either gross or microscopic hematuria and proteinuria, which may attain nephrotic levels. The peripheral blood smear may contain the findings of microangiopathic hemolytic anemia, including fragmented red blood cells and a reduction in platelets. Renal function may appear to be normal at the onset, but it rapidly declines.

Histology

Light Microscopy

The changes of malignant nephrosclerosis are frequently superimposed on those of preexisting benign nephrosclerosis. A discussion of the latter changes is found in the preceding section.

The glomerular lesions are characterized by ischemic alterations, hemorrhage, thrombosis, and fibrinoid necrosis (Fig. 12–10). Some glomeruli are small, with wrinkled and thickened glomerular basement membranes and an apparent decrease in the number of cells, whereas others are unaffected. The most striking alteration is segmental fibrinoid necrosis, affecting 5 to 20% of glomeruli. Necrosis, most easily identified using the PAS-methenamine silver stain, is recognized as a mass of fibrinoid material that has an intense pink color and is admixed with red blood cells. Destruction of the glomerular basement membrane as well as loss of definition of the local tuft architecture may also be present. Crescents are sometimes observed, particularly in association with the necrotic foci.

The changes are an extension of those in benign nephrosclerosis, although they are more extensive and severe. Rarely, small infarcts may occur as a result of arterial occlusion. Interstitial edema is commonly present.

The most characteristic vascular change is fibrinoid necrosis involving the small interlobular arteries and the arterioles (Fig. 12–11). As in the glomeruli, necrosis is recognized by the presence of a bright pink-staining, granular material within the wall of the vessel, the loss of nuclear detail, and thrombi in the lumen. Fibrin may be detected by special stains. Fragmented red blood cells are often present in the thrombi. Interlobular arteries of all sizes show intimal narrowing of three distinct patterns. The first is the so-called onionskin change, which consists of concentric layers of proliferating intimal cells (Fig. 12–12). The second, mucinous change, is characterized by expansion of the intima by an extracellular material that binds alcian blue (Fig. 12–13). There is an associated multilayering of basement membrane material in the subintimal space. The third, fibrous intimal thickening, is typical of the changes in benign nephrosclerosis, although the extent of luminal narrowing may be more severe in malignant hypertension (see Fig. 12–6). The fibrous intimal substance consists of hyalin material, multiple layers of basement membrane, and banded collagen.

Immunofluorescence Microscopy

The only difference between malignant and benign nephrosclerosis is the addition of staining for fibrinogen in areas of fibrinoid necrosis in glomeruli and blood vessels.

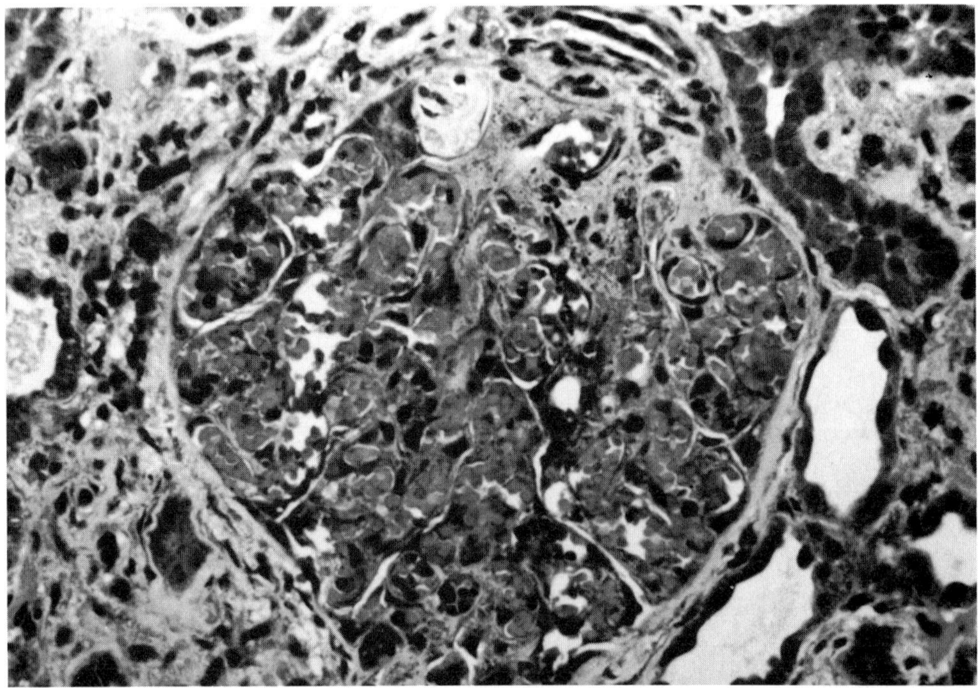

Figure 12–10. The loops are filled with red blood cells, plasma protein precipitates, and degenerating cells. These are the histologic features of fibrinoid necrosis. (H&E, ×300.)

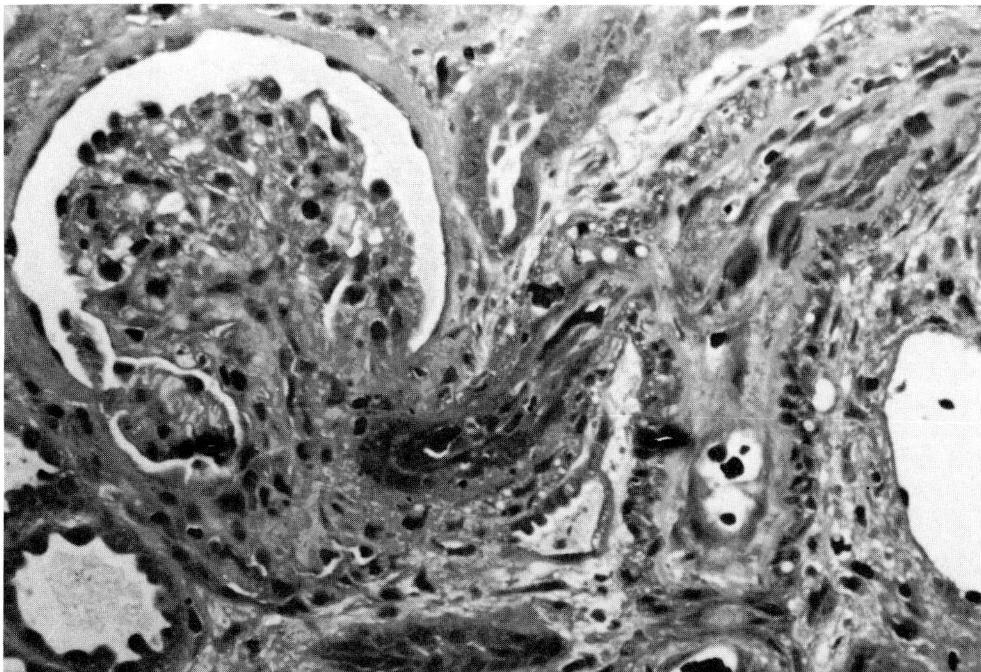

Figure 12–11. The afferent arteriole is thrombosed at the base of the glomerulus, and there is necrosis of the wall near the thrombus. The glomerulus distal to the thrombus is collapsed. The immediately proximal blood vessel is partially occluded by a thrombus. (H&E, ×300.)

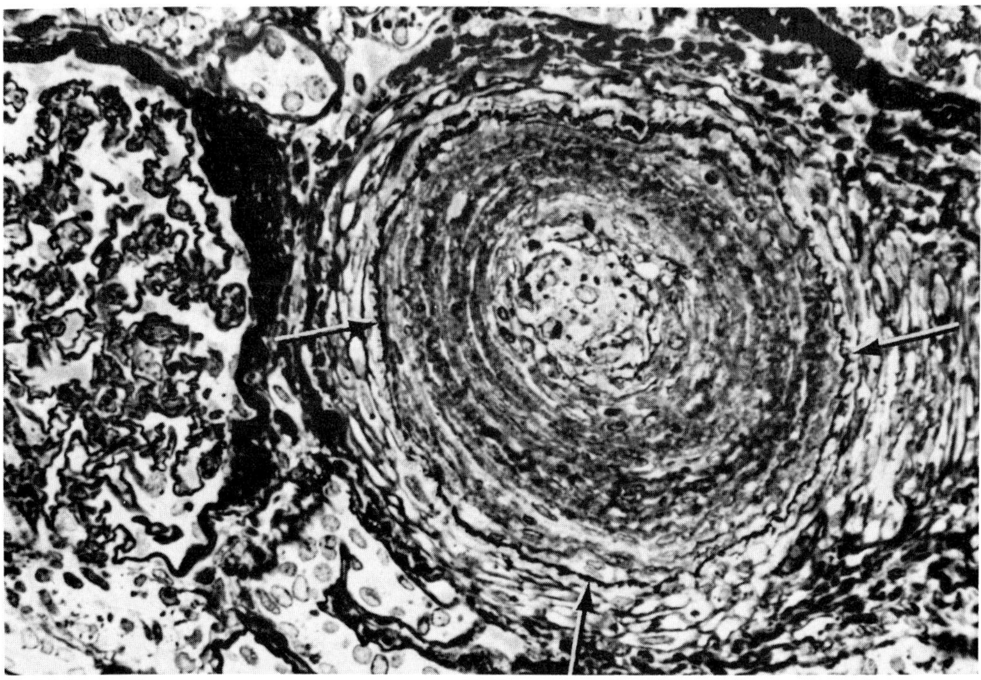

Figure 12–12. The internal elastic lamina (arrows) encircles a mass of concentrically arranged lamellae of extracellular matrix in which are enmeshed a small number of cells. The adjacent glomerulus has thickened and wrinkled basement membranes. (PASM, ×300.)

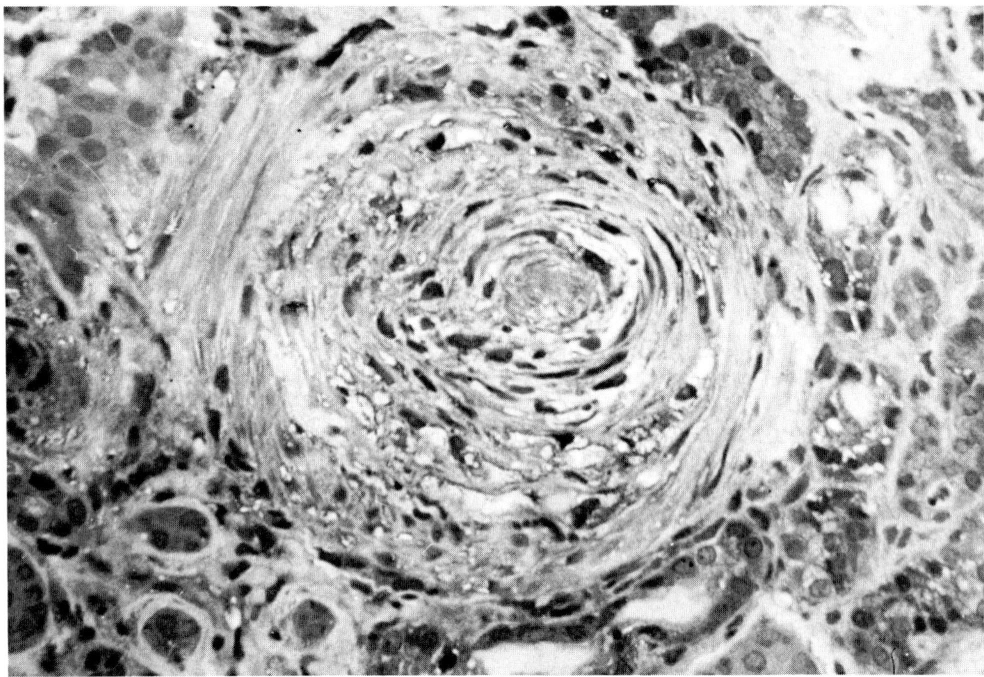

Figure 12–13. The medial smooth muscle cells appear intact. The intima is filled with concentric layers of elongated cells, some of which have many cytoplasmic vacuoles. The extracellular matrix between the intimal cells has a homogeneous mucoid appearance. (H&E, ×300.)

Electron Microscopy

The glomeruli show extreme wrinkling and thickening of glomerular basement membranes. In addition, there is subendothelial widening, often containing a granular or flocculent material. Fibrin tactoids may on occasion be identified in this space. Loss of the normal architecture of the basement membranes and mesangial matrix may be seen in areas of large fibrin deposits. Platelets and fragmented red blood cells are also frequently present. Endothelial cells show swelling and disruption and occasionally may be absent. Epithelial cells manifest focal effacement but are otherwise unremarkable. Mesangial cells are rarely interposed in the subendothelial space.

The vessels show endothelial swelling and multilamination of the basement membranes. The cells in the intimal onionskin lesions represent modified smooth muscle cells. The lucent areas contain extracellular matrix, including proteoglycans. The cells and the extracellular matrix of the media may be disrupted in the areas of fibrinoid necrosis. There usually are few changes in the media of larger arteries.

Prognosis

Before the development of effective antihypertensive agents, 90% of patients with malignant hypertension died within 1 year after the diagnosis was established. The most common cause of death was acute renal failure. This grim outlook has dramatically changed, since pharmaceutical agents are now available to control the blood pressure in most patients. Patient survival at 5 years is now 90%, and renal function remains adequate in 40% at this time.

SECONDARY HYPERTENSION

An underlying cause of hypertension may be defined in approximately 10% of patients. The two most common causes are renal artery stenosis due to arteriosclerosis, and renal artery dysplasia. A 70% reduction in the lumen is required before there is sufficient diminution in renal blood flow to lead to hypertension.

Several endocrine disorders may cause hypertension. The most common are Cushing's syndrome, pheochromocytoma, primary aldosteronism, thyrotoxicosis, hyperparathyroidism, and acromegaly. Administration of steroids may also cause hypertension.

Hypertension may occur in patients with chronic renal failure without regard to the initial cause of the renal disease.

Patient Presentation

The presentation depends, in large part, on the underlying cause. Certain features suggest a particular etiology. For instance, renal artery stenosis secondary to arteriosclerosis is the most common lesion in young white patients who develop the sudden onset of malignant hypertension or an unexpected acceleration of benign hypertension. Renal artery dysplasia is most common in young women.

The criteria for establishing a clinical diagnosis of renovascular hypertension include increased peripheral plasma renin activity, the presence of angiotensin II-dependent hypertension (good response to angiotensin-converting enzyme inhibitor), contralateral suppression of renal vein renin, and anatomic confirmation.

Histology

Light Microscopy

The appearance of the glomeruli depends on the type of renal vascular disease being considered. In the case of renal artery stenosis, the glomeruli distal to the stenotic vessel remain relatively well preserved, whereas the tubules are uniformly smaller and lined by a simple cuboidal epithelium, lacking brush borders and other aspects of normal tubules. As a consequence of the loss of tubular mass, the glomeruli appear to be more closely approximated than normal. The contralateral kidney may show changes of benign or malignant hypertension, depending on the blood pressure.

The glomeruli in patients with hypertension secondary to endocrine disorders have no special features other than those related to the degree of hypertension present.

The glomeruli of hypertensive patients with chronic glomerulonephritis or other primary glomerular diseases generally reflect the underlying disease process.

Diffuse, uniform tubular atrophy is accompanied by diffuse interstitial fibrosis in the kidneys distal to renal artery stenosis. The changes in the other types of secondary hypertension resemble those in benign nephrosclerosis.

The blood vessels in the kidneys distal to the stenotic renal artery may show fibrous intimal thickening, but unless there had been preexisting hypertension, the changes are likely to be minor. On the other hand, the blood vessels in the contralateral kidney show changes reflective of the blood pressure.

Immunofluorescence and Electron Microscopy

The morphology is identical to that described for benign and malignant nephrosclerosis and depends on the blood pressure.

Prognosis

The course and prognosis depend on the nature of the lesion causing the hypertension, its response to treatment, and the amount and degree of renal disease induced by the hypertension. For example, in a patient with renal artery stenosis, if renal ischemic atrophy is advanced, restoration of blood flow to the affected kidney by angioplasty will not result in significant return of function. On the other hand, if the renal changes are mild on both the affected and unaffected sides, reestablishment of blood flow to normal levels will result in a return to normal renal function and blood pressure.

RENAL ATHEROEMBOLIC DISEASE

Embolization of material from aortic atherosclerotic plaques can cause either acute renal failure, if the event is massive, or a slowly progressive loss in renal function, if the material is being dislodged from the plaques at a continuous but slow pace.

The potential for atherosclerotic plaques to embolize to the kidneys was not recognized until 1945, and the fact that this event might lead to significant renal functional impairment followed nearly 15 years later. Showers of plaque emboli may occur without a precipitating event but more commonly appear as a complication of an intra-arterial procedure such as angiography or vascular surgery. The frequency of this complication ranges from 1 to 5% in these procedures.

Patient Presentation

Atheromatous emboli to the kidneys occur most frequently in elderly patients and increase in incidence with age. Coexistent hypertension is also a precipitating factor. This diagnosis should be entertained in any elderly patient with acute renal failure of unknown origin, especially in the presence of other signs of advanced atherosclerosis.

Although not a common accompaniment, embolization may be suspected by the appearance of multiorgan involvement including the skin, kidneys, gastrointestinal tract, and central nervous system. Renal involvement is signaled by the onset of acute renal failure often accompanied by hypertension, which may be difficult to control. When this syndrome follows angiographic procedures, it is necessary to determine whether the renal lesion is due to contrast medium nephrotoxicity or embolization. In the former, renal failure occurs immediately and resolves within 2 weeks. However, renal failure associated with emboli may occur as late as 2 to 6 weeks after the embolic event.

The symptoms and signs may mimic a systemic illness such as vasculitis. Peripheral eosinophilia ranging between 6 and 18% may be noted, as well as signs of progressive renal insufficiency. Thus, this diagnosis must be considered in patients with renal failure appearing within several weeks after an invasive arteriovascular procedure.

Histology

Light Microscopy

The hallmark of this lesion is the irregularity of involvement. Because these patients have preexisting severe arteriosclerosis, the changes of benign nephrosclerosis are often present, and the changes induced by the emboli are superimposed on these lesions. The emboli may lodge in the glomerulus. The most common change is ischemia with wrinkling and thickening of the glomerular basement membranes.

Tubular and interstitial changes reflect the preexisting vascular disease. Those due to the embolic process vary from mild ischemia to foci of necrosis, depending on the diffuse-

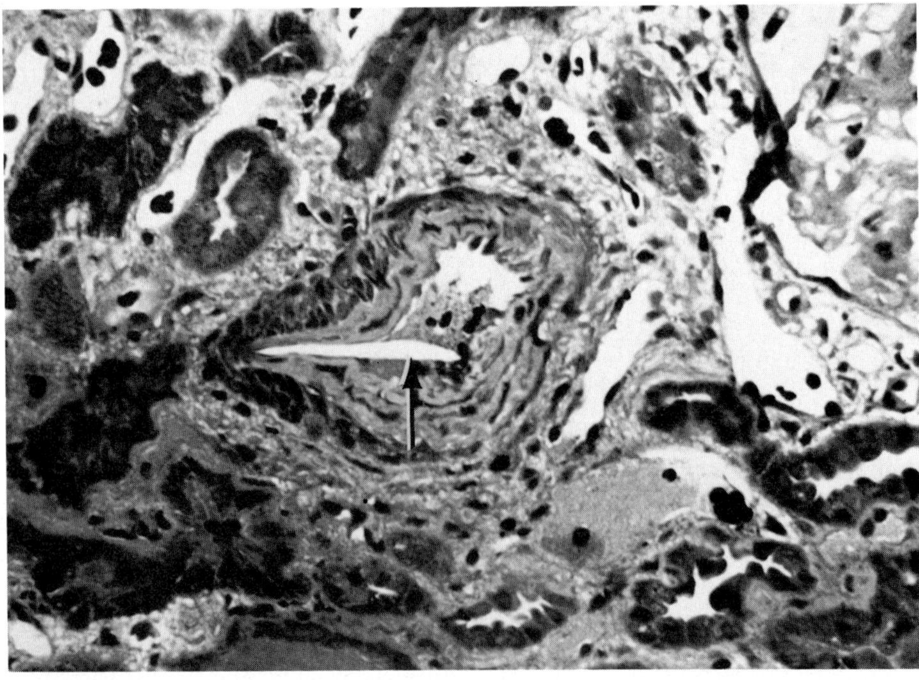

Figure 12–14. An elongated, point-shaped crystalline structure (arrow) and amorphous material surrounding it partially occlude the lumen of this small artery. (H&E, ×300.)

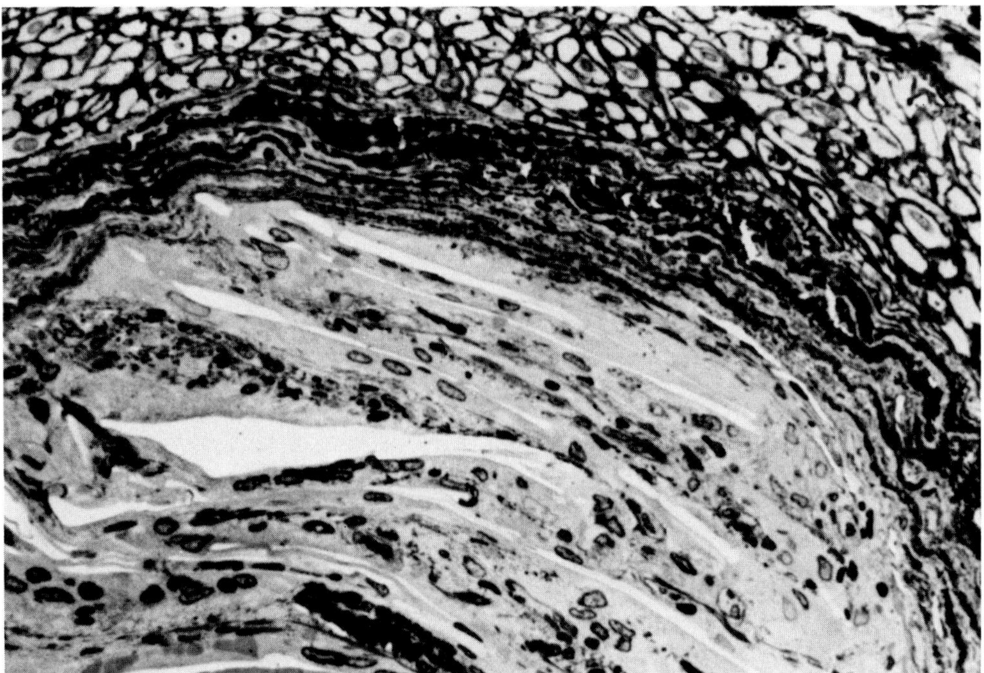

Figure 12–15. This large artery has a large mass of material occluding the lumen. The luminal material contains needle-shaped crystals surrounded by multinucleated cells and amorphous debris. (PASM, ×300.)

ness and severity of the vascular occlusion secondary to the embolization.

When a biopsy specimen is evaluated shortly after an embolic event, needle-shaped crystals, together with other amorphous eosinophilic material, may be seen occluding blood vessels (Fig. 12–14). At a later time, the embolic material is incorporated into concentric layers of proliferating cells in the subendothelium (Fig. 12–15). The crystals may be incorporated within giant cells at this stage.

Prognosis

The course varies among patients. The most ominous sign is the occurrence of renal insufficiency. Unfortunately, there is no effective therapy. Many patients eventually require dialysis.

SELECTED READINGS

1. Genest J, Kuchel O, Hamet P, et al (eds): Hypertension, 2nd ed. McGraw-Hill, New York, 1983.
2. Heptinstall RH: Renal biopsies in hypertension. Br Heart J 16:133, 1954.
3. Hsu H, Churg J: The ultrastructure of mucoid "onionskin" intimal lesions in malignant nephrosclerosis. Am J Pathol 99:67, 1980.
4. Kincaid-Smith P, McMichael J, Murphy EA: The clinical course and pathology of hypertension with papilloedema (malignant hypertension). Q J Med 27:117, 1958.
5. McManus JFA, Lupton CH Jr: Ischemic obsolescence of renal glomeruli. The natural history of the lesions and their relation to hypertension. Lab Invest 9:413, 1960.
6. Nagle RB, Kohnen PW, Bulger RE, et al: Ultrastructure of human renal obsolescent glomeruli. Lab Invest 21:519, 1969.
7. Sevitt LM, Evans DJ, Wrong O: Acute oliguric renal failure due to accelerated (malignant) hypertension. Q J Med 40:127, 1971.
8. Sommers SC, Relman AS, Smithwick RH: Histologic studies of kidney biopsy specimens from patients with hypertension. Am J Pathol 34:685, 1958.

Chapter

13

TUBULAR AND INTERSTITIAL LESIONS

Conditions affecting the tubules or interstitium inevitably lead to changes in both compartments because of their anatomic proximity and their functional interdependence. However, one is often able to determine which of the two areas is the principal or initial site of involvement. For instance, ischemic injuries primarily affect the proximal tubular epithelial cells. However, the adjacent interstitium almost always is edematous. Nonetheless, the primacy of the tubular lesion is clear on examination of the tissue and the clinical history. Similarly, in patients with drug-induced interstitial nephritis, the adjacent tubular segments are often affected.

ACUTE TUBULAR NECROSIS

Acute tubular necrosis is a syndrome that has also been called acute tubulo-interstitial nephritis. The latter designation, although technically correct because the interstitium is often affected, is cumbersome and is therefore not in common use. Another name proposed for this lesion is *ischemic acute tubular necrosis,* because this is the most common underlying cause. However, it would seem more accurate and generic to retain the term *acute tubular necrosis*, which does not imply a specific or unique pathogenetic mechanism.

Acute tubular necrosis includes lesions encountered in patients who have acute renal failure due to lesions that are primarily or almost exclusively restricted to the proximal tubules. The laboratory data and clinical history are so characteristic that renal biopsies are not often necessary to establish the diagnosis, except in very unusual cases. The utility of a renal biopsy in establishing the diagnosis has been further limited by the fact that the lesions, even those that cause anuria, may not be of sufficient severity for there to be histologic evidence of cell death at the light microscopic level.

Pathogenesis

The pathogenesis of acute tubular necrosis is not agreed on, despite considerable research effort. Clearly there are multiple causes, and the spectrum of the injury and renal response are dependent variables for the ultimate outcome. The causes of tubular necrosis are multiple (Table 13–1) and include ischemia due to hypovolemia, chemical toxins, drugs, and the precipitation of toxic proteins in the tubules (i.e., myoglobin or hemoglobin).

Patient Presentation

Oliguria or anuria is the most common presenting finding. However, non-oliguric renal failure with azotemia due to tubular injury is the most common presentation in the post-surgical period.

Histology

Light Microscopy

The glomeruli appear normal, for the most part, although they may occasionally contain

Table 13–1. Causes of Acute Tubular Necrosis

Causes
Ischemia
Shock/sepsis/burns
Rhabdomyolysis
Incompatible transfusion
Hepatorenal syndrome
Toxins
Heavy metals: mercury, bismuth, gold
Paraquat
Ethylene glycol
Phosphorus
Mushroom poisoning
Carbon tetrachloride
Drugs
Lithium
Sulfonamides
Antibiotics (polymyxins, kanamycin, cephalosporins, gentamicin, tobramycin, rifampicin)
Chemotherapeutic agents (cisplatin, streptozotocin, bleomycin, vinblastine)
Anesthetics (halothane [Fluothane])
Contrast medium
Hypertonic solutions
Chelating agents

fibrin thrombi that occlude vascular loops. More commonly, however, they appear bloodless and often collapsed, resulting in an enlargement of Bowman's space. In these cases, the parietal epithelial cells are cuboidal in shape.

The most characteristic histologic finding is that the interstitial region is widened by edema (Fig. 13–1). There are few interstitial inflammatory cells, although a few lymphocytes or plasma cells may be seen. In fact, the paucity of interstitial inflammatory cells is the single most useful feature in the differentiation of lesions that are primarily tubular in origin from those that originate in the interstitium. Thus, when acute tubular necrosis is accompanied by a dense interstitial inflammatory infiltrate, the lesion must either be considered to be both interstitial and tubular in origin or it is assumed that the initial lesion originated in the interstitium.

The tubules frequently show mild and focal lesions. In these cases there is often a complete absence of tubular cell necrosis, with sloughing into the lumen. Rather, the tubular epithelial cells may show loss of surface microvilli and flattening of the cells. The most conspicuous finding is the dilation of the tubular lumen, which is accompanied by thinning of the epithelial cell cytoplasm (Fig. 13–2). In most cases there are few casts, but cytoplasmic fragments may be visible in the lumen. When present, casts are most often seen in distal segments and contain either hyalin or granular material. Pigmented or hemoglobin casts, which have a granular appearance and a brown-orange color, are conspicuous only in patients with hemolysis or

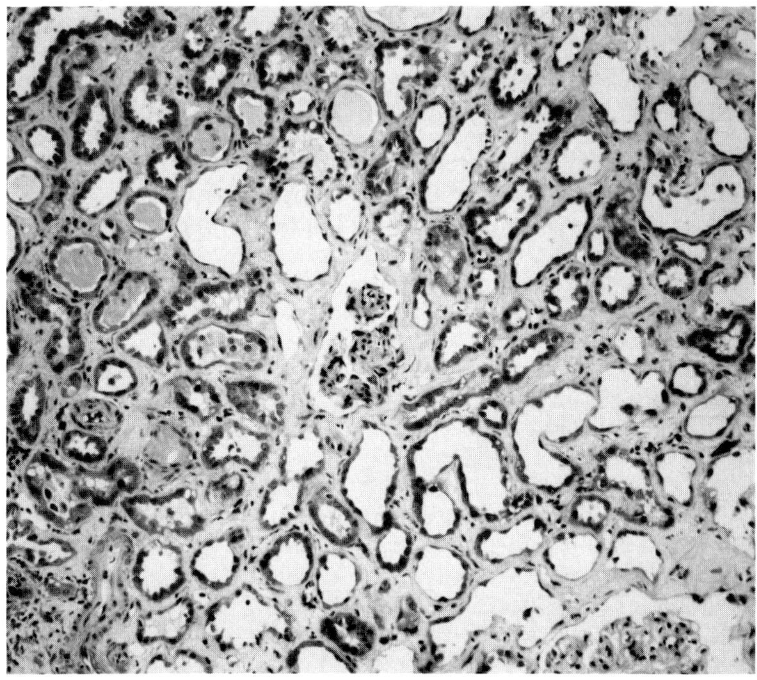

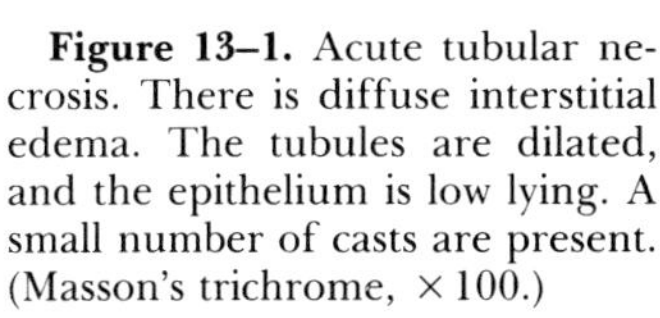

Figure 13–1. Acute tubular necrosis. There is diffuse interstitial edema. The tubules are dilated, and the epithelium is low lying. A small number of casts are present. (Masson's trichrome, ×100.)

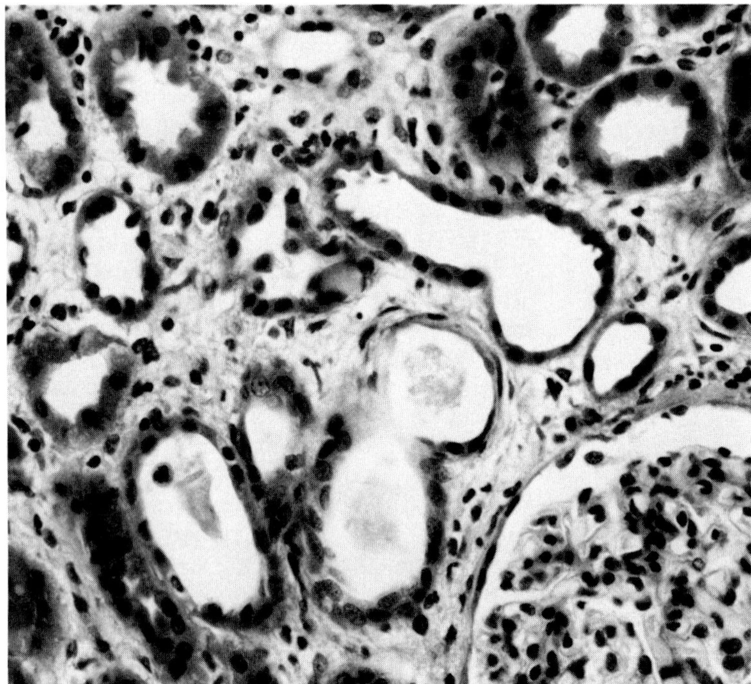

Figure 13–2. Acute tubular necrosis. There are few inflammatory cells within the edematous interstitium. The brush borders of the proximal tubular cells are absent. (Masson's trichrome, ×250.)

rhabdomyolysis. Crystals are found in the tubular lumen and in the tubular epithelial cells of patients with polyethylene glycol toxicity. The presence of large casts, multilaminated casts, or casts with a surrounding cellular reaction should signal the presence of a dysproteinemia, especially multiple myeloma (see Chapter 9).

The brush border of the proximal tubules is always altered, being either completely or partially absent (see Fig. 13–2). This is best appreciated in periodic acid-Schiff (PAS)-stained sections. Fine cytoplasmic vacuolations are most marked in patients who have received infusions of hypertonic solutions (low-molecular-weight dextrans or mannitol). This histologic lesion is called osmotic nephropathy. Occasional tubular cells may be sufficiently damaged to lead to sloughing, but true necrosis is rarely observed.

The term *lower nephron nephrosis* has been used to describe a lesion of the distal tubules following a period of ischemia. This is not a common finding in renal biopsies because it is often a terminal event, and it is almost always associated with lesions in other tubular segments. The use of this term is no longer considered appropriate to describe a tubular injury because nephrosis now carries the connotation of a glomerular change leading to proteinuria. Thus it has been replaced by the use of descriptors that pinpoint the cause and anatomic site of the lesions more accurately (e.g., post-ischemic acute tubular necrosis, involving distal segments).

Normally the tubular basement membranes are intact and continuous when examined by PAS or silver stains. However, in areas of severe epithelial cell injury with necrosis and karyorrhexis, there may be interruptions of the basement membranes. This observation is made most frequently in toxic injury and signals that the repair process will be accompanied by fibrosis.

The accumulation of leukocytes in the vasa recta of the medulla is a very common lesion at autopsy in patients with acute tubular necrosis. Since they are often restricted to the medulla, they are not commonly found in renal biopsies.

Whatever segment is involved, the presence of regeneration can be recognized by the presence of cells with hyperchromatic nuclei and basophilic cytoplasm. This may be the only feature present in biopsies performed more than 1 week after the acute insult.

The blood vessels are not affected, and changes therein reflect preexisting lesions.

Immunofluorescence Microscopy

There are no accumulations of either immunoglobulins or complement. Fibrin-related antigens may be found in the peritubular regions, in the presence of capillary injury and/or passive congestion.

Electron Microscopy

The electron microscopic findings confirm the absence of lesions noted at the light and immunofluorescence microscopic levels in the glomeruli. Although the morphology of early tubular lesions would be of considerable interest, few studies are available in humans. Therefore, in the evaluation of a renal biopsy lesion, one must rely on data from animal studies. This is especially true when there is mild injury rather than necrosis.

The proximal and distal tubular changes consist of vacuolation and swelling of the cytoplasm and loss of the brush border microvilli. There is concomitant loss of the basal and lateral infoldings of the cell membranes. Myeloid bodies are occasionally present in the cytoplasm and probably represent modified lysosomes. They are most common in patients who have received aminoglycosides.

Regenerating tubular epithelial cells may also lack a brush border and the lateral interdigitations and may also have a small number of cytoplasmic organelles. In contrast, in acutely injured cells, the cytoplasm of regenerating cells is not increased in amount and the cells tend to be low lying.

Prognosis

The prognosis is nearly universally excellent, and the renal injury almost always completely resolves without sequelae. The only exceptions appear to be those unusual instances in which the injury was of sufficient severity to result in dissolution of the tubular basement membranes and interstitial framework. These lesions heal with scarring and disruption of the architecture.

SELECTED READINGS

1. Olsen S, Solez K: Acute renal failure in man: Pathogenesis in light of new morphological data. Clin Nephrol 27:271, 1987.
2. Solez K, Morel-Maroger L, Sraer JD: The morphology of "acute tubular necrosis" in man. Analysis of 57 renal biopsies and a comparison with animal models. Medicine (Baltimore) 58:362, 1979.
3. Wilson DM, Turner DR, Cameron JS, et al: Value of renal biopsy in acute intrinsic renal failure. Br Med J 2:459, 1976.

ACUTE INTERSTITIAL NEPHRITIS

Acute interstitial nephritis is a clinicopathologic entity defined by the presence of acute renal failure and infiltration of the cortical interstitium by inflammatory cells. The syndrome has multiple causes and diverse clinical manifestations (Table 13–2).

The pathologic lesions were first described at the end of the 19th century in patients with scarlet fever. The introduction of antibiotics led to a rapid decline in the incidence of streptococcal infections and therefore in the virtual disappearance of acute interstitial nephritis for a number of years.

Acute interstitial nephritis was considered to be a curiosity in 20th century medicine until the 1960s, when it emerged again as an important entity. The reasons for its reappearance were fourfold. First, several new classes of therapeutic agents with renal toxicity were introduced into general clinical use. The drugs that initially were most commonly associated with interstitial lesions were antibiotics of the penicillin group and non-steroidal anti-inflammatory agents. Second, the use of renal biopsy became widespread, revealing interstitial lesions that had previously been difficult to appreciate. Third, a new systemic syndrome consisting of uveitis and interstitial nephritis was recognized. Finally, the group of hemorrhagic fevers initially called nephropathia endemica were discovered. The etiologic agent was quickly found to be the Hantaan virus, and, as evidenced by many subsequent cases documented in the

Table 13–2. Causes of Acute Interstitial Nephritis

Causes
Infectious
Scarlet fever
Sepsis
Leptospirosis
Legionellosis
Hantaan virus
Other infections
Drug reactions
Antibiotics
Non-steroidal anti-inflammatory agents
Sulfonamides
Other
Miscellaneous
Sarcoidosis (granulomatous lesions)
Uveitis (idiopathic)
Idiopathic
With linear deposits
Without linear deposits

current literature, this disease remains a significant cause of acute interstitial nephritis.

The true frequency of acute interstitial nephritis is difficult to determine accurately.

Pathogenesis

The pathogenesis of acute lesions of the interstitium is complex, but many lesions are thought to be immunologically mediated. The frequency of lesions in this compartment has greatly increased with the introduction of a large number of new therapeutic agents, many of which have the potential for triggering an inflammatory reaction when concentrated by the renal tubules or are capable of inciting an allergic response. In both instances, if the kidney is a major site of drug metabolism or excretion, the interstitium is often the site of the adverse reaction. Drugs in this category include antibiotics and the non-steroidal anti-inflammatory agents. A number of animal models support the concept of an immunologic cause. These include models in which antibodies to tubular basement membrane antigens induce an acute reaction, closely paralleling that in methicillin-induced acute interstitial nephritis. Cell-mediated immunity has also been considered to be a candidate mechanism, based on animal and human studies in which T-lymphocytes are part of the interstitial infiltrate. The concurrence of interstitial granulomas further strengthens the suspicion of a hypersensitivity reaction. Finally, some patients demonstrate a positive skin test to the antigen implicated in causing acute interstitial nephritis.

Patient Presentation

The presentation varies widely, depending on the underlying cause. The number and variety of drugs that have been implicated in acute interstitial nephritis are large. We have chosen to discuss and/or list only those that have been reported in a relatively large number of patients (Table 13–3). Some cases of drug-related acute interstitial nephritis are accompanied by fever, rash, and eosinophilia. These features suggest a drug hypersensitivity reaction. This symptomatic triad may be absent, particularly in hospitalized patients who may be receiving multiple therapeutic agents, some of which may mask the signs of hypersensitivity. Thus, the presence of the acute interstitial nephritis may be difficult to recognize, and even when suspected, the offending agent may be difficult to identify.

Table 13–3. Drugs Most Commonly Implicated in Acute Interstitial Nephritis

Beta-lactam antibiotics
Methicillin
Penicillin G
Ampicillin
Cephalothin
Cephalexin
Non-steroidal anti-inflammatory agents
Phenylbutazone
Fenoprofen
Indomethacin

Regardless of the actual basis of the injury, many patients with acute interstitial nephritis present with non-oliguric renal failure. Macroscopic hematuria may precede the development of azotemia, but proteinuria is either very mild or absent. The presence of eosinophils in the urine, signaling a hypersensitivity reaction, is a helpful finding in making the diagnosis of drug-related acute interstitial nephritis.

Infectious Disease with Acute Interstitial Nephritis

Sepsis

Histology

LIGHT MICROSCOPY

It is not common to perform a renal biopsy in a patient suspected of having an acute infectious renal disease. The observation of a leukocytic interstitial infiltrate and leukocyte casts suggests the presence of an acute infectious interstitial nephritis.

IMMUNOFLUORESCENCE MICROSCOPY

Although few studies have been published, our experience and that of others is that immunoglobulins are not present in the kidneys. Small, scattered granular deposits of C3 may be found in the mesangium and along the basement membranes of the tubules and Bowman's capsule.

Hantaan Virus or Hemorrhagic Fever or Muroid Virus Nephropathy

It is not clear whether this lesion should be considered to be an acute interstitial nephritis or acute tubular necrosis. Hemorrhagic fever with renal manifestations has been recognized in several countries. It was first described in Korea, but cases have been reported in North America, Belgium, France, Scotland, Scandinavia, and Eastern Europe. The disease consists of fever, loin pain, acute renal failure, and transient thrombocytopenia.

Pathogenesis

The infectious agents are RNA viruses, which have been grouped together under the heading of Hantaan viruses. They belong to the Bunyaviridae family. Previously called muroid viruses, they are transmitted by exposure to rodent excreta.

Patient Presentation

The renal signs appear 4 to 10 days following the onset of fever and loin pain. The evidence of significant renal involvement is most often short lived. Few patients have other than a brief episode of oliguria, and few require hemodialysis. Proteinuria is seldom present in more than trace amounts.

Histology

LIGHT MICROSCOPY

The glomeruli and blood vessels are normal. There are interstitial edema and scattered inflammatory cells consisting of lymphocytes and plasmacytes. Neutrophils are uncommonly a part of this infiltrate. Foci of dilated tubules associated with flattened epithelial cells are present but are not a prominent feature.

Foci of medullary hemorrhage are the most conspicuous lesions. They are not associated with significant numbers of inflammatory cells.

Drug-Induced Acute Interstitial Nephritis

There has been a sharp increase in the frequency of acute interstitial nephritis due to drugs, but the total number of well-documented cases remains relatively small. The mechanism is thought to be allergic, and the nephritis usually follows the use of the drugs in what is considered to be the usual therapeutic range. The two categories of drugs that have most often been incriminated are the beta-lactam antibiotics and the non-steroidal anti-inflammatory agents. Methicillin was the first antibiotic to be reported as a cause of acute interstitial nephritis. Since the first reports, this has been a well-documented and frequently reported association. Other derivatives of penicillin and cephalosporins are the most common antibacterials known to induce acute interstitial nephritis. Other antibiotics have also been implicated, but with a much lower frequency.

The second category, non-steroidal anti-inflammatory agents, have frequently been associated with acute interstitial nephritis.

Many other drugs have been implicated as a cause of acute interstitial nephritis, including thiazide diuretics, sulfonamides, analgesics, and phenindione. It is to be expected that as the pharmacologic armamentarium expands, the list will change. Because renal lesions are one of the significant complications of drug therapy, it is important to be alert to the possibility of kidney involvement with the introduction of each new agent.

Histology

Light Microscopy

As in other forms of acute interstitial nephritis, the glomeruli and blood vessels are normal, although they may be surrounded by an intense inflammatory infiltrate. The tubules may become atrophic.

The principal lesion in a toxic reaction to non-steroidal non-inflammatory drugs is an intense, often diffuse inflammatory infiltrate. The nature of the infiltrate varies, but lymphocytes are always a major component. Several studies have shown that the lymphocytes are mainly T cells. There is no general agreement about the frequency with which each subclass is represented. Neutrophils are uncommon components of the infiltrate. Eosinophils have been noted in a few cases. Therefore, the presence of eosinophils is indicative, but not diagnostic, of a hypersensitivity acute interstitial nephritis (Figs. 13–3 and 13–4).

We first described the occurrence of interstitial granulomas consisting of epithelioid cells and giant cells in two patients who had methicillin-induced acute interstitial nephritis (Fig. 13–5). Granulomatous lesions are also common in patients exposed to other beta-lactams. They have also been encountered in patients with sulfonamides, thiazides, phenindione, and an analgesic widely used

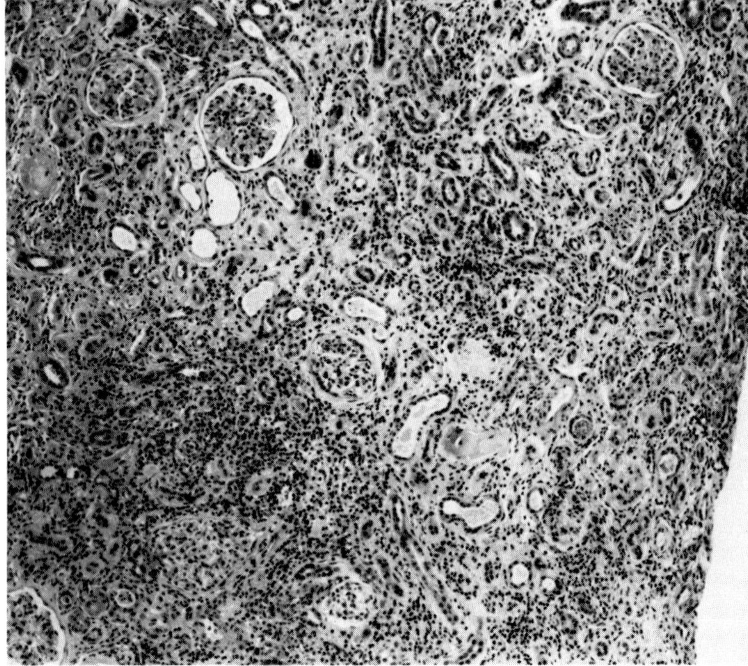

Figure 13–3. Acute interstitial nephritis. The patient had taken non-steroidal anti-inflammatory drugs in therapeutic doses. The interstitium contains a diffuse inflammatory cell infiltrate, which severely distorts the tubular architecture. (Masson's trichrome, ×100.)

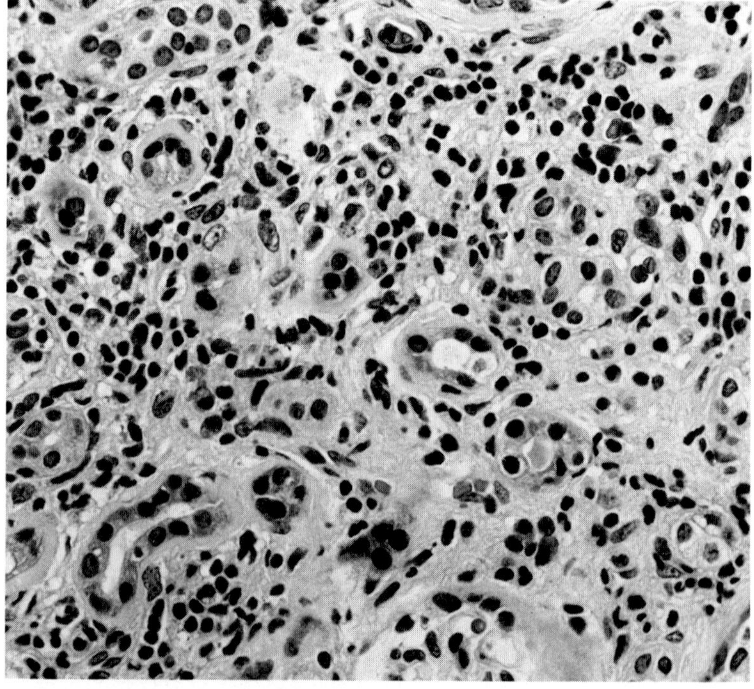

Figure 13–4. Acute interstitial nephritis. The inflammatory cell infiltrate contains principally mononuclear cells. (Masson's trichrome, ×250.)

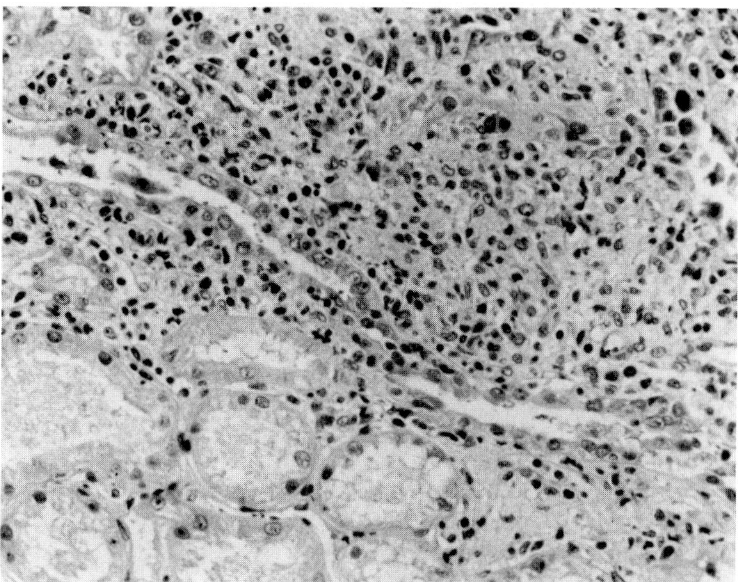

Figure 13–5. Acute interstitial nephritis. Methicillin-induced granuloma in the interstitium. (Masson's trichrome, ×250.)

in France (glafenine). The granulomas may be small and sparsely distributed, but in some biopsy specimens they may occupy the major part of the renal interstitium. In the latter case, the granulomas may be confluent and resemble the histologic pattern seen in sarcoidosis.

Some histologic features may help in differentiating lesions induced by the non-steroidal anti-inflammatory drugs from those due to beta-lactam antibiotics. In the former, the interstitial inflammation is predominantly composed of small lymphocytes and occasional plasma cells, but eosinophils are absent or rare. Arteriolosclerosis and obsolescent glomeruli are commonly present in biopsies from these patients. In addition, the lesions by electron microscopy are quite different (see below).

The interstitial lesions following exposure to beta-lactam antibiotics sharply differ from those just described. The infiltrate is more diffuse and includes a larger proportion of plasma cells and lymphocytes, and eosinophils are scattered throughout or in large aggregates. Epithelioid cells and multinucleated cells are often present, and they may form granulomas. Finally, there are often breaks in the tubular basement membranes with infiltration of the tubular epithelial cell layer by inflammatory cells.

Immunofluorescence Microscopy

Few cases have immune reactants in renal tissue. Essentially the only findings are in those patients with methicillin-induced acute interstitial nephritis in whom there may be antibodies against tubular basement membranes. In this instance there are linear, diffuse deposits of IgG along the tubular basement membranes (Fig. 13–6).

Electron Microscopy

The glomeruli in patients with lesions induced by non-steroidal anti-inflammatory drugs often have spreading of the pedicels. They do not have deposits along the tubular basement membranes. These lesions stand in sharp contrast to those in patients with a hypersensitivity reaction to the beta-lactam drugs. In the latter there are seldom podocyte changes, but there are electron-dense deposits along many tubular basement membranes.

Prognosis

If the cause of the renal lesion can be determined early in the course and removed from the patient's environment, the prognosis is generally excellent. If, however, the

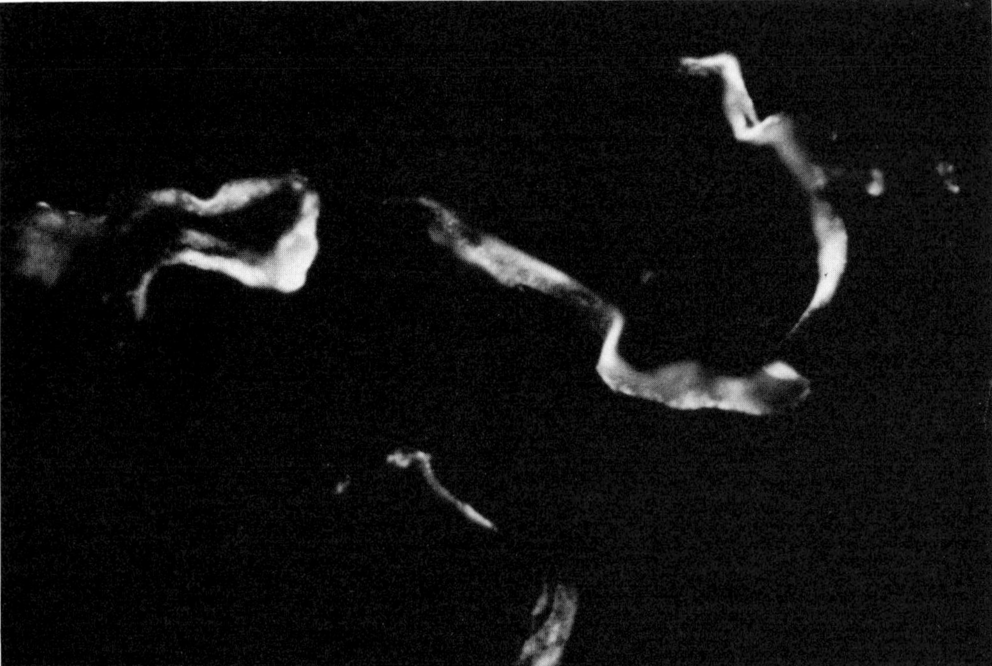

Figure 13–6. Acute interstitial nephritis. Immunofluorescence micrograph, anti-IgG. Linear deposits along the tubular basement membranes. (×250.)

lesions at onset are severe or are not recognized, renal failure may ensue. In our experience, patients with a large number of interstitial granulomas seem to be particularly prone to develop progressive renal failure.

ACUTE INTERSTITIAL NEPHRITIS AND UVEITIS

Acute interstitial nephritis and uveitis was first described in 1975, and there are now at least 26 reported cases. Eighty-five per cent of the patients are young women. The presenting symptoms are an anterior uveitis, enlarged lymph nodes, and acute non-oliguric renal failure. The renal findings may precede the onset or discovery of the ocular abnormalities.

Histology

Light Microscopy

The interstitial lesions are diffuse and are characterized by a heterogeneous cellular infiltrate consisting of lymphocytes, plasma cells, and a large number of eosinophils (see Fig. 13–7). Eosinophils, although considered to be characteristic of this syndrome, are only present in one-half of the reported cases. When present they are abundantly admixed with the mononuclear cells. Small foci of epithelioid cells with occasional multinucleated cells have also been described. They are restricted in size, and large granulomas have not been reported. The infiltrate is associated with prominent interstitial edema.

The tubular lesions (principally atrophy) parallel and appear to be secondary to the severity of the interstitial lesions (see Fig. 13–8).

The glomeruli and blood vessels are unremarkable.

Immunofluorescence Microscopy

There are no deposits of immune reactants.

Acute Interstitial Nephritis, Miscellaneous Causes

Sarcoidosis

The renal lesions in sarcoidosis are rarely of sufficient severity to cause acute renal failure.

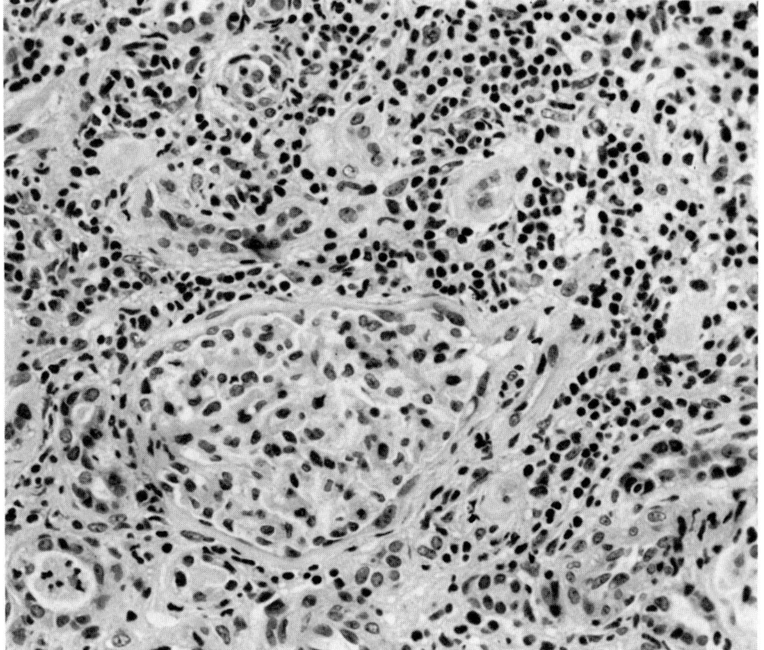

Figure 13–7. Acute interstitial nephritis and uveitis. There is a diffuse interstitial infiltrate, with considerable disruption of the normal tubular architecture. (H&E, ×250.)

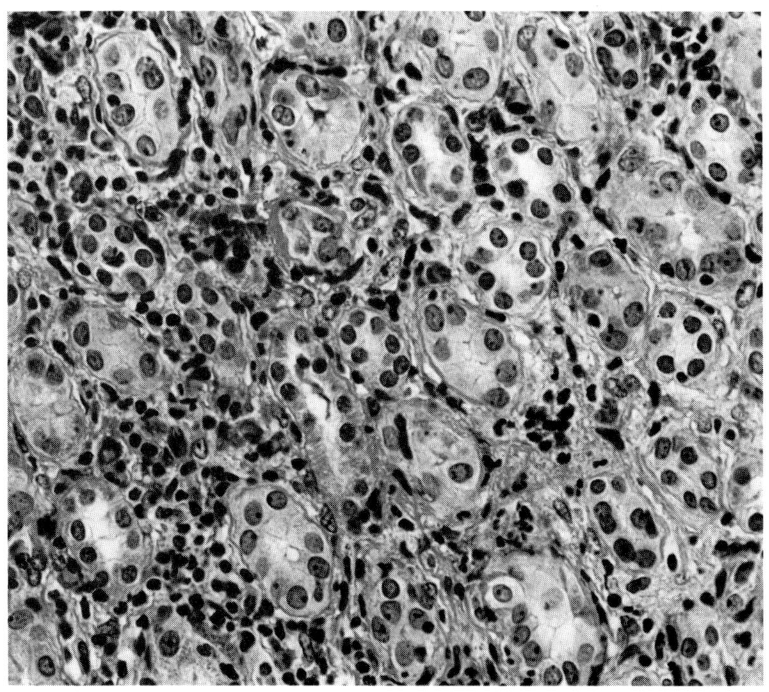

Figure 13–8. Acute interstitial nephritis and uveitis. Higher magnification demonstrating the severe tubular alterations and the polymorphous infiltrate. (Masson's trichrome, ×400.)

Histology

LIGHT MICROSCOPY

The histologic lesions are characterized by interstitial infiltrates and the frequent presence of granulomas. The granulomas, surrounded by lymphocytes and plasma cells, are identical to those in patients with drug-induced acute interstitial nephritis. It has recently been shown by immunofluorescence microscopy that some cells of the granulomas possess angiotensin-converting enzyme. The significance of this observation is unknown.

Prognosis

The long-term prognosis appears to be excellent despite the residuum of interstitial fibrosis that persists after resolution of the interstitial infiltrate.

Megalocytic Interstitial Nephritis

Although megalocytic interstitial nephritis is a rare entity, the diagnosis is readily made by routine histologic techniques. Involved kidneys are enlarged, often irregularly, by imaging methods.

Histology

LIGHT MICROSCOPY

There are nodular or diffuse infiltrates consisting of large macrophages, which may contain cytoplasmic PAS-positive inclusions. The tubules are displaced by the interstitial infiltrates but do not appear to be a part of the primary process.

ELECTRON MICROSCOPY

The macrophage inclusions are seen to be lysosomes with crystalline electron-lucent structures.

Prognosis

It has been assumed that this disorder is a minor form of malakoplakia, differing only in the absence of Michaelis-Gutmann bodies. The prognosis is unknown, but in the few reported cases, if an underlying infectious process can be treated, the lesions may regress.

SELECTED READINGS

1. Andres GA, McCluskey RT: Tubular and interstitial renal disease due to immunologic mechanisms. Kidney Int 7:271, 1975.
2. Bender WL, Whelton A, Beschorner WE, et al: Interstitial nephritis, proteinuria, and renal failure caused by non-steroidal anti-inflammatory drugs. Immunologic characterization of the inflammatory infiltrate. Am J Med 76:1006, 1984.
3. Burnier M, Jaeger PM, Campiche M, et al: Idiopathic acute interstitial nephritis and uveitis in the adult. Report of 1 case and review of the literature. Am J Nephrol 6:312, 1986.
4. Colvin RB, Burton NE, Hyslop NE, et al: Penicillin-associated interstitial nephritis. Ann Intern Med 81:404, 1974.
5. Dobrin RS, Vernier RL, Fish AJ: Acute eosinophilic interstitial nephritis and renal failure with bone marrow-lymph node granulomas and anterior uveitis. A new syndrome. Am J Med 59:325, 1975.
6. Gerhardt RE, Loebl DH, Rao RN: Interstitial immunofluorescence in nephritis of Sjögren's syndrome. Clin Nephrol 10:201, 1978.
7. Kikkawa Y, Sakurai M, Mano T, et al: Interstitial nephritis with concomitant uveitis. Report of two cases. Contrib Nephrol 4:1, 1977.
8. Kleinknecht D, Vanhille P, Morel-Maroger L, et al: Acute interstitial nephritis due to drug hypersensitivity: An up-to-date review with a report of 19 cases. Adv Nephrol 12:277, 1983.
9. Kourilsky O, Solez K, Morel-Maroger L, et al: The pathology of acute renal failure due to interstitial nephritis in man with comments on the role of interstitial inflammation and sex in gentamicin nephrotoxicity. Medicine (Baltimore) 61:258, 1982.
10. Mignon F, Mery JP, Mougenot B, et al: Granulomatous interstitial nephritis. Adv Nephrol 13:219, 1984.

CHRONIC INTERSTITIAL NEPHRITIS

As described in earlier sections, chronic lesions affecting the tubulo-interstitial compartment occur as a common consequence of many glomerular, tubular, and vascular diseases. The name *chronic interstitial diseases* should be reserved for those cases in which the lesions can be assumed to be primary in the interstitial compartment. The etiologic agents are multiple, and although some are historic curiosities, many new lesions have appeared during the past few decades as a result of the myriad new drugs and environmental toxins to which patients are exposed.

The most common cause of interstitial nephritis is the use of a therapeutic agent that has renal damage as an important side effect.

A less common cause, but nonetheless important, is the presence of a systemic disease that is immune mediated. We will describe the general characteristics of these diseases and try to identify the histologic features that are helpful in differentiating the various types of chronic interstitial nephritis.

Chronic interstitial nephritis can be classified according to the etiologic causes as follows:

1. Infection
2. Therapeutic agents and toxins
3. Metabolic
4. Systemic diseases (sarcoidosis and Sjögren's syndrome)
5. Unknown

This categorization encompasses most varieties of chronic interstitial nephritis encountered in a renal biopsy practice. We have deliberately excluded conditions that have only historic interest or are rarely subjected to renal biopsy (e.g., Balkan nephritis, tuberculosis, and syphilis).

The following descriptions consider only those findings that have general applicability to chronic interstitial nephritis. The specific etiologies will be considered after the general description, and features unique to a particular disease will be considered in the appropriate sections.

Histology

Light Microscopy

The glomeruli are usually unaffected in the early stages of this process, even in patients with severe interstitial fibrosis. The earliest glomerular lesion is thickening and multilamination of Bowman's capsule, detectable by PAS or silver stains. As the interstitial disease progresses, the glomeruli become progressively ischemic as manifested by increasing wrinkling and thickening of the glomerular basement membranes. The glomerular vascular spaces shrink, and the glomerulus slowly becomes sclerotic. Bowman's space is initially enlarged because of the shrunken glomerular tuft, and it later fills with connective tissue. The resultant obsolescent glomerulus is small and shrunken but remains recognizable by PAS or silver stains, as an ischemic glomerulus. The mesangial spaces are not enlarged in these diseases, and cellularity is normal in the early stages, becoming progressively more hypocellular as the sclerosis proceeds. The glomeruli may appear much closer together than normal as the interstitium shrinks and tubules disappear.

The tubulo-interstitial lesions are often patchy and irregular in distribution. For this reason, the renal biopsy material may not give an accurate assessment of the distribution of this lesion. The lesion is characterized by a combination of cell infiltrates and areas of sclerosis (Fig. 13–9). The nature of the infiltrate may provide insight into the pathogenesis of the disease. In the case of granulomatous infiltrates or eosinophils, for instance, a drug sensitivity reaction might be suspected.

Periglomerular fibrosis and Bowman's capsule thickening may be the earliest signs of interstitial damage. The accumulation of interstitial extracellular matrix (fibrous connective tissue) along the tubular basement membranes is a conspicuous finding in all of these diseases, regardless of the underlying etiology. It is accompanied by atrophy of the adjacent tubular epithelium.

Casts are often present in the neighboring tubules and should be carefully examined, as their appearance and composition may be of use in determining the etiology of the lesions. For instance, plasma cell dyscrasias are associated with characteristic Bence Jones casts (see Chapter 9).

Tubular atrophy accompanies the zones of interstitial fibrosis. The tubules entrapped within these areas are small in diameter, and casts fill their lumina, resulting in the histologic appearance reminiscent of the thyroid and thus the use of the descriptor "thyroidization."

The areas of interstitial fibrosis and tubular atrophy often alternate with zones where there is compensatory hypertrophy of both the tubules and glomeruli. The tubular cells are hypertrophied, and the overall tubule diameter is increased. Similarly, the individual glomerular cells are hypertrophied. These tubular and glomerular changes are the histologic markers of compensatory hypertrophy due to partial nephron loss. They are much more frequently seen in biopsies of children and young adults than in patients older then 50 years.

The blood vessels may show chronic changes consisting of medial hypertrophy, duplication of the elastic laminae, and arteriolar sclerosis. These changes parallel those of the interstitium.

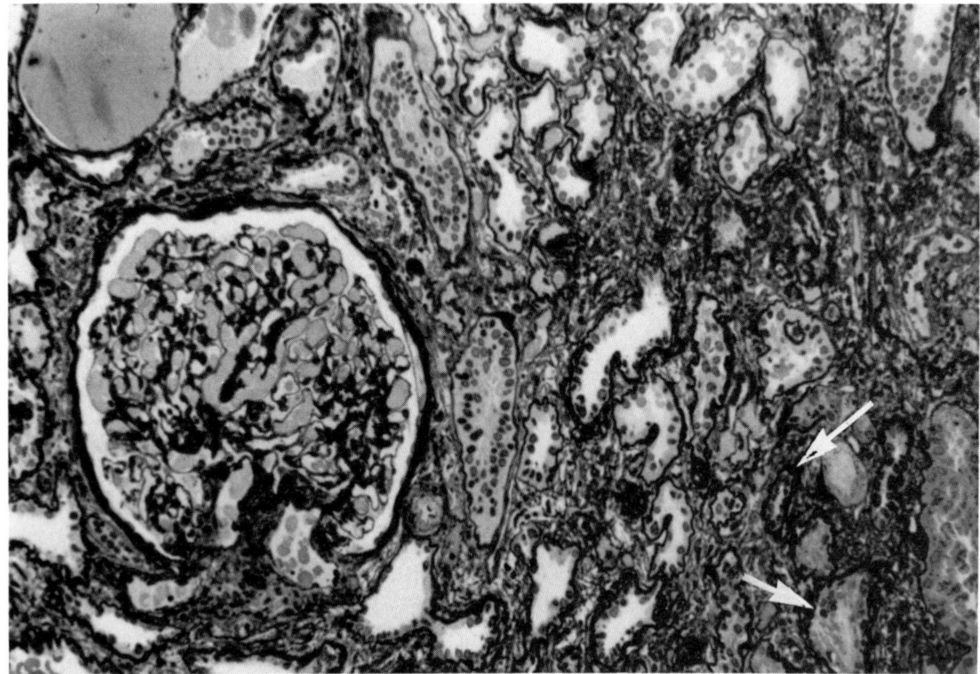

Figure 13–9. Chronic interstitial nephritis. The glomerulus appears normal, but the surrounding interstitium is densely but irregularly fibrotic. The tubules are quite atrophic in the fibrotic areas; some are dilated and contain casts, and others are very small (arrow) with thickened basement membranes (arrow). (PASM, ×75.)

Immunofluorescence Microscopy

For the most part, there are no immune reactants in biopsy specimens of the chronic tubulo-interstitial diseases, except for those associated with some of the systemic immune-mediated diseases. Immunoglobulins or complement components are restricted to the sclerotic zones and are in the amounts typical of this phenomenon in other conditions. Namely, there are small amounts of IgM and C3 within the sclerotic areas, particularly within glomeruli. Such deposits are considered to represent nonspecific trapping.

Electron Microscopy

The nature of the cellular infiltrate may be best appreciated by electron microscopy, but otherwise there is nothing further to be learned by this technique than by light microscopy.

Specific Conditions

Infections

Bacterial

Chronic bacterial infections are often associated with urinary tract obstruction and infection. A chronic inflammatory reaction is almost always present, and the infiltrate is composed of lymphocytes and plasma cells. Lymphoid follicles may occasionally be seen in the cortex.

Miscellaneous

Other forms of chronic interstitial nephritis are rare in practice and therefore uncommonly a renal biopsy diagnostic entity. They include the following:

Malakoplakia. This condition, most frequently observed in patients with long-lasting urinary tract infections, is characterized by the presence of an intense interstitial infiltrate principally consisting of large macrophages. Occasionally there is giant cell formation. The cytoplasm of the macrophages is expanded by large lysosomes, some of which contain PAS-positive crystalline inclusions that are also silver positive. They have been given the name Michaelis-Gutmann bodies and are found in no other renal condition. The particles have a unique ultrastructure consisting of lysosomes that contain structures composed of a crystalline core surrounded by a multilaminated structure.

Tuberculosis and Histoplasmosis. These infections are very rare in the Western world and are not a biopsy subject.

Drugs and Toxins

Analgesics

The prolonged, heavy use of analgesic compounds that contain phenacetin results in chronic tubulo-interstitial nephritis. It has been estimated that the patient must ingest more than 5 kg of these compounds before the lesions become manifest. Such consumption obviously requires several years to realize, and the lesions are thus chronic, cumulative, and difficult to detect because of the insidious nature of the process. One of the consequences of this abuse is the occurrence of papillary necrosis, a diagnosis that is rarely achieved by renal biopsy. However, the cortex develops irregular areas of interstitial lesions. There is prominent tubular atrophy and interstitial fibrosis (Fig. 13–10). The atrophied tubules are filled with hyalin casts, and the epithelial cells contain lipofuscin pigment in their lysosomes. There is often a modest mononuclear interstitial infiltrate.

A recent report has linked the chronic abuse of acetaminophen to chronic renal disease, but the histologic lesions have not been described. This association awaits independent confirmation.

Lithium

The existence of a renal lesion following chronic lithium ingestion is not established beyond doubt. However, some patients who have no other obvious cause of chronic interstitial disease have a history of chronic lithium ingestion. The fact that acute tubular injury may follow acute lithium toxicity lends credence to the supposition that chronic ingestion of lithium in low doses might be a cause of chronic interstitial disease.

Cyclosporine A

Renal lesions due to cyclosporine A are reviewed in Chapter 11. The use of cyclosporine A in conditions other than renal transplantation has led to the clear demonstration that it can cause chronic tubulo-interstitial and vascular disease.

Antineoplastic Agents

Many antineoplastic agents are thought to cause tubular and interstitial toxicity. The lesions are often acute, but they may also be chronic. The list of offending agents in-

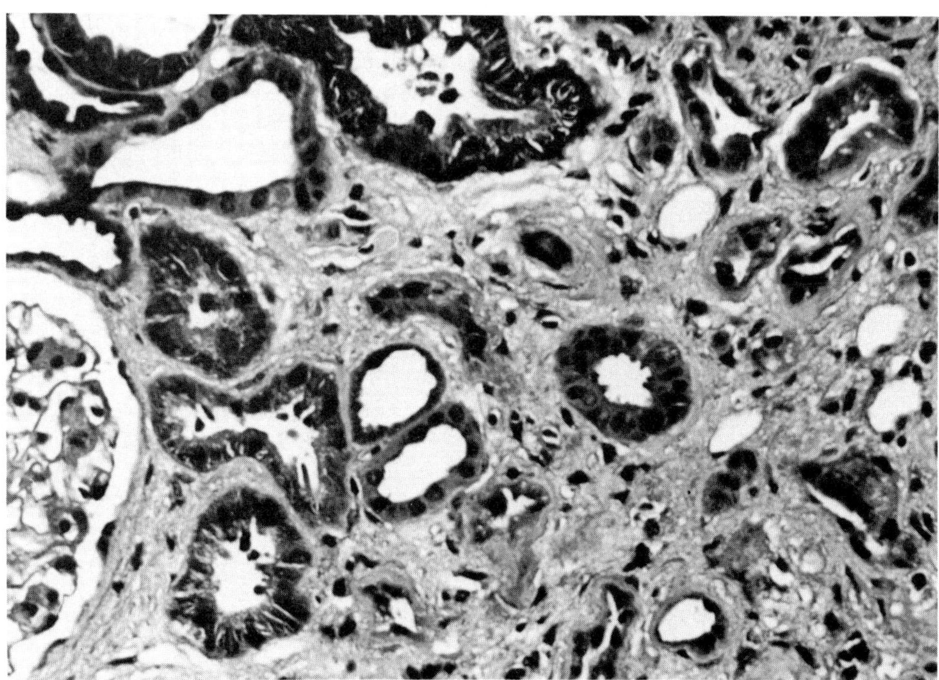

Figure 13–10. Chronic interstitial nephritis. Phenacetin abuse. The interstitium is diffusely fibrotic, and the entrapped tubules are atrophic. (H&E, ×300.)

cludes *cis*-platinum, nitrosoureas (methyl CCNU, streptozotocin), and mithramycin. The renal lesions have most frequently been observed as post-mortem findings, and the diagnosis has therefore been retrospective. In general, these agents cause acute, severe tubular injury followed by progressive interstitial fibrosis. Because most patients receive a combination of chemotherapeutic agents and are often infected with unusual organisms, it may be difficult to determine the exact agent that caused the chronic renal lesion.

Heavy Metals

Chronic exposure to heavy metals usually occurs at the workplace; this is especially true for lead. The only histologic marker of chronic lead intoxication is sparsely scattered nuclear inclusions in tubules. The inclusions may mimic viral inclusions and are best seen in hematoxylin and eosin (H&E) sections. By electron microscopy, the inclusions appear as dense, often multiple intranuclear masses. They may appear to be bounded by a single layered membrane.

Cadmium

Cadmium is a known nephrotoxin, and a tubular lesion has been produced in experimental animals. Little information is available about renal effects in humans.

Metabolic Disturbances

Several types of metabolic disturbances are associated with chronic tubulo-interstitial damage. Although they are seldom the subject of renal biopsy, they are mentioned here because they may be missed unless special stains are used in their detection.

Hypercalcemia

Calcium deposits may be found along the tubular basement membranes, the basement membrane of Bowman's capsule, and the basement membranes of the arteriolar wall smooth muscle cells. They also occur in the tubular epithelial cell cytoplasm and in the lumen of the tubules. When present in the interstitium they are surrounded by an inflammatory cell reaction that may include macrophages. Calcium deposits are recognized by von Kossa's stain.

Urates

Urates are highly soluble in water, so the tissue must be processed in absolute alcohol, including the fixation steps. The crystals have a characteristic elongated, rectangular shape and are present in the interstitium. They are often surrounded by inflammatory cells and macrophages, forming small granulomas, known as tophi. Many of these inflammatory foci are found in the medulla.

Oxalosis

These deposits are found either in patients with a hereditary primary enzyme deficiency or in those who have been exposed to certain toxins, such as polyethylene glycol. Oxalates are also soluble, and special care must be taken in the fixation and processing of tissues to ensure their preservation. The crystals have a characteristic rhomboid shape, often arranged in rosettes, and may be admixed with calcium precipitates.

Cystinosis (see Chapter 8)

Hypokalemia

Prolonged, severe hypokalemia results in proximal tubular cytoplasmic lesions consisting of vacuolation and swelling of tubular epithelial cells and interstitial fibrosis. The vacuoles are larger than those present after exposure to hyperosmotic solutions. The interstitial fibrosis is not associated with an interstitial infiltrate and is often of modest degree.

Granulomas, Including Sarcoidosis

Granulomatous lesions in the interstitium may be observed in patients with chronic tubulo-interstitial disease. Although they are uncommon, their discovery may provide important diagnostic information. We reported on 13 patients with this finding in 1983. At that time, we noted that the granulomas contained macrophages and occasional multinucleated giant cells. They were surrounded by large infiltrates of lymphocytes. Several categories of diseases were found in association with the interstitial granulomas:

Sarcoidosis

The granulomas in patients with sarcoidosis may sometimes be differentiated from those due to other causes if the multinucleated giant cells contain asteroid bodies as cytoplasmic inclusions. It has recently been reported that cells in the infiltrate stain positively when tested with an antibody to angiotensin-converting enzyme Finally, the patients are often hypercalcemic, and calcium deposits may accumulate in the interstitium.

Granulomatous Interstitial Disease

Granulomatous interstitial disease is an idiopathic entity, but before the diagnosis can be made, other causes of interstitial granulomas must be thoroughly investigated. These include tuberculosis, drug hypersensitivity, and vasculitis.

Systemic Diseases, Including Sjögren's Disease

The interstitium is affected in many of the systemic diseases. However, only in Sjögren's disease do the interstitial lesions constitute the principal renal manifestation. Approximately 20% of patients with this syndrome develop chronic tubulo-interstitial disease. It is often recognized because of the appearance of acidosis.

Histology

LIGHT MICROSCOPY

The glomeruli are normal in most instances. There have been some reports of mild mesangial hypercellularity, but this is by no means a common finding.

The interstitium contains a homogeneous, monotonous infiltrate and may be mistaken for a lymphoid malignancy. The composition of the infiltrate is almost solely small lymphocytes, with occasional plasma cells and a rare neutrophil (Fig. 13–11). There is seldom significant interstitial fibrosis. The infiltrate may displace the tubules, and those present in the areas of dense infiltrate have flattened epithelium and thickened basement membranes. There are few casts within the tubules.

IMMUNOFLUORESCENCE MICROSCOPY

The glomeruli are usually negative. It is common to find granular deposits of IgG and complement components in a coarse pattern along the tubular basement membranes and occasionally along the intertubular capillary basement membranes (Fig. 13–12). IgG may be present in the nuclei in a lightly speckled pattern. This finding of uncertain significance is shared by some of these pa-

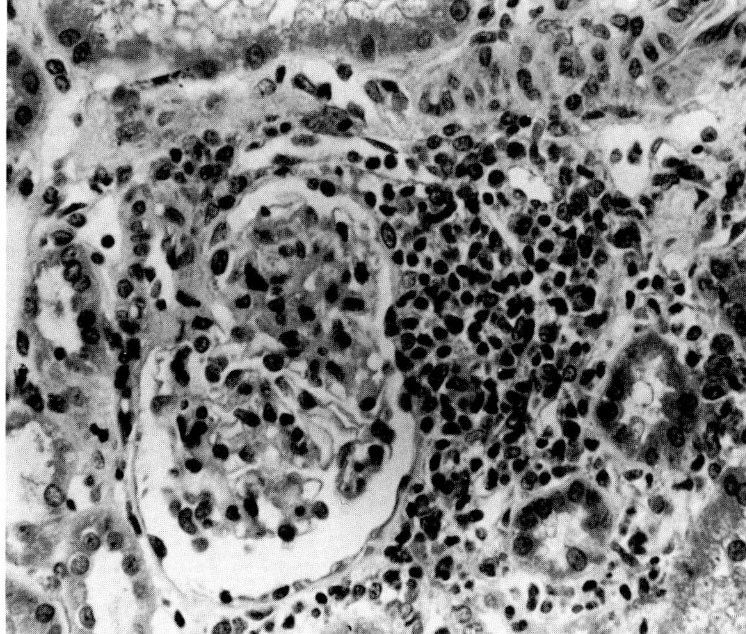

Figure 13–11. Chronic interstitial nephritis. Sjögren's disease. There is a prominent mononuclear interstitial cell infiltrate. The adjacent glomerulus is normal. (H&E, ×250.)

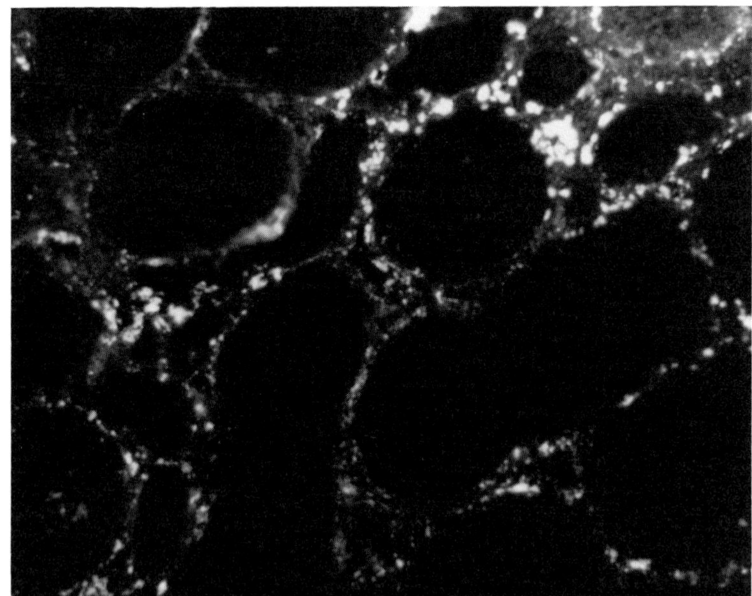

Figure 13–12. Chronic interstitial nephritis. Sjögren's disease. Immunofluorescence micrograph, anti-IgG. There are granular deposits along the tubular basement membranes. (×400.)

tients and some with systemic lupus erythematosus.

Idiopathic

A group of patients with chronic interstitial nephritis have no recognizable etiology or associated disease. These are exasperating cases not only because one is unable to establish an etiology, but also because one is obligated to consider the multiple known causes of chronic tubulo-interstitial disease.

It must be emphasized that any advanced renal disease may be associated with interstitial scarring. In these instances, there is often a sparsely scattered infiltrate of lymphocytes. This histologic picture is not the consequence of a primary interstitial disease process, and it is therefore not accurate to label it as chronic interstitial nephritis.

Histology

Light Microscopy

The lesions consist of a chronic interstitial nephritis without distinguishing features.

Immunofluorescence Microscopy

Linear or granular deposits of immune reactants may provide an indication of an immune pathogenesis, but for the most part these studies are negative.

Prognosis

The clinical course of chronic interstitial nephritis is characterized by the slow deterioration of renal function, which parallels the amount of tubular loss. Histologically, the increase in interstitial connective tissue is associated with a thickening of the tubular basement membranes and atrophy of epithelium. The accentuation of the multilamination of the Bowman's capsule, which is characteristic of the disease, also progresses. Chronic vascular lesions lead to ischemic obsolescence of glomerular tufts and tubular atrophy. In late lesions the remaining glomeruli are closely approximated due to the advanced tubular atrophy.

The rate of progression varies with the extension of the lesions and with the nature of the etiologic factors. The progression may be considerably delayed or prevented if the cause of the disease can be identified and removed. The best examples are analgesic agents and infectious diseases. It is currently thought that these disorders progress at a slower rate than glomerular diseases.

SELECTED READINGS

1. Mignon F, Mery JP, Mougenot B, et al: Granulomatous interstitial nephritis. Adv Nephrol 13:219, 1984.
2. Pirani C, Valeri A, D'Agati V, et al: Renal toxicity of nonsteroidal anti-inflammatory drugs. Contrib Nephrol 55:159, 1987.

Index

Note: Numbers in *italics* refer to illustrations; numbers followed by (t) indicate tables.

◆ MAJOR PROBLEMS IN PATHOLOGY ◆

The **Major Problems in Pathology (MPP) Series** provides current, accurate, and detailed information on specific areas of Diagnostic Pathology.

The volumes reflect the distilled wisdom of their authors, providing a scholarly review of the topic and practical guidance for the reader. Excellence of text, illustration, and referencing are hallmarks of the series.

Now—you can order the **MPP** volumes of your choice FREE for 30 days! Simply indicate your selections on the postage-paid order card, or call toll-free **1-800-545-2522** (8:30–7:00 Eastern time; in Fla. call 1-800-433-0001). Be sure to mention **DM#8974.**

Become an MPP series subscriber! You'll receive each new volume in the **MPP** series as soon as it's published—one to three titles per year—and save postage and handling costs!

If not completely satisfied with any volume you order through the mail, just return it with the invoice within 30 days at no further obligation. You only keep the volumes you want. *Your satisfaction is guaranteed!* ■

Valuable additions to your working library!

Available from your bookstore or the publisher

Complete and Mail Today for a FREE 30-Day Preview!

YES! Please send me the **Major Problems in Pathology** titles I've indicated below. If not completely satisfied with any volume, I may return it with the invoice within 30 days at no further obligation.

- ☐ W2503-7 **Disorders of the Spleen** *(Wolf & Neiman)*
- ☐ W8770-9 **Immunomicroscopy: A Diagnostic Tool for the Surgical Pathologist** *(Taylor)*
- ☐ W1359-4 **Mucosal Biopsy of the Gastrointestinal Tract, 3rd Edition** *(Whitehead)*
- ☐ W1337-3 **Pathology of Neoplasia in Children & Adolescents** *(Finegold)*
- ☐ W7493-3 **Pathology of the Uterine Cervix, Vagina, and Vulva** *(Fu & Reagan)*
- ☐ W1463-9 **Problems in Breast Pathology** *(Azzopardi)*
- ☐ W1434-5 **Surgical Pathology of Bone Marrow: Core Biopsy Diagnosis** *(Wittels)*
- ☐ W1027-7 **Surgical Pathology of the Lymph Nodes and Related Organs** *(Jaffe)*
- ☐ W1852-9 **Surgical Pathology of Non-Neoplastic Lung Disease, 2nd Edition** *(Katzenstein & Askin)*
- ☐ W5782-6 **Surgical Pathology of the Thyroid** *(LiVolsi)*
- ☐ W1224-5 **Surgical Pathology of the Uterine Corpus, 2nd Edition** *(Hendrickson & Kempson)*
- ☐ W3040-5 **The Renal Biopsy, 2nd Edition** *(Striker & Olson)*
- ☐ W3835-X **Thin-Needle Aspiration Biopsy** *(Frable)*

☐ Enroll me in the **MPP** Subscriber Plan so that I may receive future titles immediately upon publication, and save postage & handling costs! I may preview each new volume FREE for 30 days—and keep only the volumes I want.

Name______________________________

Address____________________________

City________________ State________ Zip________

Staple this to your purchase order to expedite delivery. © W.B. SAUNDERS 1989. Printed in USA. Postage & Handling additional outside the USA.

C02414 **DM#8974**

MAJOR PROBLEMS IN PATHOLOGY

- **Disorders of the Spleen** *(Wolf & Neiman)* Order #W2503-7
- **Immunomicroscopy: A Diagnostic Tool for the Surgical Pathologist** *(Taylor)* Order #W8770-9
- **Mucosal Biopsy of the Gastrointestinal Tract, 3rd Edition** *(Whitehead)* Order #W1359-4
- **Pathology of Neoplasia in Children & Adolescents** *(Finegold)* Order #W1337-3
- **Pathology of the Uterine Cervix, Vagina, and Vulva** *(Fu & Reagan)* Order #W7493-3
- **Problems in Breast Pathology** *(Azzopardi)* Order #W1463-9
- **Surgical Pathology of Bone Marrow: Core Biopsy Diagnosis** *(Wittels)* Order #W1434-5
- **Surgical Pathology of the Lymph Nodes and Related Organs** *(Jaffe)* Order #W1027-7
- **Surgical Pathology of Non-Neoplastic Lung Disease, 2nd Edition** *(Katzenstein & Askin)* Order #W1852-9
- **Surgical Pathology of the Thyroid** *(LiVolsi)* Order #W5782-6
- **Surgical Pathology of the Uterine Corpus, 2nd Edition** *(Hendrickson & Kempson)* Order #W1224-5
- **The Renal Biopsy, 2nd Edition** *(Striker & Olson)* Order #W3040-5
- **Thin-Needle Aspiration Biopsy** *(Frable)* Order #W3835-X

Enroll today!

See reverse side for details.

BUSINESS REPLY MAIL

FIRST CLASS MAIL PERMIT NO. 7135 ORLANDO, FL

POSTAGE WILL BE PAID BY ADDRESSEE

ORDER FULFILLMENT DEPARTMENT

WB SAUNDERS

Harcourt Brace Jovanovich, Inc.

6277 SEA HARBOR DRIVE

ORLANDO FL 32821-9989